Ama

A Story of the Atlantic Slave Trade

Manu Herbstein

PICADOR AFRICA

First published 2001 by E-reads, New York.

Published 2005 by Picador Africa
an imprint of Pan Macmillan South Africa
P O Box 411717, Craighall, Johannesburg 2024
www.picadorafrica.co.za

ISBN 1770100032

Typeset in 10 on 12 point Palatino by The Setting Stick
Cover design: Donald Hill of Studio 5

Printed and bound by Pinetown Printers

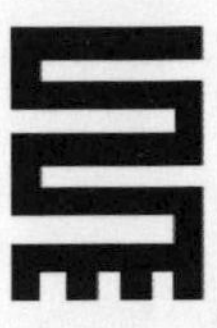

The Asante Adinkra symbol *Nkyinkyin*, signifies toughness, adaptability, determination and service to others. The corresponding Akan proverb, *Obra kwan ye nkyinkyin yimiie*, means the path of life is full of twists and turns.

AFRICA

In a pitched battle in 1772 the musketeers of the army of the Asante Confederacy vanquished the archers and cavalry of their northern neighbour, the Kingdom of Dagbon. The victorious Asante exacted from their defeated enemy an annual tribute of 200 cows, 400 sheep, 400 pieces of cotton cloth, 200 pieces of silk cloth and 500 slaves.

CHAPTER 1

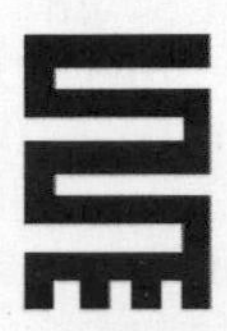

There was a puff of dust on the horizon.

Nandzi peered through the heat haze with narrowed eyes, and wondered what it might be. Then Nowu, on her back, whimpered, distracting her attention. She took his weight with one hand and tucked in the end of her cloth with the other. Nowu was her youngest brother but one. He was four. The previous day the elders had made the customary incisions on his face. That morning he had been feverish. Tabitsha, their mother, had made an infusion of roots to dress the wounds and for him to drink.

Then, at noon, they had heard the sound of distant drums, announcing the long-expected death of Sekwadzim, Tabitsha's father. The household had assembled quickly, all twelve of them, and soon Tigen, her father, was leading them across the plain.

Nandzi had been left behind to take care of Nowu.

She twisted her head and glanced over her shoulder. His eyelids were drooping but he was not yet asleep. She felt his forehead. He was still very warm. She sang a lullaby and danced him gently up and down in time with the song. Then she quickened her pace as she crossed to the deep shade under the mango tree which stood by Tabitsha's door.

It was unusual for Nandzi to be left alone in the compound. Indeed, she could not recall that it had ever happened before. At first she had been a little apprehensive, but Tabitsha had taken her aside.

"You see that I am carrying Kwadi on my back," she had said.

Kwadi was Nandzi's newest baby brother.

"Nowu is too ill to be taken with us to the burial. Someone will have to stay behind to watch over him. You are the eldest. Soon you will be old enough to go to your husband. It is time that you learned to take responsibility."

Nandzi had winced at the mention of her husband. Like all Bekpokpam girls, she had been betrothed at birth. Her husband, Satila, had been twenty at the time. He came from Sekwadzim's hamlet. She remembered the first time she had seen him. She had been five and he had come to make the first payment of bride corn, *to beat the corn,* as they say, with two large baskets of sorghum. She had giggled when Tabitsha had told her to squat on her knees before her husband. Satila had told her to rise and had pinched her cheek and then she had run away to play and had forgotten all about him.

When she was seven he had come again to *send the corn*, bringing three baskets this time. She had been too shy to answer him when he spoke to her. Each harvest time since then, he had come to *tie the corn*, bringing one tied bundle of guinea corn in the first year, two in the second year and so on. Last harvest he had brought nine. Next year he would bring ten bundles and add the bridal cloth and the bridal cowries for her father. Then it would be time for her to go to him.

Satila was approaching forty. He was an ugly, scrawny man, with an untidy beard which he had grown after the death of his father. The thought of sleeping with him made her feel sick. What was worse, she would be expected to give up seeing Itsho once she went to live with Satila. The only advantage she could see was that Satila lived in a bustling village of thirty.

Her thoughts turned to Itsho and she smiled. Itsho was strong and handsome. He made her laugh. He was forever teasing her.

Itsho would be at Sekwadzim's burial. He would notice her absence and would guess that she had been left at home. Perhaps he would make discreet inquiries. Surely, if he knew she was alone, he would come to see her. They would talk and laugh together and then they would make love in her mother's room.

At her back, Nowu sighed. Nandzi twisted her head to confirm that he had fallen asleep. Her thoughts turned again to Itsho. He would remove her cloth and stroke her body with his fingers. Itsho was so kind and gentle. Today there would be no one to disturb them, no giggles outside the door.

She scanned the higher ground to the north, but there was no sign of him.

Nandzi bent and passed through the low door of her mother's room. Tabitsha was Tigen's second wife. She had once been married to his elder brother. When his brother had died, Tigen had taken the widow, as custom demands.

Why are husbands always so much older than their wives? Nandzi reflected, not for the first time. *Itsho is young and vigorous. Why can't I marry him, rather than that old, dry stick of a Satila? If only I could marry Itsho, we could make love every day, not just when Tabitsha finds it convenient to let us use her room. Even Lati would make a better husband than Satila, though I don't love him half as much as Itsho. But then Itsho is quite poor and Lati will one day inherit his father's farms and cattle.*

Oh, it is no use thinking of it, she thought. *They will never let me marry a young man. I will have to go to Satila next year: there is no avoiding it. I must just make the most of the short time I have left with Itsho.*

But if Satila does not treat me well, I will know what to do.

The last time Itsho had come, when they were lying close together after they had made love, she had suggested to him that they run away together. He had been slow to reply. It seemed to her that the idea had not occurred to him before.

"No," he had said, "that is not possible. You know that my father has already found a bride for me. I have seen the child. She is two years old. In three years time, I will go to beat the corn. When she has reached your age she will come to me."

"But you will be old by then," Nandzi had said, "an old, dry stick like Satila. I want you to marry me, so that we can live together and I can lie like this with you every night."

"No," Itsho had repeated, "I am sorry; but it is just not possible. It is against all our customs. My father would never allow it."

"Nandzi carefully loosened her cloth and slid the sleeping Nowu round into her arms.

She had not raised the matter again, but she had thought bitterly, *what do customs matter? Are customs more important than the two of us? We are so good together.*

And she had lost a little of her respect for Itsho.

Men are such cowards, she had thought. *Just think of it, preferring a small baby girl, who will not be fit to be a wife for at least another 15 years, to me. How can that make sense?*

She had shed a silent, bitter tear at her fate.

Nandzi laid Nowu down on a mat in the darkest part of the room. She felt his forehead. He was still warm but he was sleeping peacefully. She dipped a cloth into the bowl of medicine and wiped his face. Then she sponged the rest of his body.

When she came to his small penis, she smiled and thought, *Ei, men! What pleasure they can give with this small thing, o!* and she shook her head.

When she had dried Nowu and covered him, she went outside to look for signs of Itsho, but the landscape was deserted. Their compound was isolated, alone on its low ridge, with no other human habitation in sight. Over to the east, the land fell towards the river. The level of the water in the flood plain had fallen. She looked out at the grid of raised embankments which criss-crossed the shimmering water.

Soon the flood waters will recede and it will be time for net fishing, she thought. *Then we shall eat fish until we burst.* She wondered why it was that girls were not permitted to eat meat until after they were married.

Nowu might have some appetite when he wakes, she thought. When the drums had announced the death of her father, Tabitsha had been busy making a light soup, using the antelope which Lati had brought them as a gift. The fragrance of the meat rose from the pot which was still simmering on the low fire. But that was a meat dish. She would have to cook something else for herself. She sat down on a low stool to rest for a moment. The soup smelled delicious; she was hungry; her mouth watered. She looked around. The compound was empty.

Why should I not eat some of the antelope soup? she thought. *There is no one here to see me. And, after all, when I go to Satila, I shall be able to eat as much meat as I like. Or, at least, as much as his generosity will allow.*

Satila had a reputation for meanness.

Nandzi meditated. *This is really a stupid taboo. We have so many unreasonable customs. Like marrying old men. And not eating meat. What would happen to me if I ate some meat, after all?*

She took a ladle and a small bowl and dished up some of the liquid. Then she took a sip. It tasted as good as it smelled. She put the bowl to her lips.

*****

Suddenly she felt the ground beneath her bare feet vibrate; a moment later she heard the horses' hooves.

Quickly, she rose. A large troop of Bedagbam were galloping towards the compound. They could only be Bedagbam. Only the feared and hated Bedagbam rode horses.

Nandzi was overcome by panic. She had no time to consider what the horsemen might be after, but all her instincts told her that this was no friendly visit. Briefly, she contemplated flight. But they were already too close: they would see her. On foot, there was no way she could outstrip the horses. And there was

Nowu. Nowu! She would have to hide. She put down the bowl and stumbled the short distance to the door of Tabitsha's room. Quickly she gathered a pile of skins. Nowu was fast asleep. She lay down beside him and pulled the skins over them. Her heart was pumping furiously.

That puff of dust on the horizon. If only I had guessed, I would have had time to get away and hide.

There were twenty horsemen. Their leader's mount was white. It was clad in a padded coat of intricately decorated cloth. The rider wore a heavy leather jacket. His legs were stretched out straight, pressing his high leather boots into the stirrups. In his right hand he held aloft a spear, ready to be thrown or thrust. A bow, a leather quiver of arrows and a sword hung by his side. The men bunched close behind him in a cloud of dust were similarly clad and armed. Their guttural war cries rent the air.

Under the skins, Nandzi thrust her fists against her ears to block out the fearful noise.

They reined in their mounts just in time to avoid a collision with the low mud wall which surrounded the compound. Neighing and snorting, the horses rose on their hind legs, then pranced and turned as the riders struggled to control them. Abdulai, the commander, the polished brass of his horse's accoutrements glinting in the sunlight, signalled silence. Only the horses' blowing disturbed the peace of the afternoon. The compound appeared to be deserted. Abdulai nodded to the two horsemen alongside him. Damba and Issaka dismounted, handed their reins to others and stretched their limbs.

There was only one entrance, a low door in a large round mud brick building. Tigen had adorned the thatched roof with the staves and bows of his dead forebears and skulls of victims of the hunt: antelopes, birds, a leopard.

Nervously, their spears at the ready, the two warriors advanced and peered inside. The building contained only a single room; apart from a few hoes and baskets, it was empty.

They passed through into the courtyard. Issaka saw the pot simmering on the fire. Silently he pointed it out to his companion. A scrawny hen, surrounded by her brood, scratched the ground. Damba kicked at it and it fled, screeching, its chickens in pursuit.

Under the pile of skins, Nandzi shivered.

They entered Bato's room. Rolled up sleeping mats stood stacked against the wall. There were two low wooden stools. A few pieces of indigo Yoruba cloth hung on hooks and a pile of skins lay on a padlocked chest.

The young men's room stood to one side of its own inner compound. Near the entrance there was a large granary, raised off the ground on three legs, full of sorghum. The room seemed bare. The young men who slept there had taken their weapons and drums and dancing head dresses to Sekwadzim's burial. The warriors were less nervous: clearly the compound was deserted.

"What's this?" asked Issaka in a low voice.

It was a large turtle shell. In it lay the head of a crocodile, encased in a matrix of pulped roots, wrapped in fibres and stuck with porcupine quills. He prodded it with his spear.

"Take care," replied Damba. "That is their medicine."

"Ei!" exclaimed Issaka, taking a step back. "I fear."

A third man joined them.

"What are you two up to?" he asked. "Abdulai is impatient. We have much work to do today."

"Tell him we are searching the place to make sure there is no one hiding here. Did you see the pot cooking on the fire? They can't have gone far."

He paused.

"There is a wooden chest in the next room," he continued. "Break it open and see if there is anything of value inside. That will keep Abdulai happy."

Bato's kitchen was full of pots and firewood. The smoked carcass of a small buck hung on the wall.

They passed into Tabitsha's room. It was much like Bato's.

"There is nothing here," said Damba, turning to leave.

In her refuge, under the pile of skins, Nandzi lay petrified. She heard the men's voices in the room but did not understand what they were saying. What if Nowu should wake up and cry out, revealing their presence? She placed her hand over the child's mouth. But Nowu's nose was blocked. Unable to breathe, he woke and struggled to free himself.

"Wait," said Issaka. The skins had moved. He flipped them aside with the point of his spear. Nandzi and Nowu lay revealed. Nandzi screamed and clasped her hands over her head, as if trying to make herself invisible. Nowu, still half asleep, sensed her fear and began to cry.

"Ah, what have we here?" shouted Issaka in excitement.

This was their first catch and he, Issaka, had made it. Abdulai came into the room, fuming with impatience.

"Issaka, Damba," he bellowed. "If there is no one . . ."

He cut himself short as he saw the figure of the girl cringing on the floor.

Then he repeated Issaka's question.

"What have we here?"

Striding across the room in his long red boots, he grabbed Nandzi by her upper arm, lifting her to her feet. Nowu was holding Nandzi's cloth and as she was pulled away from him, the cloth unwound, leaving her unclothed. She stretched out a hand for the garment, but it was too late.

"What have we here?" Abdulai echoed again, deliberately enunciating each word.

He relaxed his grip on the girl and at once Nandzi tried to run; but the doorway was blocked by Issaka and Damba. Moving swiftly, Abdulai grabbed her two arms from behind.

"Get out of here," he told his two lieutenants, spitting the words from between his teeth.

They fled their master's anger.

"Now we shall have some fun together, shall we not?" he said to Nandzi.

Leaving her right arm free he grabbed her waist from behind and pulled her buttocks against his penis, which had taken its stand beneath his baggy pantaloons as soon as he had seen her naked body.

Nandzi struggled, striking him repeatedly with the elbow of her free arm.

"You beast. You filthy pig," she screamed at him.

Abdulai just laughed. He was much too strong for her.

"I don't hear your language, my darling," he replied, "but I am sure that those are words of love."

Nowu was screaming uncontrollably.

"Issaka, Damba" he called.

A head appeared in the door.

"Take this child," he ordered; and then, "Get out, get out."

He struggled to hold on to Nandzi with one hand, freeing the other to release his pantaloons and lift his heavy leather armour. The pantaloons dropped to his ankles. His penis pressed on Nandzi's bare skin. He was no longer the dignified commander of a company of slave hunters. His instincts had taken control of him. He was a two legged animal bent on copulation.

He forced Nandzi down. With his left arm he pinned her shoulders to the ground. With his right hand he took his penis and guided it into her vagina, sighing as he penetrated into the depths of her body. Nandzi continued to scream abuse at him and struggle. But now he had two hands free to pin her wrists to the ground. Nandzi twisted her head and snapped her teeth over his fat index finger. She felt the bone and the warm spurt of blood in her mouth before she heard his cry.

"You bitch. You filthy, verminous bitch

He spat out the words as he dragged his hand from her.

"I will teach you to trifle with Abdulai."

He moved her wrists out of range and put the weight of his elbows on her arms. Then he began to drive into her. In and out he drove, just as he had often driven his spear repeatedly into the body of a prone victim, relishing the fountain of blood, thrusting the spear in again and again long after his adversary was dead.

He moved her hands onto the back of her head and forced her face into the polished dung floor.

"I will teach you. I will teach you. I will teach you. Remember me. My name is Abdulai. Abdulai the famous general of Dagbon."

Deeper and harder he drove. Nandzi could not control her sobs. Suddenly, as he plumbed her depths, she felt a surge of pain unlike anything she had ever before experienced. It was as if he had mounted the sharp iron head of his assegai onto the end of his penis. Each time he plunged into her, the pain rose to a crescendo. She screamed in agony but he paid no heed. Once, twice, three times. She summoned up all her strength in a superhuman effort to throw him off, but he was too strong and too heavy. Then she lost consciousness.

Abdulai completed his business inside her and rested on her prone body. As his penis shrunk, he became aware of the pain in his finger and placed it in his mouth to stem the flow of blood. Then he rose to his feet and drew up his pantaloons with his free hand. Nandzi's cotton cloth lay where it had fallen on the ground. He picked it up and with his teeth tore off a strip to use as a bandage.

"Damba, Issaka," he called, dropping the cloth on Nandzi's still body. The two warriors had been watching Abdulai's performance discreetly from a distance hoping perhaps that their commander would reward them for their discovery by allowing them to exercise their own erections, but they were to be disappointed.

"Take this hussy and put her on a horse," he ordered. "Tie her well. Then collect the cloth and skins and let's get out of here. This place gives me the spooks."

He hid his bleeding finger from them. The blood had soaked through the bandage.

CHAPTER 2

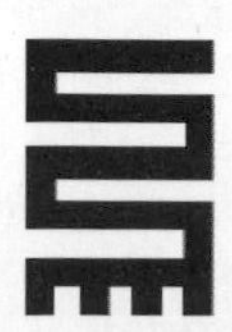

When Nandzi came to, she was lying face-down on the back of a horse, securely trussed.

Her cloth had been wrapped around her and her arms bound to her body with leather thongs. Her legs hung down on one side and her head on the other. Alongside the tethered horse stood another, piled high with the family's chattels.

Her body ached from head to foot. When she moved, she felt a sharp pain in her abdomen.

Damba emerged from the compound, carrying two hoes.

"Ah, the lady has awakened," he said, threading the shafts of the hoes through the ropes which bound the plundered goods to the pack horse.

There was no sign of the other members of his party.

"Water," Nandzi whispered, but Damba did not understand.

He untied the horses, put boot to stirrup and hoisted himself onto his saddle. Nandzi felt the animal move beneath her. She had never before been on a horse. For a moment she was overcome by terror so stark that it transcended her pain. Then she heard Nowu's wail.

"Nowu. Nowu," she cried.

She struggled to free herself but there was no escape.

"The Asante have no use for small children," Damba said, flicking his whip on the horse's withers, "and, as for you, you will have plenty of time to get down and walk, once we are clear of danger."

He guessed that Nandzi did not understand his language, but the sound of his own voice allayed his fear of being alone in Bekpokpam territory.

Nandzi moaned. Every step the horse took jarred her body and sent shooting pains through her belly. Her tongue was parched and there was a foul taste of vomit in her mouth. At first she lay limp, but the movement of the horse threw her head from side to side and up and down. She felt her neck would snap. So she raised her head as far as the thongs would allow and tensed her neck muscles. A cloud of red dust enveloped them, irritating her nostrils. She sneezed. Her hands were bound. A mixture of mucus and dust hung from her nose until the motion of the horse shook it free. Tears ran down her cheeks and soon her face was marked with red streaks. She closed her eyes and tried to concentrate. What had happened? What should she do?

The horse stumbled. Suddenly, as in a nightmare, she felt Abdulai driving into her again She screamed.

"Shut your mouth, woman," Damba told her.

Nandzi shook her head vigorously and breathed out hard through her nose, trying to dislodge a thread of mucus. *Nowu, all alone by himself in the compound,* she thought; and she despaired. *Sick as he is, he might just wander off and be eaten by a some wild beast. Tabitsha will blame me for not looking after him properly. And Tigen, my father, who speaks to me so rarely these days, surely he will not be able to contain his wrath?* Then it struck her that she might never see them again. *Where is this man taking me? What will they do with me?* She shuddered again at the thought of Abdulai. *What if he were to take me as his wife? Better to die.* With every fibre in her body, she hated him. *I will kill him in his sleep and then try to escape. If I have to, I will risk the rage of the ancestors and kill myself afterwards.*

She saw the ground through the cloud of dust and flies which kept them company. Her eyes itched and she squeezed them shut, moving through a dark void, rising and falling with the motion of the horse. The image of Abdulai returned to her again and again. He was a giant black fly, mounting her from behind. She opened her eyes to drive the spectre away.

They reached the summit of a ridge. Damba led the two horses through a farm. Their hooves kicked up the small mounds of earth, breaking the fresh yam shoots. Nandzi studied the head of the pack horse, its flaring nostrils, the shock of hair which fell forward between its ears, its mild eyes. *What does a horse know?* she wondered. She looked at the load on its back. With a shock she recognised the pattern of one of Tabitsha's favourite cloths. *They must have stolen everything they found in the compound.* She gnashed her teeth. *It is lucky,* she thought, *that they put on their best for the funeral.*

"You, our ancestors," she whispered, using words she had heard spoken by the elders, "who send us rain, and shelter our homes and our farms from winds and lightning, it is I, Nandzi, daughter of Tigen, speaking. I have no drink to give you, but you will surely know the reason."

Tears came to her eyes. She concentrated on her task.

"The Bedagbam came on their horses and stole our goods. Their leader assaulted me. They abducted me from those who nurtured me and cherish me. My small brother, Nowu, is all alone, sick with fever and exposed to the wild beasts. Father of my father Tigen, father of Tigen's father and your forefathers before you, whose names are lost in time, strike down our oppressors. Especially, I beg you to kill the cruel one who raped me, who does not deserve to live amongst human beings. Hear my call. I will give you food and drink when I am able."

Then a thought came to her. *Perhaps it is the ancestors themselves who have sent this trouble to me. It was just as I was tasting the meat soup that the raiders came. The ancestors are punishing me because I ate meat.*

So she spoke to them again.

"Father of Tigen, it is me again, Nandzi. It is true that I tasted the antelope soup, but I only took a small sip. I had no evil intent. If I have angered you by my conduct, I implore you to forgive me. I will never repeat the offence. I promise."

"Stop that mumbling," said Damba, and then, "Oh, oh. Trouble ahead."

He secured the leads of the pack horse to his saddle.

Nandzi noticed the concern in his voice and raised her head. In the distance, ahead and across to the left, a figure approached them on foot along one of the raised pathways. She recognised Itsho's familiar form.

"Itsho," she called, but the light breeze carried her voice away.

Damba said, "Shut your mouth."

He brought his bow from his back and pulled an arrow from his quiver. At the pace they were moving, their path would cross Itsho's. Nandzi raised her head again. Itsho had seen them and halted in his tracks. He, too, had his bow at the ready.

"Itsho, Itsho!" she screamed again.

This time he heard his name called.

"It is me, Nandzi," she called. "Run, run for help. The Bedagbam kidnapped me. They are many. On horses. Run, run or this one will shoot you."

Itsho hesitated. Then, slowly, uncertainly, he moved back the way he had come, watching them, keeping just out of range.

"Nandzi," he called back. "Is that you?"

Nandzi repeated her warning.

Damba shortened her horse's lead, bringing her closer so that he could pummel her on the back with his free fist, crying "Shut up, shut up!"

Knowing that Damba did not understand their language, she called again to Itsho, who had had second thoughts about fleeing and was again approaching them.

"Itsho, keep clear. It is too dangerous. Run. Get help. Follow our trail. Catch us in the night."

Damba reached down fiercely and placed his hand over her mouth. Then she remembered Nowu. She sank her teeth into a finger. With a curse he snatched his hand away.

"Itsho. Nowu is all alone in the compound. He is feverish. Go for him. Please."

Itsho stood at a safe distance and watched them pass.

"Nandzi. I have heard you. I will do what you say. Never fear. We will rescue you as soon as darkness falls. The Bedagbam are cowards. We will kill them all. To the last man."

Damba watched him uneasily, bow at the ready. When they had passed by, he kept looking over his shoulder.

Nandzi saw Itsho follow the horses' tracks back towards the compound. Her pain returned. But the encounter had given her comfort and hope. She fell into an exhausted, uneasy sleep.

*****

Nowu was lying under Tabitsha's mango tree, fast asleep. Itsho felt his forehead. He was still warm, but the high fever had passed.

"Nowu, wake up. We're going to look for your Mama."

"Where's Sister Nandzi?" asked Nowu.

"Now up on my back," replied Itsho, not knowing how to reply.

"Bad men took Nandzi away," Nowu said, to no one in particular.

"I know, Nowu," said Itsho. "And just as soon as I have handed you over to your mother, I am going to chase those bad men and beat them and bring Nandzi back to you. I promise."

*****

By the time Itsho reached the dead man's compound, the funeral party had left for the burial ground. Itsho handed Nowu into the care of Sekwadzim's wizened elder sister.

Sekwadzim's clanswomen were carrying his body, wrapped in cloth, to the grave side. As Itsho arrived, the cloths were being unwound. The dead man was laid naked on the ground, his hands over his genitals. Itsho could say nothing until the ceremony was over. One by one the elders addressed the dead man, reciting his virtues and asking him to greet their ancestors at the place where he was going. Impatiently, Itsho shifted his weight from foot to foot. *To whom should I tell the bad news*? he wondered. *Tigen is always distant when I greet him. Tabitsha, I know, is fond of me, but her father is only now being buried. It is a bad time to approach her. Moreover*, he thought, *this is a matter for men*. He moved closer to Tigen. At last the body was laid gently in the grave and the clansmen began to throw soil on it.

Itsho tugged gently at Tigen's sleeve.

"Father of Nandzi, I must speak with you. It is urgent."

Tigen looked at him in surprise. He noticed that Satila, Nandzi's husband, was watching them. It would not be wise for him to be seen talking to his daughter's lover in public. But the serious expression on Itsho's face disturbed him.

"Yes, what is it?" he asked.

Itsho drew him aside and spoke in a low voice. He came straight to the point. There was no time for the customary civilities.

"Nandzi has been kidnapped," he said. "The Bedagbam have taken her."

He told Tigen all he had seen.

"I will call the elders together," said the old man.

"There is no time," said Itsho. "If we do not start soon, we will miss their trail in the dark."

Tigen nodded. The grave was now full of earth. The women were making their way back to the hamlet. The calabash of Sekwadzim's spirit was broken and the young men pressed the pieces into the mound.

Tigen started to speak.

"Attention. Attention," he called.

Itsho asked him quietly, "Shall I go to break the news to Nandzi's mother?"

Tigen nodded. The mourners were silent, waiting for him to continue.

"This young man, Itsho, who is known to you, has brought me very serious news. A party of our hated enemies has raided my compound and abducted my daughter, Nandzi."

Satila stepped forward but Tigen motioned him to silence.

"They may have taken others. We must raise a war party of the young men immediately. There is no time to waste. They must track the marauders and attack them before dawn. I apologise to the elders for not asking their approval first, but action cannot wait for custom at a time like this. The young men should collect their weapons and meet at once at late Sekwadzim's compound. Itsho will lead them to pick up the trail. May Sekwadzim's spirit and the spirits of our ancestors guide them and bring them success. Death to the Bedagbam!"

The funeral party broke up in confusion.

Satila said to Tigen, "I will join the young men."

Tigen moved to pacify the elders, apologising for his lack of ceremony.

"No, no," said one greybeard, "you did right. The ancestors will smile upon you."

*****

For a moment, Nandzi wondered where she was.

She rubbed her eyes and then remembered: she was playing a part in a nightmare. The first dim glow of dawn was in the sky. Around the walls of the room she saw the sleeping forms of her fellow captives. She badly wanted to piss. In the doorway the guard lay snoring. She rose quietly and moved to an empty place along the wall, lifted her cloth and stood with her legs apart. The urine hit the earth floor with the sound of a cloudburst. She looked around, but no one had woken. Her beads. She noticed they were missing. Of course, that monster had ripped them from her waist. How would she manage, she wondered, when her period came in a few days' time? But so much could happen in a few days. *Maybe Itsho will rescue me and I will be home by then. What has happened to Itsho and the men? Surely they must be out there in the dark? But if they delay just a little longer, it will be light and then it might be too late.*

She strained her ears. The guard was snoring. Outside all she could hear was the hum of the crickets. The Bedagbam had talked late into the night. *They must all be asleep like the guard at the door. Itsho! Come now! Attack! Attack!* She willed them to action.

There were four in the assault party. Each wore only a loin cloth. They had smeared their naked bodies with shea butter. Their task was simple but dangerous. It depended on all the Bedagbam being asleep. Timing was critical. Too early and it would be too dark for the archers to find their targets. Too late and they would lose the element of surprise and with that, probably their lives too. Silently, taking extreme care with each footstep, they crept into the ruined compound. Quickly each selected his victim. At a signal they slashed simultaneously at the exposed skin of the sleepers with their razor sharp knives. Their aim was not to kill, but to cause as much pain and bleeding as they could. Even as the first cries of their bloody victims rent the early morning air, they slipped away into the half light.

The screaming caused instant panic. The Bedagbam, waking, believed the enemy were amongst them. They struggled to their feet, grabbing their weapons, rubbing their eyes. The wounded cried for help, but their comrades' first priority was to save their own skins. Man for man, the Bedagbam feared the Bekpokpam. They would do their utmost to avoid fighting with them hand to hand. Yet, as they grasped their swords and staffs, ready for just such close combat, there was no enemy to be seen. Their assailants might just as well have been ghosts.

Abdulai came to his senses first. A cruel man, he inspired fear amongst his subordinates; but he also inspired respect and they depended on his leadership.

"The horses, the horses," he cried. "Leave the wounded. We will come for them after."

His men grabbed their saddles and rushed towards the horses, which had been tethered by a thicket of cassia.

As the Bedagbam warriors emerged from the protective mud walls of the compound, somewhat clumsy in their heavy leather armour, they made a perfect target. Itsho and his comrades rose to their feet and fired their first volley of poisoned arrows. It was still too dark to make out the individual forms and they shot indiscriminately into the moving mass of men. Others shot at the horses. Some of the Bedagbam tried to return to the compound, but Abdulai was there, urging them on. He knew that once they were mounted, no one could match their speed and the extra range their height gave them.

"The horses, the horses," he cried, again and again.

Their leather armour was protection against all but the swiftest arrow. To achieve a kill, the poisoned tip had to enter exposed skin. The horses were a more vulnerable target, but they were tethered close together and the poison took time to act. So the horses nearer the attackers formed a protective barrier for those behind. Disturbed by the noise, the arrows, the wild whinnies of pain of those which been struck and the evident panic of their masters, the tethered beasts tried to rise on their hind legs. Their masters swore at them as they quickly and skilfully saddled up.

Again and again, the Bekpokpam loaded, drew and released. The poisoned arrows whistled through the air.

Nandzi moved from captive to captive, trying to release their bonds, but the knots had been well tied and her fingers were stiff. The first man she freed stood undecided whether to help her or to flee. Outside there was confusion. It was impossible to tell from which direction the attack was coming. Unarmed, he did not know what to do.

"Run, run," she told him. "Run round the back of our people and join them."

She was struggling with the next man's bonds.

"If only I had a knife," she thought.

Abdulai, already mounted, urged his followers on.

"Mount, mount," he cried.

His horse prancing, he glanced around. Now there was enough light to see those of his companions who lay where they had fallen, begging for help as they died a slow and painful death. There was light enough, too, to see the enemy. Impatiently, he waited until he judged sufficient of his band to be mounted.

Then he cried, "Attack, attack."

Shooting fiercely, Itsho was the first to run out of arrows. Throwing down his bow and quiver he ran towards the compound, intending in the confusion to liberate Nandzi, if that was all he could achieve.

He had chosen the wrong moment. Abdulai's horse ran him down. A hoof crushed his skull.

Seeing the horsemen approaching at a gallop, the attackers fled in disarray. The Bedagbam chased them ruthlessly, shooting from the saddle, slashing with their swords or driving their spears into their enemies as they passed. The attack had failed.

CHAPTER 3

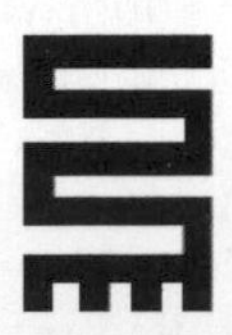

Abdulai called in his men and counted his losses.

Two were dead, victims of poisoned arrows. Another was paralysed and would die soon.

The medical orderlies, old soldiers, had already used their plant medicines to staunch the wounds of the four men who had been slashed in their sleep. One was fanning the patients with a therapeutic cowstail.

Three horses had been struck by arrows and would not survive.

One of the captive slaves had escaped in the confusion. A number of the attackers lay dead in the long grass: food for the vultures which already circled overhead; and for the hyenas.

"You, you, you and you," said the commander, "dig graves for our dead."

This was work which could not be left to the slaves.

"Damba, take two slaves and bring water from the river."

"Issaka, take another two and collect firewood."

They had not eaten a cooked meal since the previous day.

He sent men out to hunt for antelope or guinea fowl; and others to patrol the outskirts of the camp: the surviving attackers might just be stupid enough to regroup and return.

Young lads, apprentice soldiers, unsaddled and groomed the horses. Then they hobbled them and put them out to graze.

Abdulai took off his heavy leather armour. He spread his mat where the ruined building made some shade, washed his face and hands and settled down to pray. When he had completed his obeisance, he folded his legs before him and, fingering his beads, considered his position. In Yendi he would have to explain the loss of men and horses. It was a high price to pay for the twenty slaves they had captured. He knew that it was inexcusable: if the guards had not fallen asleep it would never have happened. Yet he was the commander and the Chief of the Horses would hold him responsible. Somehow he must contrive to shift the blame onto the guards. They would be tried and sentenced to death for dereliction of duty, but that would have to wait until their return to Yendi. These days it was only the Asante conquerors who had the right to carry out executions.

He might be put on trial himself. That would be wholly unjust, he reflected. He had given the necessary orders. It was not his fault that they had been disobeyed.

"There is no justice in this world," he whispered to his beads. "If they put me on trial I shall have to pay a heavy bribe to the Court of Eunuchs to secure my release."

*****

Nandzi listened to the confused tumult with mounting excitement.

Itsho had not failed her. She could see nothing of the battle: the walls were too high and a guard remained at the doorway, threatening the captives with a whip, demanding that they stop whispering amongst themselves. Then the shouting outside became less strident. The voices were still the voices of their captors. The attack must have failed. Nandzi despaired.

She sat down with her back against the wall, clasped her knees to her chest and closed her eyes. She must not give up. Itsho would never give her up. While he lived, he would struggle to free her. The man whose ropes she had unbound and then helped to scale the wall would take her message to Itsho.

Damba came into the ruined building.

"You," he said to Nandzi and signed to her to stand.

He looked around and chose a young lad. He cut the ropes that bound the boy's wrists behind his back.

"Get up," he said.

The boy rose, massaging his arms.

"Take the calabashes," he told them.

"Out!" he ordered, indicating the doorway with a nod of his head.

The boy led the way down the hill. The dew had already dried on the long grass. There was no path and he had to force his way through. The sun was hidden in the dusty haze of the Harmattan.

"What is your name?" Nandzi asked the boy.

"I am called Suba," he replied shyly, turning his head to look at her.

He turned into a crude path which someone had beaten through the grass ahead of them.

"Where are you from?" she asked. She was following in his tracks. They had left Damba some way behind.

Suba's reply froze on his lips. He halted so suddenly that Nandzi collided with him.

"What is it?" she asked.

Then she saw the body lying face down across the path. The head was all but severed from the neck. The ground was soaked with blood. She took a step back.

"What is it?" Damba asked in his language, pushing past them.

He inserted the toe of his leather boot under a shoulder and turned the body over. The head twisted to one side showing a severed artery and windpipe. Nandzi put her hands over her eyes and uttered a terrible cry of woe. Then she fell to her knees and retched. She had eaten nothing since the previous day. She tasted bile. Damba looked at her and smirked.

"Women!" he said aloud while he waited for her to get up. "Come on, let's go."

Nandzi looked up at the vultures. *It might have been Itsho*, she thought. *No! Itsho escaped. Itsho escaped. Itsho escaped.*

She repeated the words over and over again, willing her mind to control Itsho's fate. She could not bring herself to contemplate his death. *Itsho escaped. Itsho escaped.*

The river turned out to be no more than a trickle of water running in a narrow channel which meandered along a sandy bed. Soon, as the dry season progressed, the flow would stop completely. Small trees grew on the banks, an oasis of green shade in the scorched dry plain. They washed their hands and faces in the cool water. Suba dipped his ladle into the shallow stream and began to fill his calabash. Damba kneeled to make his own ablutions. Nandzi watched Suba for a moment. Then she began to dig a small pit in the sandy bed.

"What are you doing?" Damba asked.

She did not understand his question and continued to dig. When the hole was big enough she forced the empty calabash down into it. The water flowed in over the rim. Suba was still struggling to fill his vessel.

Nandzi tried to break off a handful of grass from the bank but it was too tough. She pulled and it came away with a sod of soil around the roots.

"Hold it," Damba told her and cut off the roots with his sword. He smiled at her but she did not see his face. She formed the grass into a ring and put it on her head. Suba helped her to lift the full calabash. She steadied it and adjusted the balance while Damba helped Suba in the same way.

Damba led them up the hill. Vultures were picking at the naked body. Damba slashed at them with his sword. They screeched at him, flapped their great wings and hopped aside. Damba let the captives pass. Nandzi averted her eyes, unwilling to witness the damage the birds had inflicted on the corpse. It was not custom to leave the dead unburied. The man's spirit would wander without peace and return to trouble the living. She wanted to ask Damba to let her dig a grave, but she had no means of communicating with him.

"Do you speak their language?" she asked Suba. "We should ask him to let us bury the dead."

"Small," replied Suba and added, in explanation, "from the market."

He had come to a fork. He took a rough path, made by the passage of a horse, which would lead back to the camp by a shorter route than the way they had come.

"What should I say?" the lad was asking, when he came across another prone body.

It was lying on its back, naked like the first they had seen. The impact of a horse's hoof had crushed the skull and splashed the victim's brains around. Flies droned on the fragments of flesh. (Once she had asked Itsho how it was that flies, and hyenas and vultures too, so quickly located a new source of food.) The face was unrecognisable, but Nandzi recognised the body at once. Unaided, she lifted the calabash from her head and set it carefully on the ground, taking care not to spill any water. She knelt by Itsho. The worst had happened. Deep inside her, this was what she had feared. Now she could not avoid the reality. Yet she felt that this was all a dream; and that somehow her disembodied spirit was watching the scene from a distance. She was completely calm. She laid her cheek upon his chest. The body was still warm. She lifted his arms, one at a time, and stretched them over him, placing his hands over his genitals. She looked up. The vultures were still busy elsewhere. She must cover the body. Then she felt a hand on her shoulder. It was Damba.

"It is someone you know," he said.

"Tell him," she said to Suba, "tell him it is my husband."

"I am sorry," said Damba, when Suba had explained. "Bring the water and we will come back with a hoe to bury him."

Nandzi refused to rise. She forced her fingers into the sandy soil and scooped up a handful, testing whether she would be able to dig a grave without a tool. Damba was scared of Abdulai. He would never approve the wasting of time on the burial of an enemy. It must be done without his knowledge. He looked around. They could not be seen from the camp.

"Come," he said, echoing his words with sign language, "We will go to the camp and come back with a hoe."

"Tell her," he said to Suba.

Nandzi pointed to the sky.

"You fear the vultures," said Damba.

There was a baobab tree nearby. Damba helped Suba to put down his calabash.

"Go and see if you can find branches, firewood," he said to the lad, showing by signs what he proposed to do.

*****

"Why have you been so long?" asked Abdulai as they approached.

Nandzi flinched. This was the man who had raped her the previous day. But he did not seem to recognise her.

"I stopped to pray," lied Damba. "The stream is almost dry. We need a hoe to dig a pit."

Abdulai grunted.

"The hoes are being used to dig the graves," he said.

"I think I know where to find one," said Damba.

He was thinking of the hoes he had looted from Tigen's homestead.

"Don't waste time," said Abdulai. "We must eat and leave."

They off-loaded the full calabashes and took empty ones. Cooking fires had been lit. They would eat millet porridge with a little dried fish. If the hunters were successful, the war party would also have some grilled meat.

Damba wanted to leave Suba to dig the grave but Nandzi insisted that she would do it herself.

"Itsho," she said aloud when they had left her, "you gave your life trying to save me. It would have been better if you had never met us on the way. Then, at least, you would still be alive. Itsho, I love you. I will never take another husband. You are my husband now. I am digging your grave myself, with my own hoe, which was stolen from me. I cannot give you a proper burial in keeping with custom. Even if our captors would permit it, which they wouldn't, there is no Earth Priest here. I cannot even ask the men, my fellow captives, to come. The Bedagbam would not allow. But I will say a prayer to the ancestors myself, to accept your spirit and let you rest in peace."

When Damba and Suba returned from the stream, Nandzi was still digging and still talking to Itsho. Damba put down the calabash he was carrying and signed to Nandzi to put it on her head, promising that they would return to finish the burial. Abdulai must not know what he was doing.

When Damba and Suba came back from the third trip to the stream, Nandzi was ready. She washed Itsho awkwardly with a corner of her cloth. Then the man and the boy helped her lift the body into the shallow grave.

Nandzi stood up, the hoe still in her hand.

"Oh, Ancestors," she intoned, "ancestors of Tigen my father and of Itsho's father. I am Nandzi, daughter of Tigen and Tabitsha. Forgive me that I, a mere woman, address you directly. Forgive me that I bring you no drink. You will know the reason. The Bedagbam captured me. My lover Itsho came to rescue me and they killed him. I have had to bury him in this lonely place, far from his home and mine. Protect his body from the wild beasts. Accept his spirit, I beg you, to live amongst you. Accept the spirit of Itsho. I am Nandzi. I have spoken."

She paused. Damba looked about anxiously.

"Oh Ancestors," Nandzi continued, "another matter. One of our people, I do not know his name or where he comes from, lies down there. The vultures are eating his flesh. There may be more. I do not know. Accept his spirit too and those of any others who have died in trying to rescue us from the Bedagbam. Do not let them become evil spirits of the bush. It is not our fault that they have not received a proper burial. There is nothing to be done about it."

When they had finished the filling, Damba and Suba stamped on the soil to discourage the hyenas from digging up the grave. Then they piled stones and branches on the surface. Damba was becoming more and more anxious. But Nandzi was at peace with herself. What had happened had happened. She had done her duty. Itsho would know.

*****

Nandzi touched Damba's arm and looked him in the eye for the first time.

"Thank you," she said.

Damba nodded an acknowledgement. *These people are also human,* he thought, as he sent the two of them back into the prison. He had been led to believe otherwise.

Nandzi sat down against the wall. Dry-eyed, she examined her fellow captives. One man was wearing an apron of leaves, another was dressed in bark cloth. Others wore torn and dirty cotton garments. They sat and lay uncomfortably, their wrists still tied behind their backs. She searched for a spark of rebellion, but their eyes were listless, without hope.

She looked up at the clear blue sky. Then, without warning, she felt reality strike her like the blow of a cudgel on the back of her neck. *Itsho is dead. I am a slave. No one will come to rescue me. I will never again see my mother and my family.*

She wailed a dirge. She had never been deeply moved by a death before, not even when Tabitsha had lost a new-born baby. She had hardly seen the child before it died. When the women had shrieked their customary lamentations she had smiled secretly because she thought their grief was feigned. She had always smiled at the way her mother would wail at a funeral. Tabitsha could turn her tears on and off, as if by command.

Now it was her turn to howl; but the cry came from her heart. She wept for Itsho and she wept for herself. The sobbing convulsed her and it would not stop. The men were embarrassed. Nandzi was the only woman in the cell. Their skills did not run to the comforting of a strange woman.

Then Suba also began to cry. He was the youngest of the prisoners; but Suba liked to think of himself as a man and he knew that men did not express their grief openly as women did. He was proud of his manly behaviour that morning, of how he had concealed his shock and had even helped to lower Itsho into the grave. But he too had been snatched from his mother; and the encounter with the two disfigured corpses had shaken him more than he had cared to admit to himself. Now Nandzi's wailing and sobbing broke his reserve and his tears began to flow. Once the dam had broken there was no holding his grief. He cried for his mother.

Suba's outburst penetrated the cocoon of self-pity in which Nandzi had enveloped herself. She stopped crying and wiped her face.

"Suba," she called, but he paid no attention.

She rose and went to him. She put her hand on his shoulder.

"Suba," she said, "don't cry. Suba, you are a man, you must be strong."

He paid no attention to her. She sat down by his side and put an arm around his shoulder. Still he continued to cry.

"You were so strong this morning," she said. "I could not have managed without you. I could not have explained anything to the man. If it were not for your help, the vultures would now be picking over Itsho's body. And I didn't even thank you. I forgot to thank you."

Suba looked up at her and wiped his eyes. Then he fell upon her breast and sobbed and sobbed. She held him tight. He was only a child, she realised. *And I,* Nandzi thought, *I am already an adult, ready to have children of my own, to be married. I have no right to cry: this boy needs my support.* But she could not control herself and the tears came to her eyes again. So they hugged one another and cried together; and Suba was comforted and fell asleep in her arms.

All this the other prisoners, the men, watched in silence. They were men no longer, Nandzi thought. They had all been emasculated and become the dogs of their new masters.

The guards brought in two bowls of steaming gruel. Their hands untied, the famished prisoners gathered round the bowls and pushed and shoved and struggled for a handful of the watery pap.

Nandzi had no heart to join them. Suba stirred. Gently, she moved him aside. Then she stood up.

"Will you not leave some for the boy?" she shouted at them above the hubbub.

The men withdrew. In their hunger, they had lost their dignity and forgotten the mutual obligations which custom imposed upon them. They looked at her in guilty silence, sullen and surly at having been exposed. Who was this young girl to scold them so?

"Here. Take it," said one of them, handing her the bowl.

*****

They walked across country, picking a way through the coarse reeds of the long grass, over low rolling hills, through level patches of desiccated swampland. Scattered trees and termite mounds, as tall as two men, dotted the landscape. The captives walked in a small, tight group. Most of the men wore nothing but a loin cloth. The rough grass scratched their skin. A few wore the pants and cotton smocks in which they had been captured. All were barefooted. None wore a hat.

The air was full of the fine dust of the harmattan. The sun was hidden but its fierce dry heat penetrated the haze and withered them. The men spoke little. They were turned in upon themselves, crushed by the consciousness of their new status. Only when their captors cracked their whips to make them walk faster, did they turn on them with a quick look of hatred.

Twice during the morning they came across a running stream. There they quenched their thirst and scooped handfuls of water over their grimy whitened bodies. Once they came upon a dawa-dawa tree in fruit. Abdulai paused to let Suba climb it and even allowed the slaves a share of the pods with their yellow powder.

Nandzi walked a little behind the group of men. Suba was glad to keep her company. He talked and talked. He told her about his family and about how he had been taken by the Bedagbam. Unwittingly, he chased from her mind the oppressive picture of Itsho's broken head.

All around them rode their captors, always ready to flick a whip at a straggler. They wore broad-brimmed conical straw hats, trimmed with red and black leather. There was little chance of being attacked now and they had consigned their leather armour to their saddle bags; but they carried their spears at the ready and their hide shields, swords, leather-stringed bows and quivers of iron-tipped arrows were close at hand. Most wore a long-sleeved smock of thick hand-woven cotton, dyed in indigo or black and yellow, and calf length cotton trousers. Some had covered their noses and mouths with a cloth to filter out the dust.

Their black and bay horses were smaller than Abdulai's. They had delicate ears and a short head, and were brightly caparisoned; their leather bridles and saddlery were embossed with intricate designs and their bells made a kind of music. Abdulai's stirrups were of brass, but the other warriors used iron.

Tsetse flies had infected many of the horses with sleeping sickness, making them lethargic even when they were put out to grass. Heavily loaded as they now were, they moved slowly.

The savannah was alive with game. They stepped around fresh elephant droppings, abuzz with green flies. On a patch of damp bare swampy ground, they saw the impress of the paws of great cats. The noisy passage of the party disturbed a herd of bush-buck and sent them leaping away through the reeds. Issaka released an arrow and shouted in triumph as one fell.

When the sun was at its highest, they came to a dry river bed and Abdulai allowed them to rest for an hour in the shade of the light bush, while the horses grazed.

*****

Abdulai made camp for the night under a great silk cotton tree.

By the time darkness had fallen two fires were burning. The warriors sat around one and their captives around the second, close by. When the slaves had eaten, Abdulai sent Damba and Issaka to tie their hands; but Damba left Nandzi and Suba free. Guards were set to patrol the camp in shifts throughout the night. Others would keep the fires stoked. Abdulai had little fear of another attack from humans; they had not seen another living soul during the day's march. It was animals he feared. His captives, he knew, feared them too.

"Suba," Nandzi whispered to the boy as they piled dry grass against one of the buttresses of the mighty tree, "I am going to escape tonight. Will you come with me?"

The boy nodded vigorously.

"You will not be afraid of the wild beasts?"

He frowned bravely and shook his head.

"Then let us sleep early," she whispered. "I will wake you when it is time to go. We'll just slip away quietly while the guards are not watching."

Nandzi had only just fallen asleep when she was woken by the drumming. The younger warriors were dancing in a circle around the fire, casting fantastic shadows as they dipped and spun, their smocks whirling. A drummer squeezed the strings of the hourglass drum which he carried in his armpit, beating the goat skin with a bent stick. The plaintive whine of a one-stringed gonje fiddle and the sweet tones of the hand piano echoed out into the enveloping darkness.

Nandzi pulled her cloth over her head to try to block out the sound and the chill of the night air; but it was no good: once woken she could not fall asleep again. Confused thoughts raced through her mind. She imagined the scene of her sudden return to Tigen's compound. They would surely take her for a ghost. How Tabitsha would hug her! And Nowu! She closed her eyes and saw Itsho's mutilated body; and she shuddered. *If only they had decided not to attack this morning when the ruined buildings offered some protection to the Bedagbam; if only they had followed us through the day, they might have had a better chance tonight. Perhaps the survivors of the attack party have done just that.* She sat up and peered into the dark bush. In the distance, a hyena howled. By her side Suba twisted and turned in his sleep. Then he, too, was awake.

He sat up and hugged his knees. He looked shaken.

"What is it?" she asked him.

"I had a bad dream," he replied.

The dancing had stopped. The Bedagbam were talking loudly and laughing. Abdulai rose to his feet. At once his men became quiet. He walked around the fire and flicked his fly whisk this way and that. Then he began to talk in his language. He spoke in a sing-song voice, sometimes jabbing the air. It sounded to Nandzi as if he was telling them a story. From time to time they applauded. She yawned twice and then she was asleep.

She was woken by the pre-dawn chorus of bird-song in the branches of the silk-cotton tree.

She shivered and yawned. The surroundings were unfamiliar and for a moment she wondered where she was. Then she knew. The stress of the previous morning, the forced march, the late hour at which she had fallen asleep: all had taken their toll and she had overslept. Already the camp was stirring. Her plan to flee would have to be postponed.

*****

Damba took to riding alongside them. He asked them their names and told them his own.

"Did you understand Abdulai's history last night?" he asked Suba.

The boy hung his head and made a non-committal noise.

"What does he say?" Nandzi asked him.

Suba explained, "Last night their leader, the one they call Abdulai, told them a long story, about how they, the Bedagbam, came to be living in this place. He is asking me whether I understood the story."

"Well, did you?"

"More or less," Suba replied, "but I don't know if it would be wise to admit that to him."

"What was the story?"

"He said their ancestors came on horses from a far place on the edge of the great desert, where they had lived before. Their leader was called the Red Hunter. The son of this Red Hunter married the daughter of the priest, the Tindan Na. During the annual festival, while the Tindan Na was in his tent, putting on his robes, his daughter's husband crept up behind the old man and brought a great club crashing down on his skull. Then he donned the dead man's priestly robes and declared himself the new Tindan Na. So it was, he told them, that the Bedagbam became the owners of the land."

CHAPTER 4

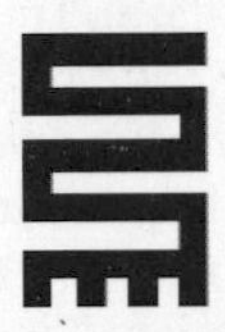

At noon on the fourth day after Nandzi's capture, they saw Yendi in the distance.

The warriors halted to put on their armour and smarten up their horses' trappings. Abdulai took the lead on his white charger. The horsemen formed up in two files with the ragged slaves on foot between them. The drummers set up a triumphant rhythm and the party entered the town.

The houses, like those in Tigen's hamlet, were roughly circular in plan, with conical thatched roofs and grouped in family compounds. The white walls shone in the sun and the thatch on the roofs was fresh and neat. Everything looked new.

As they passed the first compound children appeared as if from nowhere and fell into place, skipping and dancing after the cavalcade. A small boy called out, "Papa, papa!" to a hero on horseback, but his father passed by without hearing or recognising him. Women abandoned their domestic chores and ran to join their neighbours, merging into groups, pointing out the warriors and the slaves to one another and falling into animated conversation. Men with white beards, who had been squatting on their haunches in the shade of a mango tree to chew kola and discuss the weighty matters of the day, rose and stretched, adjusted their baggy cotton trousers and their batakaris, slipped into their sandals and made their own more leisurely and dignified way to the market square.

A woman ran up ahead of the party and halting, looked back to scan the warriors' faces. When they had all passed her, she gathered up her cloth and pursued Abdulai.

Coming abreast of him for the second time, she caught her breath and screamed, "Captain Abdulai, where is my son Ali? What have you done with Ali?"

Abdulai waved a greeting to Ali's mother.

"Later," he cried back. "Later. I will come to see you."

Ali had been struck by a poisoned arrow. He lay buried in a grave his mother would never see. Abdulai did not relish the prospect of having to break the news of the death of three of his troop to their families. Especially to the women. The men were usually understanding in such circumstances, even proud of a son who had died in battle; but the women were troublesome. "Why *my* son?" this woman would demand. What answer could one give to such a question? She would make him feel personally responsible for Ali's death: and that was manifestly unfair.

Nandzi had observed this incident. Now, as she passed, the woman collapsed into a heap of flesh and crumpled cloth by the road-side, knowing that her son was surely dead. Looking back, Nandzi felt for her, all alone with her grief in the small cloud of dust thrown up by the horses and the excited crowd. She wondered whether it was one of Itsho's arrows which had killed the woman's son.

"We must be the first party to return," said Damba to Suba, who was walking alongside his horse, one hand on the bridle. The boy had become quite attached to him and was diligently striving to expand his vocabulary.

The traders had dispersed and there was little activity in the market square. A horse was tethered to an iron hook which had been driven into a tree trunk. Small donkeys, their front legs hobbled, browsed in a patch of dry grass. Goats scavenged amongst the unswept debris. In one corner, in the shade of a tree, a class of boys droned a recitation of passages from the Holy Book under the watchful eye of a malam.

Abdulai drew fiercely on his mount's bit, forcing the white beast to rear. The small boys whistled their applause. He turned the horse to face his men.

"Damba, Issaka," he called out, "muster the prisoners under the tree over there. Check that their hands are well tied. Then let the rest of the troop fall out. The two of you remain on guard until I send you a relief."

*****

A first-time visitor to Yendi would have been at pains to pick out Na Saa Ziblim's palace. It was no more than a group of seven compounds, some larger, some smaller, disposed, seemingly at random, about an unwalled open space adjacent to the market. One of the main roads of the town passed right through the palace grounds.

The largest compound housed the private quarters of the Na. The bleached shoulder blades of a foal guarded the great entrance doorway against the passage of evil spirits. Most visitors passed no further than the first room, an imposing reception hall with a conical thatched roof. Here the King gave audience during the day and the favourite royal horses were stabled at night.

The Na reclined on cushions arranged on a lion's skin. This in turn was spread upon an ornate Moroccan carpet. He was dressed in voluminous cotton trousers and a heavy long-sleeved batakari intricately embroidered in the Muslim style. He wore silver rings on his fingers; leather amulets containing fragments of parchment inscribed with short passages from the Holy Book hung from a silver chain around his neck. Around him sat numerous chiefs, elders and officials, several of his wives and his eldest son. The Tolon-Na, Commander-in-Chief of the King's army, was there. So too were the Kumbong-Na, Commander of the Royal Archers, and the Galidima, Chief of the Eunuchs. The Owner of the Land was also present. At the periphery stood the head barber, the head butcher and the head blacksmith. The principal court musician stood ready to give the signal to his drummers. Sundry slaves and lackeys hovered in attendance, waving fans, offering tepid water in silver goblets and kola nuts on trays. This was the court of the Ya Na, King of Dagbon.

Bowing low, the Chief of the Horses led Abdulai into the royal presence.

When Abdulai had completed an elaborate obeisance, Na Saa indicated with his fly-whisk that he should rise. Saa Ziblim was not yet forty, handsome, as befitted a king, sharp of eye, in his own estimation a progressive reformer, a man who, though he relished power, used it wisely.

"Let us hear your man's report," he said to the Chief of the Horses.

The Chief of the Horses launched into a long, obsequious recitation of the virtues of the Na and his ancestors.

Na Saa cut him short.

"Are you the Chief of the Horses or the Chief of the Royal Praise Singers?" he asked, looking over his shoulder at that very person.

Those entitled by rank to be amused at the discomfiture of the Chief of the Horses expressed their appreciation of the Na's humour in a proper manner.

"Curtail the poetry and proceed with your report," ordered the King.

The Chief of the Horses was a man of the old school. He had served the previous king, Na Gariba, and had somehow survived his late master's undoing. Judging him incapable of modernising the army, Na Saa was actively seeking an opportunity to sack him.

The Chief of the Horses suppressed his anger. He had served the great Na Gariba for many years. What right had this young upstart to treat him with such disrespect? He knew what custom demanded. It was the duty of elders such as he to act as custodians of the history and culture of the people. Traditional protocol could not be so lightly dismissed. Ignoring the Na, he proceeded with his formal litany of praise.

Na Saa interrupted him for the second time. He spoke abruptly.

"Sit down, old man," he ordered.

"Commander," he addressed Abdulai, "what is your name?"

He knew very well who Abdulai was. He judged him a man of unquestionable loyalty, brave, a good leader, but brutal and, worse, obtuse. An unsuitable candidate for succession to the skin of the Chief of the Horses, he reflected.

Abdulai's peroration went on and on. He dealt with every unimportant detail of the expedition at great length. As he heard the blend of romance, boasting and equivocation issue from his own lips, his confidence grew. He contrived to tell his story without any mention of his losses.

"Have you finished?" asked the Na at length. "You say that you captured twenty slaves, a woman, a boy and eighteen grown men. Is that correct?"

Abdulai concurred. It was clear that the Na appreciated his achievements. Perhaps he would reward him with the gift of a new horse, he thought.

"What were your casualties, men and horses?" Na Sa asked him quietly.

He knew the answer. Damba had already reported to him, in private.

Abdulai felt his world collapse about him.

"Two men killed; and two horses," he replied.

"Think carefully, Commander Abdulai," said the King. "I ask you again. What were your casualties, men and horses? Tell me the truth, now. I shall not ask you a third time."

"Three men killed; and three horses," replied Abdulai.

He had made a mistake in underestimating the Na. The King must have powerful medicine at his disposal. It was uncanny how his question had addressed precisely the facts which Abdulai had resolved to conceal.

"Why did you fail to state this in your report? Why did you lie to me?"

Abdulai hung his head. He knew that an attempt to answer could only exacerbate his predicament.

"The Council of Eunuchs will sit on this matter, examine all witnesses and report to me," ordered the King. "Galidima, understood?"

The Chief of the Eunuchs nodded gravely. Na Saa looked around to gauge reaction. He had not been on the skin long and still needed to consolidate his position. Every decision he made had a political dimension to it. Support had to be earned. He would not fall into the trap of complacency which had been Gariba's downfall.

"Now send a message to Nana Koranten Péte. Tell the Asante Consul that the Ya Na invites him to join an inspection of the first consignment of slaves to arrive this season."

*****

The slaves were allocated a large compound.

In the course of time it would become overcrowded, but the first twenty captives had plenty of space. Their bonds were untied and they were free to move at will within the prison walls.

Nandzi had the small room set aside for female slaves all to herself. As the only woman she was expected to do the cooking. If the men had had their way, she would also have gathered the firewood and washed their ragged garments. They found it hard enough to come to terms with the psychic effects of capture and enslavement; that they should be further humiliated by being forced to do women's work was inconceivable. Fortunately for them their captors' views on what was proper work for men and women were little different from their own.

Suba was a great help. He was happier in Nandzi's company than in that of the grown men. It was he who every morning dumped the pots of excrement on the outskirts of the town. It was Suba who brought the calabashes of rationed water from the well near the market. And at night he slept in the open doorway of her room.

*****

Na Saa Ziblim and Koranten Péte walked hand in hand, deep in conversation.

They communicated with one another, after a fashion, in a mixture of Hausa and Asante which caused them both much amusement. It was Koranten Péte, commander of the central division, who had led the victorious Asante forces in the recent war. The Asante King had rewarded him with title to one third of the tribute which the Dagomba were now obliged to pay each year. He needed little further inducement to spend the months of the trading season watching over Asante interests in Yendi.

The King and the Consul were followed by a long procession of dignitaries and officials.

The Galidima, Chief of the Eunuchs, was responsible both for policing the city and for the administration of justice. The fines imposed by the Council of the Eunuchs, in cattle and cowries, formed a substantial portion of the royal revenues. Beardless and effeminate the Galidima was also the guardian of the King's wives.

The eunuchs, too, had wives. These women, their unions sanctioned by the King himself, were prostitutes in all but name. They bore the added misfortune of seeing their male children castrated in order that they might one day succeed their mothers' husbands.

Demonkum, already Chief of Those-who-sit-before-the-Na and shortly to be enstooled in the Asante manner with the new title of Chief of the Guns, followed the King. He was dressed in the style of the Kambonse, wearing a richly embroidered cloth, rather than the customary smock. Kambonse was the Dagbon name for the Asante; and Kambonse was the name that Demonkum had chosen for the musketeers whom he was training. Three years at the Asante court had convinced him of the superiority of their military technology and strategy and he was determined to reform the Dagbon army along similar lines. But there was opposition. He smiled wryly as he recalled the recent humiliation of the leader of the reactionary party, the Chief of the Horses, conspicuously absent from this day's inspection.

Damba, who had been put in charge of the slaves' compound, was at the entrance to meet the Na and his party. He had made an attempt to smarten up his prisoners. They had had their first proper bath since their arrival. Discarded old clothes had been found for the man who had arrived dressed only in withered leaves. Damba had persuaded his mother to let him have an old cloth for Nandzi.

The Na and Koranten Péte walked slowly down the line, stopping to inspect and discuss each slave. Speaking his own language, the Na asked a slave his name. When he received only a blank, uncomprehending look in reply, he tried again in Hausa; then Nana Péte tried Asante.

"Bush people," said the Consul to the King. "It seems that they do not hear any civilised language."

"If you please, sir," said Damba, stepping forward nervously, "this boy, he is called Suba, hears our tongue."

"Suba, is that your name?" the Na asked.

Suba was lost in embarrassment. He had become proud of his developing skills as an interpreter and was pleased at the way that Damba depended upon him, but he was just a humble village lad and quite unversed in the customs of a royal court. He was overwhelmed by the rich clothes and arrogant bearing of these nobles. Fortunately for him, he did not have to reply. Nandzi, standing next to Suba at the end of the line, had caught the royal eye.

"What's this?" he said, examining her frankly.

Nandzi dropped her eyes and looked at her bare feet. This was not the first time she had seen that look in a man's eyes. But this gorgeously robed man was a king. What could he want with her? How should she react? Was this a threat or, might she hope, an opportunity? She concentrated her mind and tried to summon up a vision of Itsho.

The King put his hand under her chin and lifted her head, giving her no choice but to return his gaze.

The Asante Consul put his arm around the King's shoulder.

"No, no, your majesty," he said firmly, "you have not forgotten our treaty, have you?

"Not just this one?" the King appealed, distracted from his projected dalliance.

"I fear not," said the Consul. "You have brought in only twenty so far. Your target this season is three hundred. You have a long way to go yet. I regret that I cannot permit any, if you will forgive me, any diminution of my master's stock. Anything in excess of three hundred, of course, is yours to dispose of as you wish, but the first three hundred: those are ours."

*****

Damba persuaded the Na and the Consul to permit him to appropriate Suba as his personal slave.

"It is because I hear their language," Suba said proudly. "Now I am going to start learning Hausa too. And when I master that, I shall learn Asante. Then I shall know all the languages in the world."

Nandzi laughed. "That is wonderful news, Suba. Now you will not be sent to Kumase. Just think, if Damba were to take you with him on one of his expeditions, you might have a chance to escape and return to your home and family."

"I hadn't thought of that," replied the boy.

Damba was treating him kindly and his memories of home were beginning to recede: he saw a career as a court interpreter opening before him.

"But I will be sad if they take you to Kumase and leave me behind," he said.

In attendance on Damba, Suba now learned all the latest news. The Council of Eunuchs had completed its examination of Abdulai and other witnesses. Abdulai had been fined twenty cows and fifty goats, which would leave him impoverished. He had been demoted and his white horse and brass accoutrements had been confiscated. The two guards who had fallen asleep on duty had been sentenced to death.

"Damba says it is a warning to the other warriors to do their work well and not be cowards," explained Suba.

The following day Nandzi was at the head of a procession of slaves, each bearing a load of firewood for the shea-butter factory. As they entered the market square there was a commotion at the far end. Their mounted warder, eager to witness what was to come, ordered them to halt.

The Na and his court were seated in the shade of a tree. Beside the Na, on a stool, sat the Asante Consul. The two condemned men, their hands tightly bound behind their backs, were led into the square. The State Executioner, his heavily muscled body bare from the waist up, called a halt. An assistant tied the prisoners' ankles and forced them to their knees before the Na. The Chief of the Eunuchs proclaimed the charge, the verdict and the sentence in his high-pitched voice. There was a great roll of drums as the Executioner raised a heavy wooden club on high and brought it crashing down on the first man's skull, felling him with a single blow. The crowd gasped. Then it was the turn of the second victim.

The warder had seen enough. He cracked his whip at his charges and they moved off again. Nandzi turned her head as they left the market square. The corpses had been laid face down upon the ground. The Executioner raised his axe on high. As she watched, he brought it down and, with a single mighty blow, severed the head from the corpse. A great cheer went up from the watching crowd, but when it died down, Nandzi heard women wailing. She felt faint and wanted to vomit. The warder cracked his whip and she pulled herself together and walked on.

"They cut the stomachs open and took out the livers to make medicine for the Na," Suba told Nandzi later. "Then they dragged the bodies into the bush and left them there for the vultures to eat. They have stuck the heads on poles in the market place."

"Suba, I don't want to know about that."

Nandzi had other matters on her mind.

"Suba can you keep a secret?" she asked.

He was the only one she could talk to.

The boy nodded energetically.

"I am going to escape," she said.

His eyes opened wide.

"I didn't want to go without saying goodbye to you. You are my brother now and I will never forget you and what you did for me."

*****

Nandzi lay on her back and stared into the darkness.

Her arms and legs ached from her long day's work in the shea-butter factory and yet she could not sleep. The small round room was packed with women. At the perimeter they lay shoulder to shoulder, but near the centre of the room there was not enough space for all their feet. When Nandzi lay down early enough to stretch out her legs on the floor, they were soon buried beneath those of her neighbours. Tonight her feet had lain uncomfortably on top of a jumble of others until she had drawn them back beneath her knees. *When the next consignment of women arrives*, she thought, *they will have to sleep outside in the courtyard.*

The room had no windows and the single door opening provided little ventilation. Their water ration was barely enough for drinking, let alone bathing. They were all filthy. There was a pervasive smell of stale sweat and shea-butter, menstrual blood, urine and farting in the room.

Nandzi was hungry. She ran her hands over her body.

I am wasting away, she thought.

She raised herself to a sitting position and leaned back against the plastered mud wall. Immediately, it seemed, adjacent bodies filled the narrow space her legs had vacated.

She squeezed her eyes shut. *Itsho*, she breathed, *Itsho, help me*. Itsho's features filled her mind. *Speak to me*, she whispered. *Itsho, tell me what to do*. He smiled and his lips moved but she heard nothing. A woman snored. Then the vision was gone. She shook her head vigorously from side to side. *Itsho is no longer in this world*, she told herself. *I am all alone; I have no one to depend on but myself.*

Not for the first time, she considered her options. There were only two: and of those acceptance was out of the question. Her present condition was intolerable and the prospect of the future seemed worse.

Yet every escape plan she considered was fraught with difficulty and danger.

Exhausted, she fell asleep and dreamed. She was alone. A row of enormous earthenware cauldrons stretched as far as she could see. Each was supported over a blazing fire. She had to keep the cauldrons on the boil. She collected firewood from a pile and ran from one fire to the next, stoking. The smoke filled her eyes but she could not pause. The boiling must not stop. She stood on tiptoe to peer into a cauldron. There should have been shea-nut kernels bouncing up and down in the bubbling, boiling water. Instead there were men's heads. Somewhere in the distance stood Itsho, naked, his body smeared with shea-butter, watching. Two men approached, arm in arm. One was the King, the other Abdulai. "Yes, that is the one," said the King, pointing at her. Abdulai grabbed her suddenly from behind, one arm round her waist, the other hand in her crotch, and propelled her up into the air, in a great, arcing slow-motion trajectory. She felt she was gliding like a bird. Then she was diving head first into the seething cauldron.

"What is it, sister?" mumbled her neighbour, woken by Nandzi's scream.

*****

Nandzi awoke with a start.

She had taken a place near the door so as not to run the risk of disturbing the other women. She looked out and saw the crescent moon.

Cautiously she rose and stepped through the doorway into the empty courtyard. Far away a dog barked. It was bitterly cold. She rubbed her arms in turn and wrapped herself tightly in her own old cloth and the one that Damba had given her for the Na's inspection. Then she made her way silently towards the entrance hall. The brass bells which hung around the necks of the tethered horses made a tinkling sound at every slight movement. A guard lay stretched across the outer doorway, asleep. Slowly, step by step, she picked a way across the room. A horse whinnied and she froze, her heart pumping. The guard turned over in his sleep. She took a careful step. Her bare foot landed on a pile of fresh horse shit. She cursed. Another step. She heard snoring: there was at least one more guard lying hidden in the dark recesses of the room. She wondered whether these sleeping guards would also have their heads chopped off when her escape was discovered. Then, at last, she had stepped over the form at the door and was free of the prison compound.

Only the drone of the cicadas and the horses' bells disturbed the silence of the sleeping town. Like a wraith she moved through the shadows. As she reached the last compound, a dog rushed out at her, snarling. She took to her heels and ran. Reaching the limits of its territory, the beast stopped and stood in the pale moonlight, barking after her. She ran without stopping until she reached the dawa-dawa tree at the edge of the thicket where they went to cut firewood. There she collapsed on the ground, her chest heaving and wet with sweat in spite of the night chill.

When she had recovered her breath, she sat up and listened. An owl hooted nearby. *An ill omen*, she thought. The bird sat on a high branch, staring down at her.

"Whoo, whoo," she whispered.

She collected her hidden treasures: an iron cutlass, presumed lost by a firewood party; and an empty drinking gourd. There was no time to lose. She looked back at the sleeping town, taking her bearings. At the well she stopped to drink and fill her gourd. *Keep the town at your back and the moon on your right*, she told herself. *Keep going straight and in three or four days' time you will walk into your father's compound.*

*****

She had not come far, yet she was already exhausted.

She could find no tracks in this bush, not in the dim light. She had started to hack a way through with her cutlass, but that was hopelessly slow. They would laugh at her, think she was mad, if they captured her, cutting traces through the scrub from nowhere to nowhere. "Where did you think you were going?" they would ask her.

But they must not capture her. They would surely kill her if they did.

The gourd was barely half full: much of the water had spilled. She stopped to take her first sip. Then she set off again, using her slight body as a ram to force a way through the long dry grass, changing course, even sometimes retracing her steps, when she met an obstacle. The brittle reeds tore at her cloth and scratched her skin. *If I step on a snake*, she thought, *that will be the end of me*. She struggled on. It was hopeless, she knew it was hopeless. She had no idea where she was or in what direction she was going. She came to a small clearing and lay down on her back to rest. The sky was dark. There were no stars. Only the pale moon had the strength to penetrate the dust of the harmattan. The cold night chilled her through and through. *I must decide what to do*, she thought.

The rasping cough of a leopard came floating through the night air. She sat up in alarm. There it was again. Fortunately, she judged, the beast was off her track and up wind and would not have picked up her scent. But if she continued to force her way through the bush, it might well hear her. Leopards have extraordinarily acute hearing, Itsho had once told her.

Then a thought occurred to her. It was the leopard, so Tabitsha had taught her, which in ancient times had brushed the path of the fleeing Bekpokpam with its tail, hiding their tracks from their Bedagbam pursuers. Perhaps Itsho had sent this leopard to protect her in the same way? Perhaps; perhaps not. It would be better not to count on it.

She forced herself to concentrate. The moon would soon set and then it would be completely dark until dawn. She had worked a full day pounding shea-nuts and had had only a short sleep before stealing out of the prison and the town. Now there was a very real danger that she might be torn to pieces by a wild beast. There was that sawing cough again. She shivered. A fire might keep the leopard at bay but she had no means of making a fire. She stood up and looked around her. Silhouetted against the waning moon there stood a tree.

*****

Damba was fond of Nandzi. He had thought of asking leave to buy her for himself, taking her as his concubine or even as a wife.

However he had been present when the Asante Consul had placed an embargo upon the Na's lust. There was no way that he could ask for that which had been denied the King.

Damba did what he could for Nandzi, though with discretion. He had given her an old cloth of his mother's and he brought her food from time to time to supplement the spare diet which she shared with the other slaves. When he inspected the prison camp at dawn each morning, at the changing of the guard, he made a point of looking for her and greeting her.

So this morning he noticed her absence almost at once. The guards knew nothing. The girl had been there the previous evening. They had all been awake throughout the night and there was no way she could have climbed the outer wall or slipped out through the entrance hall.

Then Damba saw the footprint which Nandzi had left in the horse shit.

*****

The dew was already dry when they rode up.

Nandzi was still fast asleep. She was sitting upright on a branch tied to the trunk with her old cloth.

While two men held his great white horse, Damba stood on the saddle. Leaning his body against the tree he removed Nandzi's home-made safety harness. She did not resist as he lifted her down and placed her on the saddle before him. He noticed how hot her skin was and felt her forehead. She had a high fever.

*****

Fearing that he would be punished as Abdulai had been, Damba sought a private audience with the Na and told him exactly what had happened.

"Where is the girl now?" asked the Na.

"She is very ill, delirious with fever," replied Damba. "She is in no condition to repeat her attempt to escape. I took her to my mother's house. My mother has knowledge of the use of plants and she is treating her. It was my mother who insisted that I report to Your Highness at once. As soon as she can walk, I will send her back to the slaves' compound. Unless, of course, Your Highness orders otherwise."

"She will have to be executed," said the King, "as an example to the others. I am sure that that is what Nana Péte will require. But let your mother first restore her to good health."

*****

Damba's mother looked after Nandzi well.

At first she was only pandering to the wishes of her beloved first-born, but as she nursed the girl, she became fond of her. Using Suba, who was now staying in their compound, as an interpreter, she asked her about her home and family. She fed her well and soon Nandzi began to put on weight. As soon as she was able, she insisted on sweeping the compound and helping with the cooking.

Nandzi's outward display of gratitude and humility concealed an inner turmoil. In other circumstances she would have calmly considered her position and weighed up the choices open to her. Now she was scared of thinking, terrified of what she might find in her own mind. She no longer attempted to communicate with Itsho. She no longer thought of her mother and her small brother. Inside her, she was already dead.

She was troubled by terrible nightmares, from which she awoke screaming and sweating; but by morning she had lost all recollection of their content, or, indeed, that she had dreamed at all.

Suba was a constant visitor. Somehow he sensed the change in her and realised that it would not be wise to question her about her attempted escape. He now had a good command of Dagomba and was learning Asante from one of Koranten Péte's personal slaves. He was disturbed at the silence between them. In an attempt to penetrate her reserve he started to teach Nandzi something of what he had learned. She picked it up quickly, but in a mechanical way.

"What is wrong with Nandzi?" he asked Damba.

Damba watched her with concern, troubled by his awareness that her life was forfeit. He had convinced the Na that it would be bad for the slaves' discipline to return her to their compound, but he was running out of arguments for the further postponement of her day of reckoning. He wondered whether she was aware of the awful fate in store for her.

*****

Na Saa Ziblim and Nana Koranten Péte sat side by side on their carved Asante stools, alone together in the deep shade.

A slave, standing at a discreet distance, charged their bowls with pito when summoned. The King's stool was a gift from the Consul. They were dressed casually: the Consul wore a batakari, a gift from the Na; and the Na wore cloth, a gift from the Consul.

"I should like to see this young woman," said Koranten Péte. "The case intrigues me. It takes some courage to venture into the bush all alone at night. It is not often that you find that quality in a woman, let alone a slave. Or is the girl mad, perhaps?"

"I am told that she has recovered from her illness," said the Na.

"The girl is your property, my good friend," he added. "You must dispose of her as you see fit. However, if the decision were mine, I would have no hesitation whatsoever. A recaptured runaway slave is good for only one thing."

He drew a finger across his throat and chuckled.

"To serve as an example to her brothers and sisters. Do you understand me?"

"I understand you very well, Majesty," replied the Asante Consul. He was becoming bored with the Ya Na and his dull court.

"Shall we see her now? It would serve to pass the time."

*****

Nandzi was on her knees fanning a reluctant fire when Damba came for her.

"Put on your cloth and come with me," he said abruptly, hiding his anxiety.

Nandzi looked at him curiously. He usually spoke to her more kindly. She wiped her hands and wrapped her upper cloth.

"Come," he said. She followed a respectful step or two behind.

He spoke over his shoulder, slowly and deliberately.

"We are going to see the Na. He has sent for you."

Nandzi understood the words yet she wondered what they could signify. *I shall know soon enough*, she thought. *It doesn't bear thinking about. I shall just have to deal with the situation as best I can.*

"Damba?" she said.

She had never addressed him directly before. The sound of his name on her lips moved him.

"Thank you," she said in his language.

"Thank you? What are you thanking me for?" he asked.

"Thank you," she repeated.

*****

"What is your name, child?" asked Koranten Péte.

"Nandzi, your majesty." She was pleased that Suba had started her lessons by teaching her the greetings.

The two men laughed.

"That is not the King," Damba whispered at her furiously.

"Never mind, young man," said the Ya Na.

"Will you understand me if I speak Dagomba to you?" Koranten Péte continued.

"Please, sir, I hear a little, but I cannot speak." Nandzi stuttered.

Suba was summoned. He couldn't believe his luck. The King and the Consul were using him as an interpreter. He smiled nervously at Damba and Nandzi.

"I want to know why, what's-her-name, yes Nandzi, the name is strange to me, it sounds like our word for . . ." the Consul rambled, "but never mind. What I want to know is why Nandzi tried to escape."

What should I answer? she wondered, and asked for the question to be repeated to give her a little longer to consider her reply. But there was no time to prepare an answer which her owner might favour. All she could do was to tell the truth.

"I wanted to be free, to go back to my family and my home and to live as I lived before I was captured," she blurted out.

Suba hesitated, afraid of the effect that her frank confession might have. She nodded at him and he translated.

"I see," said the Consul. He paused and decided that it would be best at this stage not to commit himself to a reply. "Were you not afraid of being all alone in the dark, with the spirits of the bush and the wild animals? I am told that there were leopard tracks at the foot of the tree in which you were found."

"I was afraid," replied Nandzi.

"Did you see the leopard?"

"I heard it. That is why I climbed the tree. I did not see it. I must have fallen asleep. I was very tired. No one has told me of the tracks."

"What you did was not clever. Don't you know that leopards can also climb trees? You are very lucky to be alive. No one in his right senses wanders out into the bush alone at night. Yet I must give you credit for your courage."

He paused. He appeared not to expect a reply. Nandzi remained silent.

"The penalty for attempted escape is death. By rights you should be executed as an example to your fellows."

Nandzi dropped her head and began to sob.

"Stop crying, girl, and listen to me," said the Consul.

Nandzi wiped her tears with her cloth. *Let them kill me*, she thought, *it would be better to die than to continue this life as a slave.*

"Because of the courage you displayed," continued the Consul, "I might ask the King to pardon you, but only on one condition. That condition is that you promise not to try to escape again. Do you agree?"

"I agree; I promise," she said at once.

Then she sank to her knees and bowed her head.

"Thank you, my lord," she said.

"I shall present this girl to our Queen Mother as my personal gift," Nana Koranten told the King after Damba had taken her away.

Nandzi smiled and, for the first time since her escape, Itsho's face appeared to her.

Ah, she breathed, *Itsho. It is you who has been watching over me.*

CHAPTER 5

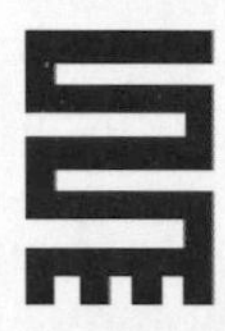

"No work, today," announced Damba.

"Today is a holiday. Not even the slaves will work. The King has proclaimed a grand durbar in the market square in honour of Nana Koranten Péte, Consul of the King of Asante. Nandzi, you will stay by my mother and serve her. Suba, you will be with me as usual."

Nandzi rubbed her tongue gently against her palate. A few days before an aged woman had appeared in Damba's compound. Nandzi had not understood a word the toothless crone had said, but Damba's mother had explained that she had come on the orders of the King. She had made Nandzi open her mouth and bite on a piece of wood. Then she had used a razor to make a small incision in her tongue. She had applied medicinal ointment to stop the bleeding and had left some more, wrapped in a leaf, to be rubbed in until the wound had healed.

"They are doing the same to all the slaves in the compound," Suba had told her.

"And you too?" she had asked him.

"No, it is only for those who will be travelling. Damba says it will be a long journey to Kumase and you may run short of food and water. The medicine they put on your tongue will stave off the hunger and the thirst."

This festival, she thought, must be another sign that they were about to leave Yendi. For the first time since her audience with the King and the Consul, she allowed herself to contemplate escape. But for the life of her she could not devise a plan which seemed more likely to succeed than her first abortive attempt. And she knew that, having promised the Consul that she would not try again, he would surely have her killed if she should fail.

There is nothing for it, she concluded. *I shall just have to make the best of it and see what the future holds.*

*****

That night Nandzi joined the family round the fire in the courtyard, as they told stories. The children, exhausted from the excitement of the day and gorged with the feasting which had followed, soon fell asleep. Nandzi helped to carry them to their sleeping mats.

"Nandzi, come and sit by me," said Damba's mother.

Nandzi squatted on her heels in the posture of respect. She saw in her mind's eye a picture of herself as a little girl, squatting just so before Tigen and Tabitsha, her own father and mother.

"My child," said Damba's mother, "you will be leaving us soon. I have become fond of you. I have tried to persuade Damba to keep you here, but he tells me that there is nothing he can do: it is a matter of politics. Politics! That is something that is the business of men and beyond the comprehension of an old woman like me. So we shall have to say our farewells. I shall remember you and I hope that you will not forget us."

Nandzi bowed her head in silence. *There is nothing for me to say,* she thought. *It is true that they have been kind to me, but it is also true that but for them Itsho would still be alive and I would still be with my own people, rather than lonely and isolated, without family or friends to trust, and bound for who-knows-where?*

"Mother, I thank you," she said formally.

*****

By the light of reed torches the guards roused the male slaves and led them out to the square.

There the blacksmiths manacled them in pairs, wrist to wrist, six pairs spaced a stride apart along a heavy chain. At dawn the female slaves brought two small bowls of gruel for each chain gang. Half the men had to eat with their left hands.

When they had finished eating, they were made to stand. The women brought the head loads which had been prepared for them: baskets of guinea corn and millet for the journey, bundles of cotton and silk cloth which were part of the tribute to be paid to Asante, a few tusks. After the loading the women and children were distributed amongst the gangs of men and the women took up their own head loads. Each gang was guarded by a horseman and two armed men on foot. The herds of cattle and sheep would follow, travelling at a slower pace, perhaps catching up with them at Kafaba. It was not until all was ready that Damba sent for Nandzi. She looked around her in amazement. The stationary caravan stretched around two sides of the market square. The free young lads who would herd the livestock flicked their whips and called their dogs, looking forward with excitement to the journey. All around them milled the townsfolk who had come to witness the departure of the slaves.

Nandzi was sent to join the leading group. She wore her own cloth and the one which Damba's mother had given her. That was the sum total of all her possessions. The other women in the group were all strangers to her. She greeted them. They responded without enthusiasm. Some wore scraps of torn and dirty cloth around their waists. Most wore only a girdle of leaves. They moved from one foot to another, adjusting their postures to the heavy head loads. A guard helped to load a basket of leaf-wrapped shea butter cones onto Nandzi's head.

"Aren't you the one who ran away?" asked a girl her own age.

"Yes," Nandzi replied, not wishing to discuss the matter.

"What happened?"

"They caught me," Nandzi replied.

There was a pause.

"My name is Minjendo," said the girl, "I am from Zabzugu."

Nandzi's reply was interrupted by the arrival of Koranten Péte and his party. They wore batakaris: one could not ride a horse wearing cloth. The Consul dismounted and Damba escorted him on an inspection. The slaves looked at him curiously, sensing that he was a person of importance.

"How many?" asked Koranten Péte.

"Three hundred," replied Damba.

"I take your word," said the Consul. "You remain fully responsible until we reach the river. There we shall take an inventory together. Now, if you are ready to move let the priests pour libation and let us be on our way; it is already getting hot."

Damba gave the signal.

"Oh ancestors, you who watch over us day and night and who know all things. We greet you with this drink. Nana greets you with this drink. Take it, we beg you. We are about to leave Yendi on a great journey to the south. Guard us, we beseech you, from footpads and robbers and wild beasts. Let no evil person meet us on the way. Let the provisions we carry for the journey be sufficient. Let us find water when we need to drink. Protect us from fatigue and preserve us from disease. Let none of us die on the road."

So sang out the priests, Dagomba and Asante, as they poured the liquor. The malam's formula was different but the sentiments were the same.

Then the drummers at the head of the caravan began the steady beat which would accompany them on their journey. The caravan moved off slowly between the walled compounds. Soon they had left the town.

"I am called Nandzi," Nandzi told Minjendo.

*****

They stopped in the heat of the day, scrambling for a patch of shade in the dry scrub.

"Woman, bring me water," said one of the men to Minjendo when she had helped him to put down his head load. He was a handsome youth, barely her own age.

"Woman, bring me water," she mimicked him. "Man, I am not *your* slave, you know."

"We are all slaves now, my sister," he said wearily, lifting his manacled hand and rattling the chain. "Please bring me water."

"No talking, there," called out one of their guards, nervous of rebellion in spite of the iron.

Nana Koranten Péte rode up to the front of the caravan with Damba.

Damba slowed his horse to a walking pace as they came opposite Nandzi. She studiously avoided looking at him, but she could not help hearing their conversation.

"I want you to meet me at Kafaba," the Consul was saying.

He had not recognised Nandzi.

"I have some business in Kpembe with the Gonja king," he continued. "I will take a small party and travel down the Daka river by canoe. The rest of my people will travel with you. My horses will meet me at Kpembe port.

"I shall need a few slaves as porters and cooks. That crazy young woman who tried to escape: can she cook? Then include her when you make your selection."

*****

Koranten Péte had hired three long dug-out canoes.

The season of floods had passed and the flow meandered sluggishly between sandbanks. Up on the high banks tall trees grew, like a row of giant spectators, watching the passing traffic. Each was different from its neighbour: one ablaze with red flowers; the next straight-boled with a head of dark green; and another top-heavy with enormous spreading branches.

The water was shallow. Soon the visible flow would stop completely and the river would turn into a series of ponds. The paddlers preferred to stand, one up front and one behind, and punt.

The sandbanks were infested with crocodiles. The only evidence of the presence of man was an occasional fishing weir, two rows of strong long funnel-shaped wicker baskets set in a frame supported by the trunk of a large tree which spanned the river.

Nandzi squatted half way along the second canoe, trailing a hand in the clear water. She could hardly remember when she had last been so idle; she had nothing to do but think. She wondered first about the trees, why no two seemed to be at all similar. Trees produced fruit and inside the fruit there were seeds. One might expect a parent tree to be surrounded by its children, but it was clearly not so. She could find no answer to that question and there was no one to ask for an explanation: the few words of Asante she had acquired were not adequate for such a complex inquiry.

Her mind turned to Itsho. Dear, dead Itsho. If only he could be sitting here with her in this canoe. He had often promised to take her on a trip like this down the Oti, to where it meets the great river she had heard talk of but had never seen. She looked up into the trees and there in the shadows she thought she could see his likeness. She waved to him.

The Asante freeman who was sitting behind her followed her gaze.

"Who are you waving to, woman?" he asked.

She turned round and smiled but she said nothing. She felt suffused with contentment. Not since Itsho's time had she felt so happy. At the back of her mind she knew that this mood could not last. All the more reason to enjoy it while it did. She would live for the present. The past, the past before her capture, held a rich store of memories, good memories, private memories to which she would return for solace in harsher times. As for the future, she refused to contemplate anything different from today's bliss.

It was late afternoon and the deep red-orange disc of the harmattan sun showed the trees in fantastic silhouette. In the leading canoe, Nana Koranten Péte was searching the banks anxiously for a site to make a bivouac for the night. The current carried his vessel into the first curve of a sharp reverse bend. Without warning, the front paddler thrust his paddle down into the river bed, bringing the vessel to a jolting halt, throwing the passengers forward. Then, almost in unison, they began to yell: "Elephants! Elephants!" The canoe had been swung round by the current and now they paddled furiously upstream, making for a mooring in the thick vegetation which grew along the bank. Nandzi's canoe, the paddlers adequately forewarned, approached slowly, soon followed by the last boat. They sat there, the three canoes alongside each other, tethered to an overhanging branch, catching their breath and watching the spectacle.

On the inside of the next meander there was a broad sandy beach. On this, and in the river itself, the mighty animals cavorted. They had been alerted by the human noises and a huge bull, with torn and punctured ears and one tusk shorter than the other, stood still, regarding them, head and trunk raised aggressively. The rest of the tribe continued their rolling and splashing in the water.

"No one knows," philosophised the man behind her, "no one knows what the elephant ate to make it so big."

Nandzi stored the words of the proverb away in her mind. She would consider its meaning later, but right now she was captivated by the sight of the calves at play. She had never seen a live elephant before.

"How I would love to have one of those babies," she said excitedly.

Nana Koranten Péte, who was nearby, turned and smiled at her enthusiastic foolishness. There was something about this young woman that intrigued him.

"The tail of the elephant may be short," he mused, recalling another proverb, "but it can still keep the flies away."

"To work, to work," he said aloud. "Soon it will be dark. You and you, bring cutlasses and cut a way so that we can climb the bank. We cannot pass by the elephants and we cannot wait until they decide to leave. We shall have to stop here for the night."

"Nana, shall I take the bull?" begged one of the Asante guards, raising his flintlock.

"No way, young man!" replied his senior sternly. "Do you not know our customs at all? Only a foolhardy hunter starts an elephant hunt without making the proper ritual preparations."

He shook his head wearily and said, to no one in particular, "The ignorance of our youth today! It makes me worry for the future of our people."

*****

It was dark by the time they had cut a ramp up the steep incline, made a small clearing in the undergrowth and fenced it with saplings.

The canoes were made fast and lashed together. Nana took his bath standing in the raft so made; and the other men followed. Nandzi and two older woman slaves busied themselves cooking a simple meal at the edge of the clearing while the men, freemen and slaves alike, sat round a roaring fire, waiting to be fed.

The forest enveloped them. A million fireflies danced in its mysterious darkness.

When the men had all been served, the women continued to hover around them, in case they were needed.

"Here," laughed Nana Koranten Péte, handing Nandzi a flaming torch, "go down to the river and take your bath. I know that you are not afraid of the bush in the dark, so you can take the lead."

He was in a generous mood, enjoying the change of scene after the boredom of the Yendi court.

"That is the girl, you know," Nandzi heard him tell the men, "who ran away from Yendi one night and was found sleeping in a tree, half dead, the next morning, with a leopard on guard below."

Vanity conquered Nandzi's fear of the unfamiliar surroundings and, gingerly, she led the other two women down the slope, offering a hand when she had stepped into the nearest canoe. She grabbed a branch with one hand and used the other to ram the end of the torch into the clay bank. Then she removed her cloth and lay back in the canoe, looking up at the flickering shadows in the lower canopy and listening to the sounds of the night. She knew the calls of most of the nocturnal animals of the savannah, but the sounds of the inhabitants of the riverine forest were strange to her.

"Are you going to sleep here tonight?" said one of the women. "Are you not scared of the crocodiles?"

They were both Asantes. Nandzi raised herself on her elbows. The women had stripped and were rubbing themselves with loofah sponges. Their wet bodies gleamed in the dim light.

Nandzi struggled to compose a reply.

"I was just resting," she said, "and listening."

*****

The elephants still occupied their minds.

When Nandzi returned to the camp, the man who had been sitting behind her was telling the story of how the elephant came to forsake the forest for the country of the long-grass. He had come to the part where the spider has defeated and killed his giant adversary in a head-butting contest. Two young men had illustrated the episode with an impromptu performance. Now cheers and laughter echoed through the forest as Ananse preened himself over the prostrate body of the elephant.

"Then the family of Elephant came to Ananse and said, 'Spider, you have defeated the head of our family. We admit it. All we ask is that you do as our custom demands.'

"'And what, may I ask, is that?' inquired Ananse.

"'The victor must provide the family with a coffin; and the coffin must be carved from solid stone, as befits a family head.'

"Ananse thought for some time. He had a cutlass and an adze and a knife. He could make a coffin of wood; but a coffin of stone? He could not see how that could be done. Nevertheless he agreed and told the late elephant's family to come back 'tomorrow next.'"

Nandzi squatted on the outside of the circle and watched the faces of the listeners, reddened, it seemed, by the fire, all their attention on the story teller.

"The next day Ananse cut down a tree with his cutlass. With his adze and his knife he carved the tree trunk into the image of a man with a musket raised to his shoulder, ready to fire. When the carving was finished, he dragged it to the front gate of his compound. He dressed the carving in batakari and trousers. Then he hid in the bush to watch what would happen.

"The family of Elephant arrived at the appointed time to collect their stone coffin, but before they could enter Ananse's compound, they saw the man-image, standing ready to fire at them. Then Ananse beat the great fontomfrom drum, making a sound like the thunder of gunshot. Panicking, the elephants at once turned tail and fled; and they didn't stop running until they had left the forest and passed into the savannah. Ananse just laughed and laughed and laughed. And then he called his wife and children and they cooked and ate the flesh of the dead elephant.

"That is my story of how the elephant came to forsake the forest for the country of the long-grass. I do not vouch for its truth. You may believe or not: that is for you, the listener, to decide."

*****

When they moved off in the morning and passed the elephants' beach, all that remained of the visitors was the disturbed ground and a few heaps of dung.

The second day was much like the first. Flocks of grey parrots with their bright crimson tails screamed and whistled at them from the treetops.

"Do you see the *nkoko-kye-na-ko*?"

The man behind her grasped her bare shoulder and squeezed. She stiffened and turned. The man pointed out the great blue turacos which had taken possession of the leafy top of a tall tree. She looked up. *What beautiful birds*, she thought. They were blue and yellow, with a black crest and a red and yellow bill. *Free*, she thought, *free to fly where they will*. At last, the man removed his hand from her shoulder.

"It is *akoko-kye-na-ko* who taught us to drum," the man told her.

In the clear sky above the river there hung a hooded vulture, its wings motionless, borne up by an unseen draft of hot air.

"Opéte," the man told her quietly, gently squeezing the soft flesh of her upper arm as he pointed at the bird.

"Opéte," he repeated, controlling his laughter and pointing now repeatedly at the leader of the expedition in the canoe ahead.

"Opéte, Opéte," he repeated with a chuckle, pointing again at the bird and his master, relishing his own profound sense of humour and making sure that his joke had not been lost on Nandzi.

"Who is calling me?" Nana Koranten Péte half rose from his seat and turned to look at the following canoes.

The ornithologist dropped his head and concentrated on cleaning his fingernails.

I am going to have a problem with this man, thought Nandzi. *He cannot keep his hands off me*.

She began to think of him as the ornithologist, the man who knows birds.

Nandzi's command of Asante was increasing rapidly. The ornithologist and his fellows were amused and flattered by her constant requests for the names of things. She would point to her head, her hair, her nose, her mouth, her teeth; and ask for the name of each. She would concentrate on committing the word to memory and then she would repeat it. They would laugh at her strange accent and coach her on the correct pronunciation and tone. Verbs and sentence structure were more difficult: though she had little concept of the meaning of grammar, she began to learn short sentences by heart, and in these she began to see patterns emerging.

A fellowship gradually developed amongst the paddlers and the passengers in each canoe. It transcended differences of language and culture and status. Conversations sprang up, often triggered by the sights and sounds of the river. A glimpse of an enormous python set the ornithologist telling the story of how Ananse had used flattery to persuade the king of serpents to allow himself to be measured.

"Ananse," he told them, "persuaded Python to let himself be lashed to a fallen tree trunk. 'Just to make sure,' the spider told the snake, 'that unstraightened sinuosities will not result in an underestimation of your great length.'"

Everyone laughed at Ananse's cheek and at the ornithologist's verbal wizardry; but Nandzi identified with the victim and saw herself trussed up like the python.

They spoke in Asante and Dagomba and Hausa or in a mixture, whichever best served their need to communicate. They sang songs. When it came to her turn, Nandzi shyly sang a Lekpokpam lullaby that she knew from Tabitsha. It was the same song, she recalled, that she had been singing to Nowu when the Bedagbam had descended upon them. *Dear mother*, she thought as she sang, *I am singing your song to these strangers. I hope that you can hear me and that you haven't forgotten me, as I have not forgotten you.* Then she wondered whether, if she concentrated hard enough, she could somehow communicate with Tabitsha over all the distance which now separated them.

She had a sweet voice. None of her companions understood the words, but somehow she succeeded in conveying the message. When she finished, there was applause and a demand for an encore.

That night, sitting around the campfire, she had to repeat the performance before a larger audience.

This young woman is certainly an acquisition, reflected Koranten Péte. *She will make an excellent gift for the Queen Mother.*

CHAPTER 6

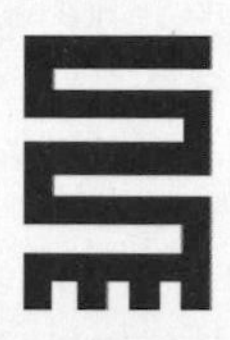

Nana Koranten Péte had business in Kpembe, important business, business of the King of Asante: kola business.

The kola 'nut' is a pink seed about the length of a man's thumb. When chewed, it is reputed to stave off hunger and thirst. It is also a mild stimulant. Many Muslims, barred by their religion from the consumption of alcohol, are fond of chewing kola, which Islam does not forbid. When pressed, some will admit that their love of kola borders on excess, even addiction. Others will protest that kola is not only harmless but that it serves a useful function in lubricating social intercourse. This it achieves not only by its narcotic effect, but also by the value attached to its use as a customary gift.

Dangerous drug or harmless nibble, the demand for kola appeared to be insatiable.

Since its forests were the principal habitat of the kola tree, Asante had a virtual monopoly in the collection and processing of the fruit, which was its principal export to its northern neighbours. In order to preserve its monopoly, the Asante state kept the northern traders out of the kola producing areas.

Kafaba was the most important international market for kola. During the harvest season, the roads from the south were crowded with porters, slaves and free men alike, all carrying head loads of kola. On the bank of the Volta River the kola was discharged into enormous dugout canoes which ferried it across to Kafaba. Asante customs officers collected an export duty of two large nuts for every hundred exported.

Kafaba was a Gonja town; but Nana Kpembewura, King of all the Gonjas, resided not in sinful Kafaba but in the quiet backwater of Kpembe, which was his capital.

"I have important business in Kpembe," Nana Koranten Péte said to his secretary, "kola business."

*****

Kafaba was a town of two parts.

The Upper Town, with its residential compounds and markets and mosques, lay above the reach of the waters of the Volta.

Each year, as the level of the river dropped slowly in the wake of the floods, a new suburb, the Lower Town, made its appearance above the receding water's edge. This was of necessity a makeshift sort of quarter. There the overflow of visiting traders, for whom there was no room in the inns and hostelries of the Upper Town, set up the depots and stockyards in which they kept their slaves and kola. Ramshackle buildings of bamboo and matting and thatch were interspersed with patches of corn and plantain, cassava and cocoyam, which would be ready to harvest before the next floods. Temporary property rights were established by rude fences which also served to protect the allotments from the depredations of the humped cattle and goats which grazed in the sweet green grass.

Through this confusion of allotments and temporary dwellings, one straight wide road was always left clear. Called the River Road, it ran from the canoe landing stage up to the principal market in the Upper Town.

Up this road, from dawn to dusk, porters with bulging calf and neck muscles jogged with their head loads of kola, returning in due course with empty baskets.

River Road was lined with small market stalls. In the morning Gonja women cooked and sold thick, sour, red-brown millet porridge; at noon and in the evening it might be grilled bream or catfish or succulent prawns in groundnut soup, served with rice, boiled yams or maize bread. Others offered spicy fried cakes of boiled beans, millet or rice. Young girls, daughters of the caterers, roamed the Lower Town with head trays of roasted groundnuts or foaming pots of honey beer.

After dark, River Road took on a different aspect. The porters, exhausted from the day's work, lay asleep wherever they could find a place to lie; but the food sellers were still there, their flickering oil lamps defining the edges of the road. Wealthy merchants from the Upper Town came out to stroll down to the river and to display, in the moonlight, their newest outfits and their youngest and prettiest wives. The men, meeting friends and associates, would bow deeply, shake hands and exchange infinitely protracted greetings and courtesies. A young wife, bathed and perfumed and dressed to show her husband's pride, her eyes expertly made up with lustrous silvery blue-white antimony, would shyly drop her left knee and touch the ground with her left hand. Then she would stand quietly by, waiting patiently for the end of the men's palaver, demurely aware of the admiration which the intricate embroidery on her wrapper and blouse and the style and colour of her headtie were attracting in the moonlight. And she would finger her gold earrings and neck chain, her bangles and her rings.

*****

When they reached Kafaba, Koranten Péte found that Damba's caravan had not yet arrived.

He paid a brief courtesy call on the Gonja chief and placed Sharif Imhammed, an envoy of the Sultan of Fezzan, who had accompanied him from Yendi, in the care of his colleague, the local Asante consul.

He left most of his party behind, in the charge of Akwasi Anoma, the ornithologist, to prepare a simple caravanserai, while they waited for Damba. Koranten Péte hastened on to Kumase with little more than a bodyguard and a party of hammock-bearers.

Akwasi Anoma staked out a site and gave orders for the slashing of the undergrowth and cutting of bamboo to make a fence. When he was satisfied that the work was in hand, he called Nandzi aside.

"Come," he said. "Take my sleeping mat and my bundle. I will show you the Upper Town."

One of the older Asante female slaves helped her to lift her burden to her head.

"Mind yourself," she warned, "that man is an incorrigible womaniser."

Nandzi trudged up the hill behind Akwasi Anoma, her feet bare, her body wrapped in her two cloths, the man's baggage on her head. Any stranger could guess their relationship. If the man ahead of her had been her father, Tigen, she would not have given the matter a second thought. If it had been Itsho, suddenly returned from the spirit world, she would have begged him to let her carry his possessions. But Akwasi Anoma was not her father and he was certainly not her freely chosen lover, dead or alive. Akwasi Anoma was a stranger to her. He was not even, so far as she knew, her owner.

When she was together with her fellow slaves, Nandzi felt hidden in anonymity. But here, as she wound her way through this great seething crowd of people in Akwasi Anoma's footsteps, it was obvious that she was the man's creature. It was obvious; yet it was so commonplace that nobody noticed. Nandzi and her master might just as well have been invisible. Of that she soon became aware, and so doing, turned her attention elsewhere.

The first slave compound they passed at once impressed itself indelibly on Nandzi's mind. Many years later, in another continent, she could still recall every precise detail of the picture. There must have been as many as three hundred slaves. They were confined within a fenced area, on one side of River Road, together with horses and asses, oxen, cows and goats. The livestock wandered freely within the kraal, seeking pasture in the overcropped bare surface. The slaves were chained in groups of ten or twenty. Some were young boys and girls. They squatted morosely, most of them practically naked, exposed to the pitiless malevolence of the sun. At night, she could see, they would have to sleep on the bare ground without mats, many without even the meanest cloth to protect them from the cold and damp. They were clearly underfed.

She struggled to catch up with her master.

Touching his arm, she said, "Papa!"

Akwasi Anoma was wondering where in the Upper Town he would locate the inn where he had once before lodged for a week. He could picture the Gonja landlord's face, but, for the life of him, he could not remember his name. Without the landlord's name, he could hardly ask for directions.

He stopped and turned.

"What?" he asked irritably. He was upset by the failure of his memory. *I must be getting old*, he thought.

With a silent movement of her head Nandzi drew his attention to the scene before them. She could not find words to express her dismay.

He looked but saw nothing unusual.

"What?" he asked again.

Near the fence sat an emaciated woman. A chain joined the manacle on her right ankle to the others in her circle. A child, a thing of skin and bones, lay on her lap, too ill or listless even to cry. Flies buzzed at its eyes and nostrils. The mother saw Nandzi looking at her and caught her eye. Without releasing her gaze, she lifted her flat, empty breasts. Then she held out both palms. *That woman could be me, it could be my mother,* thought Nandzi. She spread her hands in a gesture of impotence and despair and dragged her gaze away.

A little further off sat a tethered ring of men, quite immobile, their nakedness exposed, their eyes glazed and dull.

As she watched, one skeletal man rose slightly and, resting his elbows on his knees, lifted his bare buttocks clear of the ground. Then he began to shit. Nandzi averted her eyes.

"Come," ordered Akwasi Anoma, "I don't have all day."

A guard, with a whip in one hand and a heavy cudgel in the other, walked by on his rounds. *He looks like a slave himself,* she thought, *a callous man who has bartered his humanity for some small improvement in his food ration.* The man noticed that she was watching him. Raising the butt of his whip in a lewd gesture, he screamed an obscenity at her in a language she did not understand.

*****

The room was barely furnished: just a low bed of millet stalks and a few mats, cowskins and stools.

Akwasi Anoma stretched himself out on the bed and shut his eyes. Nandzi squatted on a mat. *What next?* she wondered.

Presently a servant brought a brass basin of hot water. She helped him to set it down on the polished clay floor.

"Papa, the water has come," she said.

There was no answer. She tried again. Then she grasped his shoulder. Akwasi Anoma woke up.

"I was sleeping," he said, rubbing his eyes. "Why did you wake me?"

"They have brought the water," she replied.

He sat up.

"I was tired," he said, examining the room for the first time. Then, "Open my bundle. Take out the soap and the sponge."

She put them down on a stool next to the basin and moved towards the door.

"Stop," he ordered. "Where do you think you are going?"

"I was going outside to let you take your bath," she said.

He looked her in the eye and smiled. Guessing the import of that smile, she dropped her gaze.

"Oh no," he laughed. "Why did you think I brought you with me? I have been working hard these past days. Now that the Vulture has left me in charge I am going to relax."

He stood up and removed his cloth and dropped the drawers which were his only undergarment. He was naked. Nandzi looked away.

"Eh, young woman," he said, "are you shy? Have you never seen a man's thing before? Look, it is even standing for you."

He washed his face in the warm water. Then he gave her the loofah and the ball of black soap.

"Start with my back," he said. "Rub hard. It is days since I had a good bath. You know we Asante are not like you northerners. It is our custom to bath twice a day."

As she scrubbed his back, Nandzi considered her position. She felt no attraction for this man. She had not been with any man since Abdulai had raped her. That rape had killed her desire. She flinched at the thought of being penetrated. But she could see no way out. Run away? To where, to what sanctuary? She knew no one in Kafaba. The man would set up a hue and cry for her and she would soon be caught. It was hard to be a slave. She had no choice.

He turned round.

"Now the front," he said, holding up his arms so that she could soap his arm pits.

She bypassed his erect penis.

"Here too," he told her, "but gently, mind you. Use your hand, not the sponge."

He pulled off her cloth and grasped a breast in each soapy hand. She flinched.

"You are covered in dust," he said. "Just rinse the soap off me. Then you had better bath too. Use my sponge."

As he dried himself, Nandzi turned her back to him and soaped herself. It was a long time since she had had a good bath and she took her time, enjoying the warmth of the water and scrubbing the dust out of her skin. Then the man came from behind and took a breast in each hand. She felt the end of his instrument against her backside. Again she flinched. He rubbed his palms over her soapy nipples. She forced her mind away.

"Itsho," she said in her own language, "there is nothing I can do. He is going to take me against my will. Help me if you can."

"What is that you are saying? Have I not taught you Asante? Speak a civilised language to me," Akwasi Anoma said to her.

When he had finished, but before he had withdrawn, he said, "What is the matter, child? Do you dislike me so much? This is a small thing between a man and woman. You must try better next time."

Then he turned his back and soon he was snoring.

Nandzi was exhausted but she could not sleep. She felt humiliated and dirty.

"Itsho," she whispered, "I could not help it."

CHAPTER 7

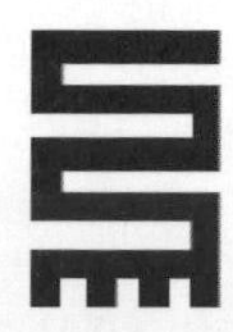

The next day, while Akwasi Anoma was in the Upper Town eating his fufu, Damba's caravan entered Kafaba from the east and passed slowly down River Road.

Damba rode ahead, scanning the compounds left and right.

Nandzi was the first to see them. She was struck at once by the condition of her fellow slaves. They were clearly much the worse for wear: emaciated, dirty, exhausted and, so it seemed to her, desperately low in spirit. She searched the column for Minjendo, but the three hundred faces were mostly obscured by the bundles and baskets on their heads.

Damba found Nandzi before Nandzi could find Minjendo. He dismounted at once.

"Nandzi," he asked, "how are you?"

Struck by the contrast with his own ragged, ill-clad charges, he continued, "You look well."

As he spoke the words, he felt suddenly ashamed, ashamed of his slaves' condition and ashamed that, in spite of his affection for Nandzi, he had not had the courage to attempt to save her from servitude. *This commerce in human beings is a bad practice,* he thought. *When the Ya Na put me in charge of the caravan, I felt honoured. Now all my ambition has gone sour: all I want to do is to go home and purge my memory of these bitter days, as I might scour my dusty body with caustic soap.*

Nandzi had not answered.

"What! Have you lost your tongue?" he jested and then, examining her face more closely, "Is there something wrong?"

What sort of answer does this man expect of me? Nandzi wondered, as she inspected her torn toe nails. *He saw me raped. He bound me to a pack horse. It is true that he permitted me to bury Itsho and kept me in his mother's house: for that I owe him; but if he and his fellows had never set out on their nefarious hunt for human beings, Itsho would still be alive and I would still be with my family.*

She was in a dark mood. The business with Akwasi Anoma had upset her. The thought that Damba might be persuaded to help her to avoid having to spend another night with the coarse bird man flitted through her mind. She dismissed it. Damba took his orders from the Asante. Even in the remote event that he might succeed in rescuing her, she would then, more likely than not, end up having to sleep with him instead. *Men are all the same,* she thought. *Only Itsho was different. And Itsho is dead.*

Damba tried again.

"Where is Koranten Péte?" he asked.

"Kumase," she answered curtly, raising her head and looking him straight in the eye.

"And who is in charge then?"

Akwasi Anoma had been sent for. Now he was approaching them.

"That man," she said, pointing at him and spitting out the words as if they were some rotten food.

Akwasi Anoma saw and heard her.

"Bush woman," he said. "You forget your status. Just remember that you are a slave. Point at me like that just once more and I will have some civilised manners whipped into you."

Nandzi turned, expressed her contempt with a hiss, and went to search the column for Minjendo.

*****

Minjendo was in a bad way, haggard and evidently ill.

She did not acknowledge Nandzi's greeting. Nandzi led her to the makeshift shelter by the cooking place. Her head load removed, Minjendo sank to the ground. Nandzi had to drag her into the shade. She sat with her head hung down between her knees. Nandzi brought her a bowl of water and helped her to drink. She spread one of her two cloths on the ground and made Minjendo lie on it. She took the corner of her other cloth, which she wore around her waist, dipped it in the water and wiped Minjendo's face.

The days which followed were a time of unceasing labour.

The three hundred slaves who had travelled on foot from Yendi had to be fed. The sick had to be nursed; wounds had to be dressed. Water had to be fetched from the river. Baskets of millet had to be carried down from the market. The shit of the chained men had to be collected and buried. Firewood had to be collected. The gruel which was the slaves' principal diet had to be cooked. The dying had to be comforted and the dead had to be buried.

Akwasi Anoma, nominally in charge, was of little help. He visited the encampment in the morning principally to give orders to the guards. The welfare of the slaves was of no concern to him. He regarded the responsibility which Koranten Péte had laid upon him as a license to indulge himself. He was often drunk by noon. Every afternoon he selected a different girl to service him. *At least*, thought Nandzi, resisting an impulse to intervene, *he has lost interest in me*.

Of Damba there was nothing to be seen.

The weakest of the slaves, the oldest and the youngest, died. The survivors responded to rest and to more regular meals, inadequate, unappetising and lacking in nourishment as they were. As the women regained their strength, more of them were able to share the work. There was no one to give them orders. The women who were willing, seeing Nandzi's example, came to her to volunteer their help. The men were a problem. She bullied the guards, persuading them to unshackle them in batches to let them have some exercise; but they were not allowed to help with the heavy work, for that would mean leaving the camp.

As darkness fell, Nandzi would wrap herself in her cloth and instantly fall into a deep dreamless sleep. At the first glimmer of light, she would be back at work.

I am working, she thought with a grim smile, *like a slave*; but as the work force grew, she found that she was spending much of her time giving orders, not by choice, but simply because there was no one else to do so.

One day, when the sun had reached its zenith, she called a halt to all work and told her fellows to find some shade and rest until it was cooler. The guards did not interfere.

Minjendo watched her.

"Once you ran away. Now you are doing our masters' work for them," she teased Nandzi.

She was stronger now, but Nandzi would not let her work.

"What else can I do? Our men are in chains. If we women do nothing, we shall all perish from hunger and thirst," she answered.

She was secretly astonished at the role which circumstances had laid upon her shoulders. She had never before had to give orders, except to children.

"What are you thinking of?" asked Minjendo.

"Nothing, nothing. At least, nothing important," replied Nandzi. "Perhaps some day I will tell you; but not now. Rather there is something you should tell me. I have not wanted to ask until now because you were not well. But now you seem much better."

"What is it?" asked Minjendo.

"What happened on your journey to this place? You were quite strong and well when we parted outside Yendi; yet when you reached Kafaba you were so weak and ill that you didn't even recognise me."

Now it was Minjendo's turn to be silent.

"You don't have to tell me. But maybe it will do you good to talk. We are all in this together now. None of us have family. We have to rely on one another."

Minjendo looked up at her. There were tears in her eyes.

"There was a bush fire," she said. "It started behind us, perhaps where we had camped the night before. The wind blew the fire in our direction. Suddenly it seemed that the whole world was alight. We were enveloped in smoke and ashes. The heat was unbearable. All manner of bush creatures came running past us. They were so intent on fleeing from the fire that they didn't seem to notice us: zebra and antelopes, grass cutters and porcupines, even snakes. And a whole family of lions, with small cubs, quite nearby, all running for their lives. Then we were all running too. For the men it was most difficult: if one fell, his chains dragged the whole gang down with him. I tried to balance my basket on my head as I ran, but it was impossible. Others just let their loads fall, so I did the same. I ran for a while, tripping and stumbling. All the time the fire was coming closer, catching up on us. I was tired out, and with the smoke, it was difficult to see. I was terrified. I thought I would have to give up.

"Then, then . . . " she sobbed.

"Take your time," said Nandzi, putting an arm around her shoulder. "Take your time. You had a terrible shock. But you are all right, you survived, you are alive. That is all that counts."

Nandzi's calm was a disguise which she couldn't sustain. Minjendo's story had upset her. She saw a terrible vision of Itsho's crushed skull, with his brains spilling out and she too began to sob. She hugged Minjendo and they clung to one another and cried until they had no more tears.

"I was pregnant," said Minjendo when she had wiped her face and recovered her voice. "I lost the child. There in the bush, with no one to help me. Nandzi, my sister: you cannot imagine the horror and the pain. And then everything went black. They told me afterwards that it was that Bedagbam man, the Master of the Caravan, the one they call Damba, who saved me. He had been riding up and down behind us, urging us on. I suppose that he wanted to make sure that he did not lose any of his slaves. He dismounted, threw me up across his horse's neck, and rode on. It was all done in a flash, they told me. I don't remember a thing: I might have been dead. Dead. Poor dead Minjendo, roasted alive without so much as a decent funeral. Her spirit wandering, wandering, but never finding her ancestors. Think of it.

"When I came to there was no more fire and we were in a new camp. We rested there for a few days, but we had lost most of our food and our water containers so Damba made us press on. Miraculously, no one had died in the fire; but some of the older ones and some of the children died on the road from hunger and thirst. Some had been burned in the fire and the burns turned bad so that they couldn't walk any more. They were left behind. I was lucky that I wasn't left behind too. Sometimes they let me ride on a horse when I was very weak."

"Poor Minjendo," said Nandzi. "What you have all been through. I didn't know."

She looked around. Akwasi Anoma was coming down the hill. From his shambling gait it was clear that he was drunk. He was singing to himself but his speech was so slurred that they could not make out the words. They watched him. Others saw him too. Soon three hundred pairs of eyes were focused on him. He halted and tried to crack his whip but he could not give his wrist the necessary flick and the thong would not do his will. He cursed. Then he looked around him. Through his blurred vision, he seemed to realise that he was the object of close observation.

"What!" he cried incoherently. "Resting? Slaves resting? Get to work! Get to work! Guards! Do you hear me? Guards!"

The guards came running up. Some of them were slaves themselves, some the sons of slaves.

"I want a woman. Line up the women so I can make my choice."

"I can't see him performing in that condition," Minjendo nudged Nandzi.

The guards rounded them up, dragging and pushing them into a reluctant ragged row.

"Your mother!" Minjendo abused a guard who laid a hand on her, but she said it in her own language and he did not understand.

Akwasi Anoma swaggered up the line, inspecting his prey, prodding with his whip end, weighing a breast.

A woman's voice called from behind his back, "Besotted fool!"

He didn't understand the language but he heard the laughter. He turned round, and this time succeeding in cracking his whip. There was silence and he continued on his inspection. He arrived at the end of the line and started back.

Half way along, he made his choice. It was a young girl, no more than a child. He pointed at her. A guard grasped her hand and pulled her after him. She resisted and began to cry. At the same time there was a murmur of protest from the women. The guard dragged the girl away. His drunken master followed.

"Akwasi Anoma," Nandzi called out, raising her voice above the hubbub.

On hearing his name the man stopped and turned.

"Who called my name?" he demanded.

Nandzi stepped forward.

"Akwasi Anoma," she called out again and, before he could react, added, in his own language, using a word which he himself had taught her: "Beast!"

Then she walked calmly to the guard and took the girl by the arm.

"Release her," she ordered.

The guard was used to taking orders. He did as he was told.

Akwasi Anoma called out, "Fool, fool. Take her," and then "Guards, guards."

The other guards, who had been watching these events with barely disguised amusement, now came to the rescue of their master.

The shock of Nandzi's challenge had sobered him. His attention had been diverted and he hardly noticed that the girl had made her escape.

"Bind the woman," he ordered.

The guards grabbed Nandzi and, handling her roughly, bound her hands behind her back and tied her ankles together.

"I will make an example of her for all of you to see," he announced. "No slave woman insults an Asante man with impunity. The rest of you, watch."

Nandzi recalled the execution she had seen in the market square at Yendi. The victim had been bound in the same way. But she knew no fear, only mad, uncontrollable rage.

"Akwasi Anoma," she called out yet again.

"What?" he asked, expecting a plea for mercy. The idea of commuting her sentence to one of judicial rape, inflicted by himself, crossed his mind.

"You are a drunken beast, a stupid drunken beast. I curse you," cried Nandzi. "We all curse you."

"Stop that witch's mouth!" ordered the enraged man.

*****

Minjendo sat by Nandzi's side, doing her best to comfort her. Jaji, the girl whom Nandzi had saved from Akwasi Anoma's clutches, attached herself to them, ever ready to show her gratitude by carrying out any task assigned to her. Minjendo left her with Nandzi while she went to search for medicinal leaves and then set her to soak them in boiled water. Nandzi lay face down. All day Minjendo dribbled one infusion over Nandzi's wounds and persuaded her to sip another. For a while she had a high fever. Then, gradually, the open wounds on her back and buttocks began to form scabs. The itching drove her to distraction but Minjendo knew that the worst was over.

Early one morning, Koranten Péte stepped out of a canoe, followed by two musketeers.

He strode up River Road, searching for a familiar face.

One of the guards caught sight of him and called out, "Nana, Nana; we are here!"

Koranten Péte strode into the camp.

"Where is Akwasi Anoma?" he demanded.

Akwasi Anoma had not put in an appearance at the camp since the day he had had Nandzi whipped.

"He is in his house," replied the guard.

Koranten Péte searched the man's face.

"In his house, is he?" he mimicked. "Then go to his house at once and tell him I want to see him. At once. Do you understand? Wait! Mensa, you go with him," he ordered one of the musketeers.

The camp was filthy. Human excrement lay uncollected. The slaves were clearly dispirited. As soon as Nandzi was able, she had told Minjendo what orders to give; but Minjendo had earned no leadership status, as Nandzi had. She was just another young woman who happened to be Nandzi's friend. The women paid little attention. They carried out only the most essential activities. For the rest, they sat around consumed with self-pity.

It took Koranten Péte little time to get the camp cleaned up. He put each guard in charge of a squad of women and gave each squad a task. His company of musketeers arrived and he quickly set them to work too. He inspected each chained group of male slaves. Then he came upon Nandzi's prone, naked body, with Minjendo and her young helper by her side.

"What's this?" he demanded. "Why are you not at work with the rest?"

Minjendo did not understand the question but she read his body language correctly. She stood up and pointed mutely at Nandzi's back. After a restless night, Nandzi had been dozing when Koranten Péte had arrived and Minjendo had not seen fit to awaken her.

Koranten Péte called the nearest guard. By chance it was the very man who, on Akwasi Anoma's instructions, had flogged her.

"Who did this?" asked Koranten Péte.

Uncertain whether he was about to be rewarded or punished, the guard hesitated. Then he saw Minjendo pointing at him and decided it would be better to own up. At that moment Nandzi woke, and, lifting the cloth to cover her nakedness, sat up. Koranten Péte looked at her in astonishment.

"You!" he said. "Did you ignore my warning and try to escape again?"

Nandzi was still dazed. She ignored his question and said to Minjendo, "Please give me some water."

Koranten Péte watched her drink and then wet the corner of her cloth to wipe her face. Suddenly there was a roar from the squad of women nearest the road. Akwasi Anoma was approaching, led by the musketeer who had been sent for him. The women all stopped their work and hooted and jeered at him.

"I'll talk to you later," Koranten Péte said to Nandzi.

He signalled to the squad leaders and the pandemonium ceased almost immediately. He cut Akwasi Anoma's greeting short and led him to the far end of the camp, out of earshot but, since there was no private place in the camp, not out of sight. The slaves watched their conversation with increasing glee as they interpreted their body language. Their guards showed no less interest. Work came to a stop.

"It looks as if your bird man is in trouble," said Minjendo to Nandzi.

*****

Koranten Péte gave himself a week to prepare the slaves for the twenty day journey to Kumase, leaving the livestock to follow at a more leisurely pace.

The Asantehene had instructed that they arrive in Kumase in time for the next

Akwasidae. Should they arrive in poor condition, Koranten Péte's reputation would suffer. And Koranten Péte had a reputation to preserve: he was a royal prince, son of Oduro Panin, King of Nsuta, one of the seven founding nations of the Asante confederacy; his wife, Abena Saka, was the Queen Mother of Mampon, another of the founding states. His name was a by-word for bravery. It was Koranten Péte who had led the Asante army which had defeated the Dagomba. And Koranten Péte was a rich man. The Asantehene had rewarded him generously for his military exploits: he was entitled to collect a one-third commission on the Dagomba tribute. So it was a small thing for him to bear the cost of fattening up his charges for a few days and providing each slave with a cheap new indigo cover cloth.

Once he had delivered his caravan into the hands of Akwasi Anoma, Damba had deliberately kept clear of the camp. He no longer had any stomach for the slave business. While waiting for Koranten Péte's return to Kafaba, he had spent his time studying the market and doing such business on his own account as his limited capital would allow.

Now he came to greet Koranten Péte and to join him in taking an inventory.

When they came to Nandzi, Koranten Péte turned to him and asked, "You know this young woman, of course?"

"Of course," replied Damba, managing a smile.

He was still smarting from the rude reception she had given him when they last met and expected another rebuff. But Nandzi felt some remorse for her behaviour and smiled back.

"Show him your wounds," Koranten Péte told Nandzi.

Slowly, reluctantly, she turned her back to them and dropped her cloth.

"She saved a young girl from Akwasi Anoma's clutches and he took his revenge," said Koranten Péte.

"I am sorry," said Damba lamely.

Those were the last words he spoke to her.

"That is a remarkable young woman," he said to Koranten Péte when they were out of earshot. "I hope you will look after her well."

"Have no fear. She will be going into the household of the most powerful woman in Asante, the Queen Mother herself."

*****

Nandzi had seen the river from the slave camp. She had been astonished at its great width: even in the dry season it was far, far wider than the Oti in flood. Koranten Péte established a temporary camp on the far bank.

He devoted a day to ferrying the tribute goods across. At dawn on the second day, the slaves were moved. The women went first, ten in each canoe, with ten paddlers to make sure that the swift current did not carry them downstream, and two guards armed with muskets.

When the women and children were all across, the men were unchained, one gang at a time. Secured only by manacles, they were marshalled down to the canoes under the eyes of an armed escort, carrying their loose chains with them. The humiliating conditions in which they had spent the last weeks had so sapped their spirit that tight security was hardly necessary. But Koranten Péte was taking no chances. Once they were safely across, they were again shackled together.

By nightfall the river crossing had been completed. Last to arrive were Sharif Imhammed and his small party.

At dawn, Koranten Péte stood before the assembled slaves. His spokesman called for silence.

"Yesterday we crossed the great Volta River," Koranten Péte told them. "Today it lies between you and your old homes. If yesterday you had not yet given up all hope of returning to your own people, today you must do so. This river is not like other rivers. This one has no bottom. Other rivers turn into a trickle in the dry season: this one never. No man has ever waded across it. If you think you might swim across it, you are welcome to try: the crocodiles will make a meal of you. And if you contemplate stealing a canoe, remember the strength of the current which you have seen today: consider that it took ten strong men to steer a straight path across from the other side."

He paused and watched as fresh palm wine was poured from a calabash into a cup. He took the cup and poured a silent libation. Then he took a draught of the sweet liquid.

He licked his lips, wiped his beard and continued his homily.

"If you behave well and work hard," he promised them, "if you learn our language and adopt our customs, you men will be given wives, some from your own ranks, but others even from amongst our own Asante women. If you marry an Asante woman your children will be Asante."

"So I say to you all: welcome to Asante. Turn your backs on your old lives. Look to a better future.

"We set off early tomorrow. I have purchased a new cloth for each of you. You will receive it the day before we arrive in Kumase. In Kumase you will be handed over to your new masters and mistresses. Your chains and shackles will be removed. You will join the families for whom you will be working. I wish you an uneventful journey and success in your new lives."

*****

At first light, the slaves were shepherded into their assigned positions.

A band of drummers led the caravan. Next came a small squad of musketeers.

Koranten Péte followed, with his guest, Sharif Imhammed. Each sat in a hammock, borne aloft on poles by four bearers. The horses had been left behind in Kafaba. There were too many tsetse flies in the forest.

The male slaves followed in groups of twelve, manacled wrist to wrist in pairs and spaced a stride apart along a heavy chain, just as in their journey from Yendi. Two armed guards marched before and behind each chain gang with some of the women and children between them. Each slave carried a head load, tribute goods from Yendi or luxuries from Kafaba.

Another squad of musketeers brought up the rear.

Koranten Péte's secretary poured libation and invoked the blessings of the ancestors. Then the royal horn was blown, the drummers struck up a rhythm and the procession moved off.

Nandzi and Minjendo were now both well enough to carry a load. They walked together, with Jaji their constant companion.

As they moved off, Nandzi began to hum a traditional dirge. In her mind she sang the words she remembered, inserting the names of those whose death she was lamenting, first Itsho and then, in turn, everyone else whose death she could recall. Then new words begun to form themselves. Dimly, she sensed Itsho's unseen presence. Her eyes were open but she seemed to be dreaming. Her spirit left her body. She floated weightlessly and saw the whole caravan from a great height.

"Why are you humming a dirge?" asked Minjendo.

Nandzi continued humming.

"Nandzi, don't you hear me?" Minjendo asked her, but Nandzi appeared to be in a trance.

She began to sing new words, softly, tentatively, adapting her rhythm to the beat of the drums.

"Oh you our ancestors, our grandparents

"And their parents; and their parents and grandparents:

"Hear our voice,

"Hear our lamentation.

"Oh you our ancestors, all those who in the dim mists of the past

"Have lived upon this earth and have gone before us into the world of the spirits:

"Hear our voice,

"Hear our lamentation.

"Advise us, help us,

"Succour us.

"Hear our voice,

"Hear our lamentation."

As she sang her voice gained power. Minjendo turned her head and looked at her. *The spirits have possessed her*, she thought; and she was afraid.

"We too have died and yet we live still.

"We are as walking corpses.

"Hear our voice,

"Hear our lamentation.

"We have no drink to offer

"But we beg and beseech you:

"Hear our voice,

"Hear our lamentation."

One of the older women began to join the chorus, "Hear our voice, Hear our lamentation," and then another.

Soon all the women in the group were singing the chorus. Minjendo was the last to join.

"Our freedom has been taken from us

"Our spirits are chained to our dead bodies.

"Hear our voice,

"Hear our lamentation.

"Who will perform the rites which will free our spirits

"And send them to your world?

"Hear our voice,

"Hear our lamentation.

"Hear us, advise us, fortify us,

"Give us back life; give us back hope.

"Hear our voice,

"Hear our lamentation."

Nandzi paused.

"Again," the older woman called to her. She began again from the beginning.

Again and again they sang the dirge until they knew all the words. The song passed up to the beginning of the caravan; and it passed down to the end. Even the women who did not understand the words were moved to join in. The guards did nothing. One does not lightly interfere in matters concerning the spirits of the dead.

The singing of dirges is women's work. At first the male slaves listened in silence, like the guards. But the words of the song captured their misery and one or two began to join the chorus. The rules of the old society were losing their power.

Soon the lament had been taken up throughout the length of the caravan and the singing echoed across the plain as they trudged on. Again and again they sang it until the words were inscribed in every memory.

Only when they came to a river was the rhythm interrupted. The musketeers fired volleys into the air to frighten off the crocodiles and they waded across waist deep without incident. For the time being the spell had been broken.

*****

Once they learned that Nandzi understood a little of their language, the guards were eager to boast of the greatness of the Asante state and to share some gossip

"Our King," one of the musketeers told her, "has three thousand, three hundred and thirty three wives."

Nandzi struggled with the figure. It was clearly a large number.

"They are the finest, the most beautiful women in the nation. If the King sees a beautiful woman, he will take her, even if she is another man's wife, or if she is a slave. Now you are quite a pretty girl. If the King sees you, he might well marry you. But be forewarned: no other man may sleep with one of the King's wives. To do so is to court terrible torture and certain death, both for the man and for the wife. Only the highest in the land can avoid this punishment."

He looked around and dropped his voice.

"Let me tell you a story. This happened during the reign of our last king, Kusi Obodum. One of the King's own sons, Adabo, fell in love with one of his father's wives. The scandal became known. Adabo was a favourite son of his father, but the King's counsellors demanded that he be handed over to the executioners. It was only with the greatest of difficulty that the King was able to extract a compromise from them. The errant wife was executed but Adabo's sentence was commuted to castration. Do you understand, his balls were cut off?"

This was dangerous gossip. The man slowed down and walked beside Nandzi, speaking so softly that she could barely hear him. She opened her eyes wide and turned to look at him.

"Adabo survived the operation," he continued, "and our present King, Osei Kwadwo, has created a special stool for him. He is the Chief Surveyor of Nuisance and Master of Those Who Keep the Roads Clear. We might well meet him on the way. You will recognise him by his gold sword and the gold and silver whips he carries."

He looked around again to make sure that no one was monitoring his conversation. He dropped his voice almost to a whisper.

"Now do you know why the King created that job for Adabo? No? Well I'll tell you. When he was a young man, Osei Kwadwo committed the same offence, not just with one, but with four of the King's wives. Four. Can you believe it? Osei Kwadwo was Kusi Obodum's nephew and the heir to the Golden Stool. They couldn't kill him. He got away with no more than a scolding. They tried to hush the whole thing up, you know, but it is difficult to keep secrets in Kumase. They got Duedu, who was the captain of the harem, to confess and he was executed to save Osei Kwadwo's reputation. But the women in the palace have okro mouths, they gossip even with their slaves. So I warn you, in Asante there is one law for the nobles and another for the common people, especially slaves. If the King marries you, even if he never touches you, and you take a lover, you must expect to be tortured and to die."

"Are you not afraid to tell such stories?" Nandzi asked him.

He looked around.

"Nobody heard me," he said.

"My name is Mensa," he continued, "what is yours?"

She told him.

"Nandzi," he said, "I like you. How about it tonight? I mean when we camp. You and me. I mean, before the King marries you and it becomes too dangerous?"

Nandzi laughed. "Thank you but they tell me that I am already the property of your King. I would rather not take the risk."

*****

A few days later, they came to the customs post at the border of Asante proper.

Beyond the border the tree cover became more dense. Almost before they were aware of it, they found themselves enveloped in the rain forest. In that vast primeval wilderness the great road to Kumase, hacked through by the labour of countless slaves, was the only evidence of the puny genius of mankind.

The slaves surveyed their surroundings with awe.

Great multicoloured butterflies and moths flitted across the patches of bright dappled sunlight which reached the road. On either side, beyond the undergrowth, lay a domain of alien gloom. Tangled ropes, some as thick as a woman's wrist, hung from the highest branches, twisted into strange contorted shapes as they descended. The scent of rotting vegetation filled the air. Tiny shrill-voiced birds, with bright red and yellow and blue breasts and long curved beaks, swept out of the darkness to suck the nectar from the wild flowers which grew in the tangled roadside jungle.

"Everything seems different," Nandzi told Minjendo.

The road was aligned to suit pedestrian traffic. It meandered this way and that, hugging the slopes of the small, closely-spaced, steep-sided hills which filled the landscape, skirting the great buttresses of a silk-cotton tree, sometimes plunging into damp, flat areas which would become impassable swamps during the rains. It was just twelve paces wide. Left untended for only a single rainy season, the forest would invade it and recover its lost territory. But this road had not been left untended. It was an important artery of the Asante economy and Adabo's maintenance gangs were forever slashing away with their cutlasses to keep it clear.

The slaves from the northern savannah were unused to the humidity. Their bodies and clothing were drenched in sweat and their wet black skin glistened in the speckled light.

The forest pressed in on them. From its depths came strange discordant sounds, a chorus of screeching, howling and wailing.

Minjendo gripped Nandzi's arm: "What's that?"

"Oh, it must be some kind of animal," replied Nandzi, feigning calm indifference. "Jaji, leave go of me."

"What kind of animal? I have never heard a noise like that before."

"Well, maybe the animals that live in the forest are different from the ones we know."

Minjendo was not satisfied.

"There it is again," she cried. "Nandzi, ask the guard. I am afraid."

"Papa Mensa," Nandzi asked the musketeer who was her suitor, "I beg you, what is making that frightful noise."

Mensa laughed.

"Those are the spirits of the forest. They are screaming abuse at us because they are angry that we have cut a road through their kingdom. Do you understand? Spirits, cruel, vindictive spirits."

He laughed again.

"What did he say?" asked Minjendo.

Nandzi translated as best she could.

"But don't mind him," she added. "He is just telling us that to make us scared."

"How can you be sure?" asked Minjendo.

Nandzi had no reply.

She said only, "Spirits or no spirits, one thing is clear: it would be madness to try to run away and hide in this forest. You would get lost in no time. And if the spirits did not kill you, there must surely be wild animals there which would."

"You are always thinking of escape," said Minjendo.

*****

In the late afternoon they passed a clearing planted with corn, plantain and cassava, all plants which were new to them.

"We must be approaching a village," said Nandzi.

A old woman who had been hoeing straightened her back and took a break to watch the extraordinary procession.

"*Adwúma óo*!" cried the first rank of Asante musketeers as they passed.

"*Adwuma yé*," she replied, "the work is good."

"*Adwúma óo*!" Nandzi echoed the greeting.

"*Adwuma yé*," the woman replied again.

Then the slaves behind followed suit and the greetings and replies rippled through the forest like the wind in a corn field.

Koranten Péte had sent a runner ahead to give notice of their coming.

For the villagers the arrival of such a large party of northerners was an event which would provide material for conversation for weeks to come. This was some recompense for the cost which they were obliged to incur in entertaining the party. The young scouts who had been on the watch all day came running in to announce the imminent arrival of the caravan. The chief put on his best cloth and the panoply which was the privilege of his office and, with drummers and umbrella bearers in attendance, he and his elders proceeded slowly to meet the oncoming party. The caravan's drums were heard in the distance and the village drummers replied. At the boundary of the village territory, the welcome party waited with quiet dignity. A swarm of small boys and girls ran this way and that, aware that some great event was about to happen, but unable to conceive what it might be and unable to contain their excitement.

A camp ground had been cleared and newly fenced. The slaves were served with water as if they were honoured guests. Palm nut soup was cooking in as many pots as the village could muster. And when the guests had eaten their fill the children, only dimly aware of the distinction between slave and free man, circulated shyly amongst the visitors, intrigued at their manacles and chains, offering them the bananas and pineapples, pawpaw and sweet limes which they had picked especially for this occasion.

Tired as she was after the day's march, Nandzi organised the female slaves to serve the men, to bring them water to drink and wash, to bring them food and to dress the festering wounds which many of them suffered from the constant friction of their manacles. When the women, too, had washed and eaten, one of them started singing Nandzi's dirge and they all joined in, singing themselves to sleep.

By day they trudged on; through Mampon, home of Koranten Péte's wife; through Nsuta, where his father was the monarch; through Agona with its wide straight streets and well built houses; through Effiduase with its busy market, and on to the very outskirts of Kumase itself.

CHAPTER 8

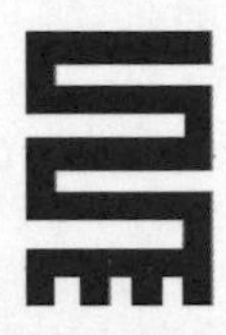

Koranten Péte had had a secure camp prepared just beyond the city limits.

His men had roofed the simple bamboo sheds with plantain and palm leaves to give the newly arrived slaves some relief from the sun. The male slaves were released from their shackles and chains. Their beards and heads were shaved and their wounds were treated with herbal balms and wrapped in medicinal leaves. There was hot water; and balls of black soap and loofahs and shea butter. There was plenty to eat. And each slave was given a large piece of indigo cloth., as Koranten Péte had promised.

"This is too good to be true," said Minjendo as she combed the knots out of Nandzi's hair. "I can't remember when I last bathed with hot water and oiled my body."

"Too good to last, I fear," replied Nandzi. "Remember, we are slaves. They must be fattening us up to some purpose."

Musketeer Mensa was passing by on patrol.

"Sir, Sir," Nandzi called to him, "Nana Mensa."

"Oh, it is you is it?" he said. "Have you changed your mind? Tonight is probably your last chance, you know. By tomorrow you might have joined the King's harem."

"Nana, don't you have a wife?" she asked.

"Several," he replied, "but what has that got to do with it?"

"Oh nothing, I suppose," she answered. "What I wanted to ask you was this. Do you Asante always treat your slaves as well as we are being treated here?"

"Of course, of course," he said. "But tomorrow is Akwasidae, a special day. Listen: can't you hear the talking drums announcing it? Tomorrow you will be presented to the King."

*****

Dressed in their indigo, each carried a basket or parcel of the tribute goods on his head. Nandzi had been given a bundle of silk fabric, Minjendo a load of Hausa men's tunics. Others carried cotton cloth, shea butter, iron tools.

The musketeers had had a chance to slip into Kumase and change into their dress uniforms.

"Good morning, Miss," said one of them.

Nandzi returned the greeting casually. Then, recognising the voice, she took a second look at the face.

"Nana Mensa!" she said in surprise. "How fine you look, and how fierce! I didn't recognise you at all. At all!"

Projecting from Mensa's forehead was a pair of gilded rams' horns. Above this rose an enormous head-dress of eagle feathers, shimmering in the early morning light. The musketeer's face and upper arms were adorned with stripes of white clay designed to terrify the enemy. His heavy red vest was embellished with countless silver and gold amulets and tiny brass bells.

Mensa did a little war dance and the amulets flapped and the tintinnabula tinkled as he sprang up and down. He spun around and the spotted tail which was attached to his cowrie-studded leather neck band swung after him.

Nandzi recalled the night she had spent in a tree in the Yendi bush with a leopard circling below and shuddered.

"Did you kill the beast yourself?" she asked him.

He answered by raising aloft his shining musket. Its haft was bound with gold wire and hung with red tassels. Then he took mock aim, miming the single shot with which he had dispatched his prey.

Nandzi continued her inspection.

"You are as beautiful as a bird," she teased him, "and as musical."

Koranten Péte approached, inspecting the ranks of his charges and their guards. He was simply dressed in a rich green, yellow and red silk kente cloth, thrown over his left shoulder. On his way back down the line, he recognised Nandzi. He took her by the arm.

"Come," he said, "and you too," signing Minjendo to follow.

"You and your friend will lead the procession today. I shall tell you what to do and you will pass on my instructions to those who follow you."

He took his place and at a sign his seven horn blowers lifted up the elephant tusks which were their instruments and blasted out their strident fanfare.

Musketeer Mensa, who had taken up his station beside Nandzi whispered, "Do you hear what the horns are saying?"

She shook her head.

"It is Nana's own horn call. Listen: *'ase ase ayo, ase ase ayo!'* That means that Nana has achieved everything he promised. Like defeating the Dagomba in war."

The drummers took over and the procession set off. The musketeers walked alongside, just in case one of the new slaves should take it into his head to attempt some foolhardy act.

Another party entered the road ahead of them. Behind the horn blowers and the drummers, a chief and his attendants walked in the shade of an enormous silk umbrella with a carved gilt pinnacle in the form of a deer's head. Behind him, a slave carried a brass-studded carved armchair on his head and twelve small boys danced and waved the tails of elephants.

They passed through the city gate, a tall tower constructed of bamboo. Looking up through the red cloth buntings fluttering in the light breeze, Nandzi saw the carcass of a sheep hanging in a red silk sling. She stretched out her arm and poked Mensa's shoulder. His eyes followed hers as she looked up again.

"It is just an offering to the gods and the ancestors," he explained.

Noisy parties joined them from left and right. The road became congested with people, all heading towards the great open square before the Asantehene's palace. Bearers plunged and spun their masters' umbrellas as each sought to outdo his rivals in dexterity and skill. Others flourished Dutch, English and Danish flags, swinging their short poles this way and that in ostentatious display. Prancing musketeers raised their flintlocks in one hand and fired carelessly into the heavens above. Explosions of firearms rent the air; countless bands of drummers competed with the harsh message of the horns and a confusion of animated chanting and singing and shouting. Minjendo coughed and sneezed as the dust and smoke and smell of gunpowder filled her nostrils. She gripped Nandzi's arm in alarm. Ahead of them, Koranten Péte pressed on regardless.

At last they entered the square. Koranten Péte led them to the space which had been set aside for them. They put down their loads and squatted on the ground in their indigo ranks. It was already hot and they began to sweat. Koranten Péte sat before them on an armchair in the shade of a large umbrella. A small boy fanned him with a fan of ostrich feathers. Immediately behind him sat a row of musketeers in their splendid attire.

The dignitaries moved to their allotted places, the kings and chiefs under their umbrellas, the less important delegations under temporary awnings. The general populace milled about behind. The noise sank to a respectful murmur, then rose again to a crescendo as horn players and drummers led each new chiefly party into the square. A group of Hausa clerics and businessmen took their seats. Nandzi thought she caught a glimpse of Sharif Imhammed amongst them.

The four sides of the square were full, except only the place of honour before the palace gate. For a long time nothing happened. They sat patiently in the sun and sweated. Then the gates of the palace opened and out tumbled the red-shirted palace dwarfs, cartwheeling and rolling on the ground, leaping and twisting. The assembly greeted them with loud cheers and rapturous laughter.

Some of the dwarfs had tiny bow legs, others huge bellies; some grotesquely distorted heads; others bodies as thin as a skeleton. They held hands in pairs and in unison whirled each other around like so many demi-human spinning tops. They fell flat on their faces and flat on their backs; they somersaulted backwards and forwards; they rolled on their sides in the dust, over and over; and then head over heels; they wrestled and boxed; they made concerted mock attacks on the ranks of the executioners and the musketeers. Every new trick was greeted with rollicking applause.

Nandzi's attention wandered. She wondered idly whether, when these court dwarfs died, their spirits were transformed into dwarfs of the forest, *mmoatia*.

Sensing some restlessness in the assembly, a group of horn players exercised their right, hallowed by custom, to issue a summons to the King.

"The horns speak," said Mensa. "Like our drums, our horns speak. They are saying, 'Oh, mighty King. We are impatient to see you. Please come. Protector of Asante, scourge of our enemies, please come.'"

A parody of a royal procession, complete with a King in his miniature palanquin, spinning umbrellas and scaled down fontomfrom drums was parading around the square. The dwarf Queen Mother acknowledged the cheering with a curtsy that took her forehead to the ground. Minjendo dug her nails into Nandzi's arm. She was so completely absorbed in the mummery that she was quite unaware that she was hurting her friend.

"Poor wretches," muttered Nandzi.

She turned to scan her fellow slaves and the audience nearby, wondering whether she would see in any other face a reflection of her own confused feelings.

Slaves, dwarfs, she thought, *dwarfs, slaves.*

She was surprised that these poor caricatures of human beings had been permitted to survive. Once, at home, when she was still young and free and a bit wild, before she had even met Itsho, she had eavesdropped on a whispered conversation between her mother and Tabitsha's rival, Tigen's senior wife. A woman in the next hamlet, she had heard, had been delivered of just such a monster. The infant's life had been snuffed out before it had had a chance to become a human being. No one had ever spoken of it again. It was as if it had never been born. *Why are such creatures ever born at all*? she wondered. *Are they sent by the ancestors to punish their parents for some misdeed?* She recalled how she had broken a taboo by tasting meat. Was her slavery a punishment for that transgression? Might the ancestors send her a dwarf child to punish her once more? She shuddered. *The minds of the ancestors are inscrutable,* she thought.

At long last, from the depths of the palace, the deep voices of the *atumpan*, the talking drums, signalled the approach of the real royal procession. The dwarfs' gyrations came to an abrupt halt and they melted away unnoticed. All rose to their feet. Koranten Péte turned and raising his upturned palms, signalled to the slaves to follow suit. Both men and women dropped their cloths from their shoulders and rewrapped them around their waists or under their armpits, leaving their shoulders bare.

Nandzi and Minjendo were in the front row of the slaves, just behind Mensa. As the procession entered the arena, he whispered a running commentary to them over his shoulder.

"The Blowers of the Golden Horns," he said, as the gates opened and the royal procession entered the arena.

The elephant tusk at the head of the procession was larger even than the one Nandzi had seen in Yendi. It was sheathed in gold and would clearly be too heavy to hold up and blow without assistance. The larger end was decorated with what looked like jawbones. Nandzi shuddered. Once Itsho had found a human skeleton lying on a lonely, unfrequented hillock. The scattered bones had turned out to be the remains of a hunter who had disappeared without trace many years before. Moved by a curiosity she could not control, Nandzi had ignored Itsho's dire warnings and picked up the whitened skull. The lower jaw had dropped and the sudden opening of the mouth had given her such a fright that she had let the skull fall to the ground. She thought she recognised the jawbones on that golden tusk. They looked suspiciously human.

Six horn players followed, each blowing into a gold mouth piece. One horn spoke first, another answered and then the other five sang out a chorus in different tones. The sound of the horns left no one in doubt that the King would soon emerge from the palace gates.

"The horns are speaking the words of our second King, Opoku Ware, 'Kotoko, Asante porcupine, remember me,' and indeed we do still honour his memory."

"Now they are speaking to our present King. 'Osei Koawia,' they are saying, 'While you reign over us, our enemies can do us no harm. The rain may beat the rock but it cannot make it move.'"

"The Master of the Royal Music; the Manager of the King's Markets; the

Keeper of the Royal Mausoleum; the Captain of the King's Messengers . . ." Mensa continued.

Each official was distinguished by the magnificence of his attire and some solid gold symbol of his office, hung around his neck, a sanko, weighing scales, a skeleton, a ceremonial sword.

Next came the fat eunuch who was the Manager of the Royal Harems.

Minjendo gasped. She squeezed Nandzi's arm again, to make sure that she had also seen the object of her astonished attention. Coming out of the gate was a man of enormous size, a veritable giant. He wore only a flimsy cloth, wrapped around his waist. His oiled body bulged with muscles. A solid gold axe hung from his necklace, both the symbol and the tool of his office. The stool which was borne aloft before him was black with the blood of his victims. An awed murmur rose from the crowd.

Then "The King," Nandzi whispered, overwhelmed in spite of herself by the magnificence of the Asante monarch.

The Asantehene was in his early forties, somewhat heavily built. His manner was majestic, yet Nandzi thought she caught a kindly look in his eye. He bent his head slightly in acknowledgement of the cheers.

"His stool name is Osei Kwadwo," whispered Mensa, "but we call him by his nickname, Osei Koawia, He Who Fights in the Afternoon. Our fathers gave him that name for his great valour and many victories. Now listen to the horns. They are saying, 'Nana, most excellent King. We will follow wherever you tell us. God spare you to lead us for many more years.'"

A great roar of welcome rose from the assembly.

The King wore a plain cloth of dark green silk and simple white leather sandals with gold and silver charm-cases on the straps. There the simplicity stopped. From head to ankles, he was adorned with the finest gold ornaments: on his head a crown of black velvet decorated with solid slabs of gold and the mysterious multicoloured aggrey beads. Just below the crown a red silk ribbon encircled his forehead. At his neck he wore a chain of imitation snail shells cast in solid gold; hanging over his right shoulder a silk cord on which hung three golden charm-cases; his arms were covered with bracelets of gold and aggrey beads; there were several gold rings on every finger; his chest was covered with a golden breastplate in the shape of the unfolding petals of a flower; around his knees hung bands of aggrey beads and around his ankles strings of exquisite tiny gold ornaments in the shape of coins, musical instruments, weapons, animals and birds. From his left forearm hung lumps of unformed solid gold, in the same raw state in which they had been wrenched from the earth.

Weighed down by this enormous burden of gold, the King walked slowly and with difficulty, supporting each wrist on the head of a page boy. Attendants surrounded him, ready to grip his elbows and his waist, should he stumble. What with the fan bearers waving their ostrich feather fans and the umbrella bearers, he could move neither left nor right.

Nandzi studied him as he passed. *This man is ill,* she thought. He has a serious illness. She pitied him. She recalled a day when she and Itsho had broken open a termite mound to look for the queen and of her disgust when they had at last found the distended immobile body. This king seemed to have as much freedom to move as that termite queen. And yet his subjects seemed just as loyal. Itsho.

The thought of Itsho kept coming back to her this afternoon. She looked up at the cloudless sky.

A slave followed, carrying the King's armchair on arms outstretched above his head.

"Is that the famous Golden Stool?" whispered Nandzi, somewhat disappointed.

"Shh!," replied Mensa. "No one, not even the King, sits on the Golden Stool of Asante."

Next came more slaves each bearing on his head an enormous royal fontomfrom drum. The elephant skin was stretched tight against a frame work of what were surely human thigh bones. Certainly the decorations were human skulls. Nandzi opened her mouth to question Mensa, but she thought better of it and swallowed her words.

The Royal Drummers who followed the drum bearers, raised their arms and beat out the praise names of the King and his predecessors, "Osei Tutu, Opoku Ware, Kusi Obodum, Osei Kwadwo. Conqueror of Banda. Conqueror of Wassa. Master of Dagomba. Osei Koawia it was who vanquished them all."

A short distance behind followed a group of women, shaded by an umbrella which was only a little smaller and less grand than that of the King. Through a gap in the silk screens which a retinue of young girls held up to protect their mistresses from public gaze, Nandzi caught a glimpse of women of such beauty, regal pride and elegant attire as she had never seen before. They were dressed simply, all in the same deep red cloth, but their earrings, necklaces, bangles and bracelets were all solid gold.

"The King's wives," she whispered.

"Shh!" warned Mensa. "You will get us into trouble."

"Well, aren't they?"

"No," replied Mensa. "No man may look on the face of a wife of the King and live. That is the Queen Mother, Konadu Yaadom."

"Which one?"

"Can't you see? The young woman in the centre, with the gold head-dress."

"Come, you are teasing me. That woman is young enough to be the King's daughter and you tell me that she is the Queen Mother? She is not much older than I am."

"The Queen Mother is not the mother of the King. And she is already a widow. Her husband, Prince Adu Twum, died less than a month ago. That is why they are wearing mourning cloth," whispered Mensa hoarsely. "If you will just be quiet, I will explain to you later."

"Then where are all the wives?"

"Shh!" Mensa warned again.

The Asantehene and his party made one circuit of the square. With his right hand the King acknowledged the cheers of his subjects. His armchair was set down. The members of his party ranged themselves around him. His supporters helped him to his seat. A squad of young men sat on the ground before him, gold handled scimitars raised high. Before them sat a crowd of small boys, the older ones proudly brandishing elephants' tails which seemed to have been dusted in gold; the youngsters waving ostrich feathers.

Immediately behind the King stood a bodyguard of handsome youths wearing leopard skin waistcoats, embellished with numerous gold and silver sheaths in each of which was a small knife with a blue agate handle. To one side were the *akrafó*, the King's souls, identified by the gold plates hanging on their chests. Pretty young girls, each carrying a silver basin, stood behind the chairs of the dignitaries.

The king clapped the tiny gold castanets which he wore on his forefinger and thumb. At a signal from the Chief Linguist the horns played a fanfare and the drums rolled. In the ensuing silence the Linguist poured libation, calling on the ancestors for their blessings.

Then the Chief Crier and Eulogist rose to his feet and, to the accompaniment of extravagant gestures, sang out the encomiums of the King for all to hear.

"Oh mighty Monarch,

"Son of Osei Tutu,

"Son of Opoku Ware

"Son of Kusi Obodum

"Who in the world can stand comparison with you?"

After each phrase he paused and the drums answered.

"The Bandas and the Wassas felt the heat of your fire

"And fled.

"The cavalry of the Dagomba heard the sound of your muskets

"And fled in panic.

"All the world's monarchs place their necks beneath your feet.

"The whole world is yours.

"Who can equal your wealth and power?

"It is not for nothing that you are called Osei Koawia,

"He who fights in the afternoon."

Then a fearsome war-cry rang out from his lips.

"*Asante Kotoko, kum apem, apem beba.*

"Asante Porcupine. Should our enemy kill a thousand warriors, would not another thousand immediately come forward?"

Every Asante man and boy rose to his feet, and the women too. Punching the air with their fists, they repeated the Crier's words, drowning out the reply of the drums; but the newly arrived slaves, ignorant and uncommitted, remained seated.

While the roar of the crowd was at its height, a company of the younger executioners rushed into the arena, flying here and there like a brood of frenetic headless chickens, hurtling through the air, spinning, swirling around in frenzied gyrations, chanting their own distinctive nasal warnings and from time to time raising their swords and clashing them in unison against those of their fellows. As the drumming and dancing reached a crescendo, the giant Chief Executioner made a fearsome entrance, cow's tail in his left hand, bloody knife of his office in the other. His face and body and the horns of *sasabonsam* which stuck out from his forehead were painted in red and black, the colours of death. He danced in a more measured style than his minions, but the threat of his vocation was apparent in every movement. The human skulls suspended from his waist struck one another as he lunged this way and that. Nandzi was not alone in shuddering at the menace of this chief of licensed killers. Then, suddenly, the drumming stopped and the death dancers were gone.

The Criers called for silence. In the ensuing hush, the Chief Linguist announced that the distinguished army commander, Koranten Péte, would now deliver the annual tribute of the King of the Dagomba, the Ya Na. Mats were laid out before the royal party. Koranten Péte signalled to the slaves to take up their loads. Nandzi and Minjendo took their places behind him as he made his way slowly to the royal podium and the other slaves followed in twos.

Koranten Péte came to a halt. While he waited for the King to complete a private conversation with the Chief Linguist, Nandzi had an opportunity to take a closer look at him and at the Queen Mother, who sat nearby.

"Nana Okyeame," Koranten Péte addressed the Chief Linguist, "it gives me great pleasure to deliver to Nana Asantehene the annual Dagomba tribute. The Ya Na has particularly asked me to convey to Nana assurances of his loyalty and fidelity and of his high personal esteem.

"The tribute comprises the goods which will now be laid before Nana, the slaves who bear these goods and herds of cattle, sheep and goats which are at this moment being driven to Kumase and which, I understand, have now reached Mampon."

The Linguist repeated Koranten Péte's words to the King.

Koranten Péte continued, "I beg leave to deliver the goods."

The King indicated his consent. Nandzi and Minjendo deposited their head-loads. Then, on Koranten Péte's instructions they helped those who had followed them to do the same.

While this was under way the Royal Musicians kept the assembly entertained with their sankos and flutes, drums and gongs and bells.

The King rose to make a formal inspection of the goods and then he shook hands warmly with Koranten Péte.

The Chief Linguist clapped his hands for silence.

"Nana Asantehene has asked me to remind you that he rewarded the distinguished leadership, great personal bravery and unquestioned loyalty of General Koranten Péte in the conquest of Dagomba with an entitlement to one third of all tributes collected. At the invitation of Nana Asantehene, Nana Péte has already made his selection."

Nandzi whispered a translation to Minjendo.

"I hope that he has chosen us," said Minjendo. "Nana Péte would not be a bad man to work for. At least we know him."

Though it was already late afternoon and the shadows were lengthening, the most important business of the day was yet to come.

Accompanied by horns and drums, the first of the visiting Kings now led his retinue of supporters to greet the Asantehene. Again, as earlier in the day, umbrellas spun and flags waved. Bare-headed and bare-chested, the visitor approached.

"Nana Asantehene," he said, "please accept my assurance of my utter devotion and that of my people. As proof of our allegiance, I should be honoured to receive your foot upon my neck. We are as nothing before you. All our property, our gold and slaves, our very lives, are yours to command."

Then he sank to his knees and placed his forehead on the ground.

The Asantehene stretched out his hands which the visitor grasped in his own. They exchanged a few private words and then, Asum Adu, Minister of Finance and Keeper of the Royal Treasury, handed the visitor a small brass chest containing a valuable gift of gold dust.

The visitor made an appropriately fawning speech of thanks and took his leave, to be followed by the next in the queue.

Nandzi yawned. She had had enough of this pomp and ceremony for one day. Moreover, she badly wanted to piss. Just as she was wondering whether the guards would let her steal away to the outskirts of the crowd to relieve herself, Koranten Péte gave the signal. He had received permission to leave.

*****

CHAPTER 9

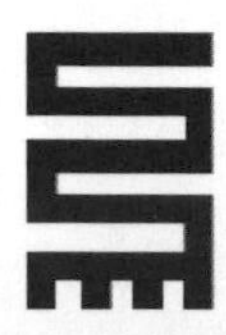

In the days which followed various strangers appeared at the camp and took parties of slaves away. Nandzi and Minjendo watched nervously but no one came for them.

The next Saturday, Mensa appeared. He was not in a good mood.

"I've been sent to fetch you," he said. "You had better put on your good cloth."

"Where are you taking me?" asked Nandzi.

"To your new mistress."

"My new mistress?"

"Yes, the Asantehemaa, the Queen Mother. You saw her at the Adae, do you remember? You thought she was one of the King's wives. Nana Koranten Péte has sent me to take you to her."

"Can my friend come too?"

"Young miss," said the musketeer, "Remember who you are. You have been brought here to work, not to spend your time gossiping with your girl friends."

He held up his right hand to still Nandzi's protest.

"And while I'm on that subject, let me give you some friendly advice. You are going to live and work in the royal palace. The palace is a dangerous place. If you value your skin, be humble. Learn to keep your mouth shut. Never speak unless you are spoken to. Never draw attention to yourself. Listen and learn. We have a proverb which says that at another's hearth, you do not have the same freedom you might have in your mother's kitchen. Remember that and you will have a better chance of surviving."

"What do you mean, 'a dangerous place' and 'a better chance of surviving?' Why?"

"There you go again. I have already said more than I intended. I was a fool to offer you the benefit of my wisdom. Now gather your things, say goodbye to your friend and let's go."

*****

In the shade in the far corner of the courtyard sat a man and a woman, each on a low stool. The woman had dropped her cloth around her waist. A baby was feeding at her breast.

The man called out to Nandzi, "Young woman, come."

She recognised the voice: it was Koranten Péte's. Could this woman be the Queen Mother? she wondered. In her confusion she tried to recall Mensa's advice. She crossed the courtyard, stopped in front of them and curtsied. They both looked at her.

"Nananom," she said, "my grandparents, I give you the morning greeting."

Koranten Péte nodded approvingly.

"Nana," he said to the woman, "you remember I mentioned I would be bringing you a gift. Well, here she is."

He turned to Nandzi.

"You told me your name but I have forgotten."

"They call me Nandzi," she said.

As the woman moved the child to the other breast, Nandzi saw it was a boy.

"She had better have a good Asante name. It is Saturday today. I will call her Ama. Ama Donko. Do you understand?"

She turned to Koranten Péte. "Does she hear Asante?"

He nodded.

"From today your name is Ama," said Konadu Yaadom, speaking slowly and raising her voice as one does to foreigners. "Ama is a good Asante name. We give it to a girl who is born on Saturday. Today you have been born again as an Asante girl. Do you hear me?"

"Yes, please, Nana," Nandzi replied.

She thought, *the woman must be deaf; and she thinks I'm stupid and deaf too.*

The child had fallen asleep at his mother's breast.

"Esi," the mother called.

There was no reply and no one came.

"E-si!" she called again.

"Typical Fanti girl," she said to Koranten Péte, "lazy, untidy, never there when you need her."

"Here, Ama," she said to Nandzi, wrapping the sleeping child in a cloth. "Do you know how to hold a baby?"

"Nana, please: yes," Nandzi replied again.

"Then take my child and sit with him there on that stool until Esi arrives to show you your duties."

She turned to Koranten Péte.

"Wofa," she said, half rising to shake his hand, "thank you for the gift. I hope she turns out as well as you promise. Slaves are so unreliable these days. Just look at Esi. She has probably gone off to the market on some pretext. The real reason will no doubt be to meet her lover."

Just then a lad burst through the gate, followed by a crowd of younger playmates. He was brandishing a wooden musket.

"Bang, bang," he cried as he rushed in, aiming his toy gun successively at Konadu Yaadom, Koranten Péte and Nandzi.

"Kwame," shouted Konadu Yaadom, "stop that nonsense at once and come and greet Nana properly. Opoku, you too."

She raised her finger to show the other boys the gate and they fled.

"Oh, Nana Péte," said Kwame, putting down his gun and using both his hands to shake Koranten Péte's right, "I didn't see it was you. You are welcome. You are always welcome. How are things in Nsuta and Mampon? Have you been in any more wars lately?"

Without waiting for a reply he took up his gun and took aim at Nandzi. "Bang, bang. Another dead Dagomba," he said and then noticing that his victim was a stranger, "Hallo, who's this?"

"Kwame Panin!" threatened Konadu Yaadom, "mind your manners, or you'll know what's what. Now go and play. Opoku, you too. I have matters to discuss with Nana. Wait, where is Amma Sewaa?"

"Looking after the girls," the boy shouted back as he skipped and jumped on his way out to rejoin his friends.

Konadu Yaadom looked after him and said, "Tchtt! The boy is wild. Wild! Sometimes I have difficulty controlling him. He is forever fighting with his elder sister and bullying my poor little Opoku."

"He'll settle down," said Koranten Péte. "Just give him just a few years and he'll be mature enough to start attending Court."

"That is just the trouble," replied Konadu Yaadom, "I very much doubt that we have a few years."

The child slept on Nandzi's lap. She listened to the conversation attentively, but carefully maintained a blank expression on her face. *If my new mistress thinks I am dumb,* she thought, *then I will act dumb.* However, her performance was unnecessary: they talked on as if she did not exist.

"What do you mean?" asked Koranten Péte, carefully putting his beaker of palm wine down beside him. There was a look of concern on his face.

"Nana is ill, seriously ill," said Konadu Yaadom. "Did you not see him at the adae? He could scarcely walk. I have tried to persuade him to go to Okomfo Tantani for advice, or even to the Muslims, but he refuses. He says it is a small thing and it will pass. I hope he is right, but I fear otherwise."

She paused.

"I am telling you this in the utmost confidence, do you understand?"

"Of course, of course. I noticed that he was not his old vigorous self, but I must say that it didn't strike me that it was that bad," said Koranten Péte. "I thought that it was just concern about the news from Akuapem that was troubling him."

"No doubt that is a factor, but I fear that there is much more to it than that. Wofa, with you of all people, I know I can be quite frank."

She paused again.

"I don't think Nana has long to live."

Koranten Péte rose from his seat and took a few steps. He covered his eyes with his hands as he considered the implications. Then he sat down again.

"His death would cause a major crisis," he said. "The boy is hardly ready to take over."

"What is more," added the Queen Mother, dropping her voice, "I have intelligence that the Bremanhene, Ntoo Boroko, has got wind of Nana's illness. Immediately Nana dies, so my informants tell me, he plans to use force to enstool Kyei Kwame, the Kokofu king, as Nana's successor. The sudden death of our young Kwame Panin, I am told, is a key element in his plan."

"I had no idea," said Koranten Péte, shaking his head. "How long have you known this?"

"Not long. If you hadn't sent me a message that you were coming to see me today, I would have sent for you."

"What do you propose to do?"

"I want you to smuggle Kwame out of Kumase. Take him back to Mampon. Brief Nana Mamponhene thoroughly about the situation. Let him make discreet preparations to march on Kumase at any time at short notice, bringing Kwame with him. I will keep him informed of the condition of Nana's health and warn him at once if there is any sign of a sudden decline."

"Who will look after Kwame in Mampon?"

"Definitely not, I repeat not, his natural mother, my dear elder sister, Akyaamah. She has already done enough harm to Asante. In fact, Kwame's presence in Mampon must be concealed from her. It is not beyond her to side with the Kokofus against her own son, just to spite Nana. But I leave that decision to your own best judgement. Kwame will accept whatever you decide. The boy worships the very ground you walk on, you know. He has done, ever since your great victory in the north."

"Well, I am fond of the boy. I believe that he will make a great ruler of Asante one day."

"Your good wife, Abena Saka, Nana Mamponhemaa, might be the best person to take charge of the boy. I know that she would not tolerate any nonsense from him. But of that you must be the best judge."

"Mama, mama."

Kwame Panin came running in at the gate.

"Nana is coming. Get ready, get ready!"

Nandzi thought, *every one around here seems to be called Nana.* Could this really be the King coming to pay such an informal visit?

It was indeed Nana Osei Kwadwo, fourth Asantehene, descended on his mother's side from Opoku Ware, second Asantehene and on his father's side from Osei Tutu himself, the founder of the Asante nation. He walked slowly and with a stick. Several attendants hovered behind him but he brushed them off impatiently as he passed through the gate, allowing only one to accompany him.

"*Àgòo,*" he called, giving notice of his arrival.

Konadu Yaadom and Koranten Péte rose to their feet and Nandzi followed suit. As she did so, the baby pissed, wetting himself, his cloth and Nandzi's too. Then he woke and began to cry. Her child's cries threw Konadu Yaadom into a state of confusion. She tried to get a stool for the King, to welcome him, to help him to the stool and to deal with the baby all at once. Osei Kwadwo waved her away; Koranten Péte went to get the stool and Konadu Yaadom took the baby from Nandzi, giving her a look which said it was all her fault. As soon as the King had taken his seat, she sat too and gave the child her breast.

"Nana," she said, "you are welcome. Please excuse this fellow's bad manners."

Koranten Péte had remained standing.

Osei Kwadwo motioned him to a stool.

"Nana, I have already presumed on Nana Asantehemaa's hospitality too long. May I ask your permission to leave?"

Nandzi was still standing. She felt that she could hardly sit down uninvited in the presence of the King. She felt acutely embarrassed standing there in her wet cloth, an uninvited guest. The King's attendant looked at her with undisguised curiosity, but no one else seemed to notice her so she remained where she was, wishing she could make herself invisible.

"Sit down, my son," said the King. "Why should you attempt to leave just as I come in? How is your wife? And Nana Mamponhene?"

He turned to Konadu Yaadom.

"Nana Asantehemaa," he said with a smile, "I need a drink. That short walk from my quarters has left me thirsty."

"Nana, of course," she replied.

The child had gone back to sleep. She handed him to Nandzi, who took that as a signal to sit down again.

"What will you take? I have some fresh palm wine. Cool and refreshing in this hot weather."

"My child, I am old enough to be your father, and then some. Stop mothering me. Give me some European liquor."

"Nana, are you sure you should . . .?"

He cut her inquiry dead with one look and she went to bring the drink.

"E-si!" she called, but Esi had not yet returned.

When Konadu Yaadom came back with a bottle and two glasses on a silver tray, Osei Kwadwo was on his hobbyhorse.

"The walls will be of stone: I have people searching the kingdom for a good source. It is not easy to find. The stone must be strong but the pieces must not be too heavy to carry. Then the roof. These our thatched roofs leak too much. What I plan to do is to bring plenty of brass pans from the coast and have them beaten flat. I will make a framework of carved elephant tusks and lay the brass sheets over them with a good slope so that the rain water runs off. I shall have the doors and windows sheathed in gold, like my niece's there upstairs."

He pointed up to Konadu Yaadom's first floor window.

"And that is not all. When the house is finished, I shall mark the occasion by giving each of my ministers a large loan to improve his own house. I want Kumase to be the finest city in the world."

Konadu Yaadom had heard all this before, not once but many times. She changed the subject.

"Nana, do you see what Wofa brought me?"

She indicated Nandzi.

The King peered at her and then beckoned.

"Does she understand Asante?"

"A little," said Koranten Péte. "That is one reason why I chose her for Nana. Less trouble to train."

Nandzi approached, overtaken with embarrassment and confusion. She felt weak at the knees as she stood before the King and she was afraid she would drop the child. She sank to her knees and bowed her head.

Osei Kwadwo chucked her under the chin and raised her head so that he could look at her face.

"A pretty girl," he said. "A few years ago, I might have taken her as a wife. I still have half a mind . . . What is your name?"

"Please, Nana, they call me . . ."

She paused, caught her own name at her lips, and said, "Ama."

She was aware of Konadu Yaadom's nodded approval.

The Queen Mother said, "All right, Ama, you can go back to your seat."

"Wait," said the King, "let me look at the child."

"Opoku Fofie," the child's mother said, in case the King had forgotten his name.

"A handsome boy. One day he will surely occupy the Golden Stool," said the King.

"By the grace of God," replied Konadu Yaadom.

"It is this child I have come to talk to you about," said the King.

"The child?" asked Konadu Yaadom, puzzled, as Nandzi made her way back to her seat, still trembling.

"Yes, the child."

He made an attempt to stand up. The lad hastened to help him but Koranten Péte intervened.

"Nana, let me," he said, taking the bottle of Dutch schnapps from the King and pouring a silent libation to the ancestors.

"The child," repeated the King. "It is not good that he should grow up without a father. Every boy, especially a future Asantehene, needs a father to look up to, to train him in manly ways. And a young woman like you needs a good man. I want you to marry again."

"But, Nana, it is barely a month since Adu Twum Kaakyire died. I am still in mourning."

"Nana Konadu, do you remember what I told you six years ago when I fetched you from Mampon and had you enstooled as Asantehemaa on your own new stool? We royals are not like common people. Our noble birth imposes certain obligations upon us. This is one of those obligations."

"Does Nana have some one in mind?" asked Koranten Péte.

"Yes," replied the King. "My son, Owusu Ansa. It is time he settled down. Otherwise he might get himself into trouble. You see," he continued with a twinkle in his eye, "I know the nature of young men. It is not all that many years since I was one myself."

They knew that he was referring to the adulterous relations he had had with not one but four of the wives of his predecessor, Kusi Obodum. It had only been his royal uncle's indulgence and the brave sacrifice of his own life by the harem-keeper (what was his name now?) that had saved Osei Kwadwo's skin.

"Is that settled then?" he asked.

"If Nana says so," replied Konadu Yaadom.

"Not 'If Nana says so,'" said the King. "Rather, 'Nana, I should be happy to marry Owusu Ansa.'"

"Nana, I should be happy to marry Owusu Ansa."

"Now that's better."

He took a deep draught of the alcohol.

As Osei Kwadwo licked his lips, Kwame Panin rushed in. Seeing the King, he came to a sudden halt and then proceeded to walk forward with a measured pace.

"Ah, Kwame, my boy, come and greet me," said the King.

When the customary pleasantries had been exchanged, he introduced the boy to his attendant.

"This is Opoku, Opoku Frede-Frede I call him. He is a fine boy. Take him away and get to know him. In future he may serve you well."

"Who is the lad, Nana?" Koranten Péte asked when the two youngsters had retired.

"He came to me as part of the death duties of the late Oyokohene. He is a smart fellow; he has a nimble mind: that is why I call him Frede-Frede. When he has completed his military training I am going to send him to the Treasury. I am always on the look-out for talented youngsters to recruit into the public service, you know. Asante has grown too large for the King to run on his own. Authority must be delegated. That creates a demand for servants of the state who are clever and honest. When I find a lad with potential, I snap him up, even if he is a slave."

"Is this lad a slave, Nana?" asked Koranten Péte.

"No, no, just an ordinary commoner. But he has an excellent memory and a good logical mind. He knows how to reason and argue. And he can count. I see a great future for him."

He paused. He squeezed his eyes and bit his lower lip as if in pain. Konadu Yaadom exchanged a look with Koranten Péte. Then the spasm seemed to pass.

"To change the subject," he said when he opened his eyes, "Nana Konadu, I have been thinking over your kind advice. I know, that if any one has my true welfare at heart, it is you."

"Nana it is true."

"I have decided to consult Okomfo Tantani."

"Nana, I am pleased. The gods speak through Okomfo Tantani. He is a powerful healer. And if any one knows the uses of medicinal herbs it is his wife. Shall I send for them? When will you see him?"

*****

Esi was short, fat, untidy, irresponsible and irresistibly ebullient.

When she laughed, as she did frequently, her eyes lit up and she showed a mouthful of fine white teeth with the gap between the front two which the Akan regard as a sign of beauty. Incurably inquisitive, she was a repository of all the most confidential and up-to-date court gossip; but there was not a tittle of malice in her. Nandzi lost her heart to her irretrievably at first sight.

"First, let me tell you the sad story of my life," Esi said as the two of them bathed Opoku Fofie in a brass basin. "Then you will tell me yours."

"My mother is Asante and so, of course, am I. But my father, bless him, is a Fanti man. That's how I come to have a Fanti name. In Asante, Sunday-born girls are called Akosua, not Esi.

"As a young man Papa was taken prisoner in one of the wars. He was made to join the Asante army and sent to fight in the north. He acquitted himself so well in the first Dagomba war, that, as a reward, he was given some land to farm; and my mother to marry.

"What happened next is a famous event in Asante history. Can you guess?"

Nandzi shook her head.

"I was born!"

The baby chortled as if he had understood Esi's joke and they both smiled at his babbling.

"Hallo my little chuckle-and-snort," Esi told him and gave him a kiss.

"Well, to continue, though I dearly cherish my beloved Papa, I have to admit that, except as a soldier and as a loving father, he has not made much of a success of his life. You see, in Asante, money is everything. Papa's ambition has always been to make a quick killing, to make his fortune through a single stroke of genius, white man's genius. He is forever talking about how clever the white man is.

"Have you ever seen a white man? I mean a real white man, like those who live on the coast? No? Well, neither have I, but Papa has and to hear him talk of them, you would think they were gods."

Esi paused as she ladled up water to rinse the soap off the baby. Nandzi was glad to be able to relax her attention for a moment. Esi spoke so quickly that it was a struggle for her to keep up.

"Now where was I? Ah, Papa and the white men. As I was saying, to him the white man is next to God. Then come the Fantis. We Asante follow a poor third. As for northerners . . ."

She gripped Nandzi's wrist with a soapy hand.

"I'm sorry, nothing personal. I certainly don't share my good father's silly prejudices."

She laid the baby on a soft towel which she had spread across her lap.

"You must be very particular about how you dry grandfather Opoku Fofie's royal bottom. Maame Konadu will give you a proper beating if you leave a single speck of dampness on his aristocratic little body."

She lifted him up in his towel and gave him a hug. He responded with a gurgle of joy. Nandzi remembered her little brother Nowu. *I wonder whether my mother has had another baby yet*, she mused.

"Well, to return to my father and his white-man schemes. Cut down Odum trees and send them to the coast. The white man will pay anything for good wood. Build a dam across the village stream and grow fish in the pond behind the dam. Go to Kumase and bring white man's cloth and liquor to sell in the village market. One thing after another. After a while my mother began to make bitter fun of him and his dream-world. After all she was not only growing the food that we ate, all eight of us (and some more that died young) but also giving him pocket money to drink his palm-wine."

"Now mister pisser," she said to the baby as she tucked in the little cloth which she had wrapped around his nether regions, "will you just try to keep dry while Ama and I have something to eat? Ama, will you please bring the soup and the fufu, while I get this fellow settled?"

"To cut a long story short," she continued, as she tore a small finger-load off the ball of fufu and dipped it into the palm soup, "Papa began to borrow money to finance his crazy projects. As time went by, he got deeper and deeper into debt. Eventually there came the crunch. The creditors were themselves in debt and they were demanding immediate settlement. To save Papa's skin, I volunteered to be pawned. What I didn't know then was that Papa's creditors owed money to our dear mistress, Maame Konadu, bless her. So Papa's creditors pawned me, in turn, to her. So here I am and here I stay, worse off than a slave like you, until Papa's unlikely miracle happens or until I can find a rich man who will pay off the debt and marry me. End of story."

She blew on a spoonful of the soup to cool it and then fed it to the baby. He pulled a wry face at the pepper. Then he licked his lips, kicked his little legs and waved his arms about. Esi smiled.

"Now what about you?" she asked. "First, how do you come to be called Ama? Do your people use the same names as we do?"

"My real name is Nandzi but Nana said she didn't like it so she called me Ama."

"Tchtt! Typical of the woman! You cannot even call your name your own in this place. However," and here, somewhat out of character, Esi paused to think, "however . . . I advise you to accept it. In our situation we have to take care to choose our battles. Otherwise . . ." and she chopped at the back of her neck with the edge of a flattened hand.

"Do you understand?"

Nandzi thought she did.

"Let's shake on that. I'm Esi," laughed the owner of that name.

"I'm Ama," said Nandzi as she took the proffered hand; and from that moment, Ama she became, to others, and, in due course, to herself.

*****

"I love going to market," said Esi. "Don't you? Even though I never have any money of my own to spend. Nana said to 'show you the ropes.' You know why, of course?"

They were standing in the shade of one of the mighty trees which lined the square, next to the stall of a gold-weigher. Lined up on his table was an array of tiny brass castings, each in the shape of an animal or a plant or some human activity. Ama watched with fascination as the man used his brass scoop to pour his customer's gold dust into one of the pans of his scales and added a selection of his brass weights to the other until the two pans swung freely.

"Have you never seen gold dust weighed before?" asked Esi.

Ama shook her head.

"Then remember the weights," Esi said, counting with her fingers. "Six *ackies* make one *tokoo*; and forty *ackies* make one *peredwan*."

"One *peredwan*," she mused, "if I had one *peredwan* I could buy my freedom. Can you count?"

"Of course. In my own language up to a thousand; but in Asante I have only learned up to ten."

"Never mind, I'll teach you the rest. But remember, it is better to have the gold weighed at home before you come to market. If you have it weighed here you could be cheated. And Nana is very suspicious; she will assume that you have stolen some. Of course, I always do."

"You always do what?" asked Ama.

"Oh my little innocent," replied Esi, "I always steal some of her gold dust, of course. I tell her that prices have gone up. She is too aristocratic to go to the market herself, so she can't check whether I am lying. But I never take more than a few *tokoo* at a time. And I hide it well. It is not beneath our mistress to come and search our room, you know."

Ama needed some time to think about all this.

"Is that right?" she asked. "Stealing, I mean."

"Right? Is it right that we should work for her for nothing, the mean thing? Last week I showed her this old cloth I am wearing: it is worn right through from washing with cheap soap. Do you think she would give me a small dash to buy a new one? No way! How will I ever find myself a husband to buy my freedom when I have to dress like this?"

"But to steal . . .?"

"Ama, in Asante only money counts. Without it you can do nothing."

She continued, "You didn't answer my question. Do you know why Nana wants me to 'show you the ropes'?"

Ama shook her head. They were wandering amongst the meat vendors. Fowls and guinea fowls, dead and alive, were on display, deer meat, dried and smoked; spiced monkey flesh; great forest snails strung on grass ropes.

"Well, she is dissatisfied with me. 'Esi is stupid, Esi is lazy,' et cetera, et cetera. She wants to use you to threaten me. If she finds she likes you, she might have me dispatched at the next royal funeral. I hope you won't play her game. We must stick together."

"What do you mean, she'll have you dispatched?"

Esi stared at her in disbelief, but the innocent, questioning look remained on Ama's face. She took her hand and led her to a quiet corner. They sat down with their backs against two buttresses of a silk cotton tree.

"Ama, it is time you learned the facts of life in Asante, the facts of life and death. Tell me first, in your country, do you worship your ancestors?"

"Of course."

"And when your kings die, do you not send slaves to serve them in the world of the ancestral spirits?"

"Esi, in my country, we have no kings; and no slaves either."

"No kings? Who rules you then? I thought every country had kings."

"We have no rulers, only Elders and Priests of the Earth."

"So that is why you seem so innocent! Well, now you are going to have to grow up. For your own good, you are going to have to hear the truth. Listen to me well.

"In Asante, as you know by now, we do have a King; and many other royals too. No Asante royal goes into the next world alone or empty-handed. We dress our dead in the finest cloth and provide them with gold, food, anything that might be useful in the land of the ancestors. We commoners do that too. But the royals fear that the ancestors will not recognise them as important people unless they arrive with many servants. So when a royal dies, they kill, kill, kill. They slaughter at random. If it is a king who has died, they can kill as many as a hundred slaves, even a thousand. When a king dies, no one is safe. They use some of the corpses to line his grave. Look across the valley there. That is what they call the Bush of Ghosts, where they dump the surplus bodies. All they keep is the blood and the head and sometimes, they say, the internal organs to make medicine."

For a fleeting moment she thought that Esi might be pulling her leg. Then she recalled the execution she had witnessed in Yendi, and the human jaw bones and thigh bones and skulls she had seen in Kumase; and she remembered too how frightened the populace seemed to be of the giant Chief Executioner. It all fitted. Esi could not be lying. She thought, *if they kill me, I shall refuse to serve their King in the next world. I shall escape and search for Itsho.*

She said, "Esi, the King, Osei Kwadwo, is ill. He will die soon. Do you mean that they will kill us when he dies?"

"How can you know when the King will die? Take care. If you tell that to anyone else but me, you will be called a witch."

"I am not a witch. But I read the sickness in his eyes the first time I saw him.

"The other day, the day I came to the palace, when you were out: Koranten Péte was visiting Nana and they were talking about the King. Nana said Osei Kwadwo was seriously ill and that she thought he wouldn't live another year. Wait! Hear me out. Then the King himself came to visit and before he left he agreed to consult an *okomfo*, I forget his name, but Nana said that this *okomfo's* wife was the best herbal healer in the country."

"Ei! My father and my mother! I am sure you are right. Ama. I am too young too die. I will run away before they kill me. They say it is an honour to go and serve the Asantehene in the next world; but, as for me, I have served the Asantehemaa quite enough in this world. Ama, Ama, Ama. We must plan. We must prepare. We must find a place where we can hide when the day comes, a place where they will never find us.

"You know, it is as if they all go mad. There is such an orgy of bloodletting. Yet once the burial and the funeral are over, they act again as if nothing terrible has happened. They forget it all as you forget a dream when you wake up. But I wonder, I wonder sometimes whether the horror of it does not come back to haunt them after dark, when they are asleep. Sometimes one hears strange screams in the palace at night, as if some one were afflicted by a nightmare."

Esi was sobbing.

"Ama, trust me," she said when she had pulled herself together. "We shall find a way. Together we will find a way. I am glad you have come. You give me strength. Let me think about it and then we will talk again. Ei, my dear father!"

*****

As they entered the Queen Mother's courtyard, Kwame Panin, hiding behind a column in the gloom of the veranda, drove a spear into Ama's basket, spiked an orange and was gone. Ama felt the impact but couldn't see its cause. Only Esi caught a glimpse of the mischief's perpetrator.

"Kwame Panin!" she called after him, but he was gone.

"He is so naughty, that boy. What he needs is a good beating. I don't understand why his mother tolerates such behaviour," said Ama when Esi had helped her to put her basket down.

"His mother?" cried Esi. Then she dropped her voice. "Oh, you mean Nana. But didn't you know? Konadu Yaadom is not his real mother."

She looked around before she continued, "Kwame is the son of her elder sister, Akyaamah. Same mother, Aberefi Yaa, who was also once Asantehemaa, but different fathers."

"And where is this Akyaamah now? Is she dead?" asked Ama.

"In a way," replied Esi, relishing the prospect of sharing a scabrous piece of gossip with possibly the only person in the palace who had not heard it before. "Take a seat and I'll tell you."

"This Akyaamah, as you call her, Kwame's natural mother, was the Asantehemaa in the reign of Kusi Obodum. His successor, our present King, Osei Kwadwo, came to find her occupying the Asantehemaa's stool. I wasn't here at the time but I have heard from others who were that, from the very beginning, Akyaamah and Osei Kwadwo didn't get on. Some say that Akyaamah had advised Kusi Obodum that Osei Kwadwo should be executed for dallying with his uncle's wives and that Osei Kwadwo never forgave her. You know about that?"

Ama nodded.

"Akyaamah's husband, and father of our young Kwame, was Safo Katanka, who was then the King of Mampon. While he was alive, Safo Katanka managed to keep some sort of peace between his wife and Osei Kwadwo, but he was already an old man and after three years he died.

"Soon after Safo Katanka's death, matters came to a head between the King and the Queen Mother. The woman started to rebuke him openly at Court. Now the Queen Mother has that right. Indeed she is the only person who may do that. However it seems she did it in such a nasty way and so relentlessly that Osei Kwadwo was publicly humiliated. They say that she threatened that if he refused to raise an army to attack the Fanti, she would do so herself.

"Nana Asantehene made a last attempt to resolve their differences. He invited Akyaamah to a private meeting. Only their personal slaves attended them, no one else; not even their closest advisers were present. Even at that meeting she insulted him. She called him a small boy; she told him he wasn't fit to sit on Osei Tutu's stool; she branded him a coward. Osei Kwadwo tried to keep his calm. He told her that the blood of both Osei Tutu and Opoku Ware ran in his veins and that she should not take his revered grandfather's name in vain. He told her that he was the Asantehene, not she and that by her behaviour she was undermining the authority of the Golden Stool. He told her that war was the business of men, not women. 'It is the business of a woman to sell garden eggs, not gunpowder,' he told her.

"Akyaamah persisted with her insults. Osei Kwadwo became angry. He told her that he would no longer tolerate her abuse. He said that she wasn't fit to be Asantehemaa. She called him stupid and ignorant. She threatened to start destoolment proceedings against him on the grounds of his adultery with the wives of his late uncle Kusi Obodum. He replied that she had lost her senses, that she was mad. That infuriated her. In a fit of uncontrollable anger she slapped his face.

"Now in our custom, the Asantehemaa is supposed to be the mother of the nation. She has the right to say practically anything to the King. But that privilege does not extend to inflicting violence upon the King's person. It is unheard of for anyone to slap the Asantehene, just as it is unheard of for him to beat any subject."

"So what did he do?"

"What could he do? He had no alternative. He called in the guards and had her placed under close arrest. Then he sent for Nana Asumgyina Penemo, Safo Katanka's successor as Mamponhene, who happened to be Konadu Yaadom's father and Akyaamah's step-father. They agreed that the matter should be hushed up. Akyaamah was sent into exile in Mampon and there she has remained since. The two slaves who were present were executed."

"The slaves were executed? For what?"

"For having been present. They had seen and heard too much. It was not proper for the story of such events to be told by slaves."

"Not proper!? And was it proper to kill the slaves on such flimsy grounds?"

"Ama, calm down. I am telling you the story as it happened. I didn't say they did right."

Ama shook her head from side to side in disbelief. She massaged her arms as if that would in some way assuage her anguish.

"What a country! Those slaves who were executed could have been me, or you. What a travesty of justice! What mindless cruelty!"

With a note of urgency in her voice, Esi said, "Ama. My sister. Get a grip on yourself. If you want to survive in this place, you have to learn to control your emotions. Remember that slaves have few rights and that the Asantehene is not only the King but also the highest judge in the land.

"Please, I beg you, remember too that you have never heard the story I have just told you. By order of the Asantehene all reference to Akyaamah has been expunged from the history of the Golden Stool. It is a capital offence to speak of her."

"But then how is that you know exactly what happened?"

"Every one knows the story and at the same time no one knows it. It is difficult, perhaps impossible, to keep anything a secret in this palace. But if you want to survive, particularly if you are a slave, or a pawn like me, you must learn to exercise the greatest discretion in choosing whom you speak to and what you say. Do you understand?"

"That's what Mensa told me," Ama mused.

"So what happened to Kwame Panin?" she asked.

"They took him away from Akyaamah, him and his elder sister, Amma Sewaa, and gave them to Nana Konadu. I guess that Nana Osei Kwadwo made that a condition for recognising Akyaamah's son as his successor. Anyway they are all family: Akyaamah and Konadu Yaadom are both his nieces."

"Do they know all this? Do they talk about it?"

"Who? Kwame and Amma Sewaa? I have never heard either of them talk about it. They treat Nana Konadu as if she were their natural mother. Perhaps they have been warned that if they take Akyaamah's part they will be denied the succession."

"I will ask them," said Ama with a mischievous glint in her eye.

"You will stir up a hornet's nest and the wasps will sting you to death if you do," said Esi.

*****

Ama dreamed. She stood beside a deep pit. Red-shirted dwarfs ran towards her, each bearing a basket on his head.

As each dwarf reached her he tipped the contents of his basket onto a bloody heap of severed human heads. Ama's job was to throw the heads into the pit. The Chief Executioner stood by, bare-chested, displaying his muscles and cracking his whip. Ama worked faster and faster but the pile continued to grow.

The scene changed. Before her lay another pit, shallower, but much larger. It was full of naked bodies. They were dead, but they continued to writhe like snakes in a sea of blood. The royal procession approached, led by the King under his umbrella. Drums beat and horns screeched.

"Yes, that is the one," said the King, pointing at her.

The Chief Executioner grabbed her suddenly from behind, one arm round her waist, the other hand in her crotch. The horns blared out again as he propelled her up into the air, in a great, arcing slow-motion trajectory which would take her into the pit. She screamed.

Ama awoke, drenched in sweat, with the sound of her scream still on her lips.

She was awake, but the horns were still screeching. She was sure she was awake. She could not still be dreaming. Here was Esi snoring beside her. Ama shook her friend.

"What's the matter?" asked Esi sleepily.

"The horns," said Ama.

"The horns? Have you never heard them before? Just the King's horns. They play every night at about this time. They are saying,

'King Osei thanks all officers and men,

'Of his government

'And of his army.

'He thanks all his people

'And wishes them a peaceful night.'

"Now go back to sleep."

CHAPTER 10

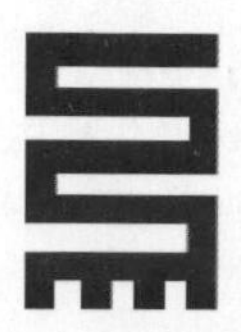

Osei Kwadwo was dying of cancer.

Okomfo Tantani, priest and servant of the river god Tano, tried his whole gamut of cures. None had any persistent effect upon the King's condition. At last the priest called for a white ram and a white ewe from the King's flocks. Konadu Yaadom contributed a white cockerel. The priest slit the throats of all three and daubed their blood on the door posts and window frames of the King's bedroom, on the royal bed and on the solid gold foot stool which a predecessor in royal office had acquired from the vanquished King of Denkyira. When these measures, too, failed to drive off the malignant spirits which were troubling the King, Tantani succeeded in persuading his patient that he was the victim of human malevolence in the person of one of his discarded wives. Only by allowing the Okomfo to discover the individual responsible, could Osei Kwadwo hope to return to good health.

The eunuch who managed the Street of Old Wives co-operated by preparing a short list of his most troublesome charges. Six old women were paraded before the ailing King. They were all his wives but he could recall neither their names nor their faces.

An ordeal by poison and the death of the unfortunate victims had no effect upon the health of Osei Kwadwo, whose condition continued to deteriorate.

The State Councillors went into caucus with the Queen Mother. It was decided, as a desperate last measure, to call in the Kramos, the Muslims. Sharif Imhammed welcomed this opportunity to demonstrate the superiority of the occult powers of Islamic prayer, over those of animist superstition. In anticipation of this invitation, for which his small community had lobbied vigorously, he had delayed his departure on his long return journey to Fezzan. Or so he persuaded himself. Truth was that no foreign visitor was permitted to leave the Asante capital without the say-so of the King and the King was in no condition to deal with such administrative matters. Until the King recovered or until he died and his successor was lowered three times onto the Golden Stool, Sharif Imhammed would remain a virtual prisoner in Kumase.

*****

"Esiii, Amaaa, where are you two? Come here at once."

Konadu Yaadom rushed into her courtyard in a state of all too evident consternation. Esi and Ama dropped the yams they were peeling, wiped their hands and came running to meet her.

"Where is Opoku Fofie? What have you done with my baby?"

Esi considered replying, *We have eaten him, you bitch*, but she said only, "Please, Nana, he is sleeping."

"Put his things together and bring him. Both of you. I may not be able to come back here tonight and I shall have to feed him there when he wakes up. Do you understand?"

Esi and Ama exchanged a nervous glance.

"Yes, Nana," they replied in unison and went to do as they had been told.

The baby grumbled a little as Ama put him on her back and tucked in her cloth, but he soon fell back into a deep sleep.

"Eat-and-sleep, eat-and-sleep," said Esi, giving him a kiss on the cheek. She was fond of him. He was only a baby after all and hadn't yet had time to acquire the royal arrogance which so offended her.

Konadu Yaadom was giving instructions to her other servants. Her first-born and his two small sisters had to be fed and put to bed. It was not easy to be a wife and mother, to manage such a large household of slaves and at the same time to perform her exacting royal duties. The imminent death of Osei Kwadwo placed great responsibilities upon her young shoulders and she was nervous. She wondered what could have happened to Koranten Péte. He should have been back by now. She needed his support. Her new husband, the royal prince Owusu Ansa, was next to useless in such matters. He was probably out drinking while his father lay dying.

She had sent Kwame Panin, the heir apparent, to Mampon for his own safety. She had no illusions: her survival hung entirely upon his. If the Kokofuhene were to succeed in his plans to take the Golden Stool, her fate would be in the balance. She would be lucky to escape with her life as her sister Akyaamah had.

Kwame Panin's elder sister, Amma Sewaa, had gone with him to Mampon, but her aunt had soon recalled the girl. Amma Sewaa was now fourteen. It was more than a year since her menarche and her nubility rites were overdue. A husband had already been selected for her, a son of the late Asantehene Kusi Obodum. More pressing matters, however, had intervened.

"Amma Sewaa, you come with us, too," said Konadu Yaadom.

Amma Sewaa was Konadu Yaadom's most obvious heir as Asantehemaa and it was important that she should be by her aunt's side in these trying times. That was the best way to fit her for her future office.

Konadu Yaadom gave strict instructions to the captain of the guards at the gate. She strengthened her personal bodyguard and then they set off, waiting for the opening of locked gate upon locked gate, until they reached the inner courtyard of the King.

Flaming torches lit every corner of the King's quarters. Courtiers sat in small groups and conversed in low tones. There was a constant flow up and down the stairs to Osei Kwadwo's first floor bedroom. Konadu Yaadom took Amma Sewaa with her to keep watch by the bed of the dying monarch.

Ama looked around. In one corner of the courtyard stood a forked *Onyame-dua*, the tree of God, with its brass bowl of rainwater, God's water, in which resided the King's favoured deities. As she passed it, Konadu Yaadom paused.

She drew aside the red and white cloths which covered the vessel and flicked water over her face. Amma Sewaa followed suit.

In another corner there was a group of Hausas. Amongst them Ama saw, to her surprise, the unmistakable figure of Sharif Imhammed, the same Sharif Imhammed who had accompanied Koranten Péte's party of slaves from Yendi to Kumase. *What*, she wondered, *could he be doing here*? She pointed him out to Esi, who, intrigued by the appearance of this gaunt, bearded stranger, plied Ama with questions about him. But Ama could tell her only that the man was reputed to have come from far across the Great Desert and that he appeared to speak no tongue other than his own. Only the most learned of the local Muslims were able to interpret his dialect of a language which they knew principally from their by-rote study of the Koran.

Ama and Esi talked quietly about their secret plan which, it seemed, they would soon have to implement. The Hausa men were washing their hands and feet, passing from one to another a curious metal vessel with a handle and a spout. When they had finished, they stretched their mats on the ground and arranged themselves in two rows, each with his legs tucked under him. Sharif Imhammed led them in a chant in the same language which Ama had heard them use for prayer before. They had only one god, Damba's mother had told her. They prayed only to him and to one powerful ancestor who was the servant of that god. It was this ancestor, whom they called Mohammed, who conferred on them their many occult skills.

"See how they count their beads," said Esi. "It looks as if they fear that that one will be lost or stolen if they don't keep checking the number."

The men changed their posture, kneeling and touching the ground with their foreheads. Then, after a moment's silent meditation, they had finished their prayers. All this Ama had seen before, though Esi had not. But what came next was new to Ama too. They craned their necks to watch. A young assistant brought Sharif Imhammed a smooth wooden board, about two spans long and one span wide. He laid it on his lap. The assistant put down beside him a small clay pot with a lid. He then produced a long white feather and appeared to slice off the end of the quill at an angle with a sharp knife. Ama and Esi exchanged incredulous stares. Others had moved closer to watch, blocking their view. They rose to join the spectators. On Ama's back, Opoku Fofie whimpered and then went back to sleep. Up in the royal bedchamber, a torch was extinguished. Perhaps the light was disturbing the ailing King.

Sharif Imhammed removed the cover of the clay pot. He dipped the sharpened quill into the pot and then removed it. Then he began to chant in his language. While he did so he held the feather in the space between the thumb and first finger of his right hand and began to scratch the board with it. Ama pushed her head between the shoulders of two of the watching men and strained to see the marks. She could make nothing of the twists and curls. The small crowd began to murmur, but Sharif Imhammed paid no attention, chanting and dipping and scratching. Once he paused and handed the quill to his assistant for sharpening. Then he resumed his chanting and the making of marks until he had covered the board with them. The assistant took the feather and the pot and put them both away.

"It is Kramo magic," said someone.

There was a murmur of awe at the man's secret knowledge; and puzzled anticipation of what was to come.

Esi said, "I fear."

The assistant rose and went to fill the kettle with water. Sharif Imhammed held the board upright within a brass basin and the assistant poured a trickle of water over it. The marks on the board became blurred and indistinct as the black liquid was washed down. The master dampened a clean white handkerchief and wiped and washed the board until all the sanctified ink had passed into the vessel. The assistant emptied the kettle onto the ground. Then he held it as his master poured the liquid from the bowl into it.

"Now I remember. I have seen it before," said the same man who had spoken earlier, "They will make Nana drink that liquid and that, by the grace of the ancestors, will heal him and make him well again."

"Saa?" asked the watchers. "Is that really so?"

"Ampá. Indeed it is," came the reply as Sharif Imhammed and his assistant rose to climb the stairs.

"Intshallah," said the assistant, who had heard and understood.

*****

Konadu Yaadom came down to feed her baby.

Ama watched her mistress as she moved Opoku Fofie from one breast to the other. Suddenly, she felt a longing to have a child of her own, to love and be loved by. But the only father she could have considered for her child was dead. Itsho. She hadn't thought of him for a long time. Had his spirit abandoned her, she wondered. She closed her eyes and concentrated fiercely, trying to summon up a vision of his face.

Opoku Fofie had fallen asleep at his mother's breast.

"Here, take him," she said to Ama. "Try not to wake him when you change his cloth."

She covered herself and rose to her feet. Amma Sewaa made to follow suit.

"No," said the Queen Mother, "stay with Esi and Ama. Try to get some sleep. Tomorrow may be a long day."

They lay down on the mats. The torches flickered fitfully. Even the soldiers on guard dozed.

In the distance the midnight horn players sounded their message to the citizenry.

"I excel all kings in the world," they proclaimed.

"Whilst I live no harm can come.

"I am a mighty king.

"No one dares trouble me."

They had not been informed of their monarch's critical condition.

Time passed.

Suddenly a piercing shriek disturbed the peace of the night. Ama sat up. No one else seemed to have heard.

"Esi, Esi," she whispered, shaking her friend.

Esi turned over. Ama tried again. Esi sat up, immediately wide awake.

"What is it?" she asked.

"I could swear I heard a terrible cry," Ama replied.

They looked up at the bedroom window. Shadows moved. There was a murmur of conversation.

"I don't know what you heard," Esi said, "but I think it's time to go."

The baby lay snuggled up against Amma Sewaa, who slept on. In the courtyard, there were signs of movement. Others had noticed the activity upstairs.

As they slipped out of the gate, they saw torches being lit in the late King's apartment.

"Pity the resident wives," said Esi as they made for the next gate. "They will be the first to go. Do you think they will be crying for the King or for themselves?"

There was someone approaching them across the dark courtyard. Esi drew Ama aside. They waited for the drunken man to lurch past. He was singing to himself.

Ama recognised the voice.

"Nana's husband," she whispered to Esi, "Oheneba Owusu Ansa."

"Blind drunk from the sound of him," said Esi. "And well he may be."

The guard was fumbling with his keys in the dark as they reached the gate.

"Queen Mother's slaves," said Esi. "We have been sent."

"Hurry up then," said the guard, angry at having had his sleep disturbed by the drunken prince.

In the next courtyard they paused and held a whispered conference. They were reluctant to wake the guards and thus leave evidence of their passing, but there seemed to be no alternative. Just as they had come to a decision, there was a banging on the far side of the gate. Still half asleep, a guard demanded identification. It was Koranten Péte. They hung in the shadows as he strode by with his bodyguards. Again, Esi and Ama were allowed to pass before the gate was locked.

The guard on duty at the gate to the Queen Mother's courtyard knew them well. Generally they steered clear of his roving hands, but tonight Esi put her arm around his waist and whispered in his ear.

"You never saw us pass this way. Do you understand?" she demanded.

"What's in it for me?" he asked.

"A bowl of Esi's special fufu and light soup," she replied.

"And what else?" he asked.

She rubbed her body against his for a moment.

"We shall see," she promised.

Pulling herself away, she took Ama's hand. As they passed this last barrier, she called out in a hoarse whisper, "Remember, now: forget you ever saw us."

"Remember your promise," he called back.

*****

There was a small store room under the steep stairway which led up to Konadu Yaadom's bedroom.

Over a period of weeks they had removed the rubbish which had found its way there: cracked pots, an old fufu pestle and a mortar which had split in two. Then they had bribed a carpenter who was repairing a leak in the roof to fix the hinges and install a heavy Hausa latch on the inside of the door. They paid for the latch with some of Esi's savings from the illicit commission which she levied on her market money.

There was no space to stand upright and barely enough to lie down side by side. Inside the tiny room, it was pitch dark and the air was dank and still. They had laid in a stock of water and dry food; but they would have to steal out at dead of night to dispose of their waste. Two small peepholes through a stair riser gave them a narrow view out into the courtyard.

"Nothing to do now but wait. Let's try to get some sleep," whispered Esi.

"How long do you think we'll have to hide?" asked Ama.

*****

The late King's quarters were ablaze with light and activity.

The slaughter started without delay. Two of Osei Kwadwo's 'souls' were decapitated first. Their severed heads, still dripping with blood, were given to a third 'soul'. With one head firmly held in each armpit, this messenger bore the official news from the Chamberlain to the Chief Executioner. The word 'death' was not spoken, for the founder-priest, Okomfo Anokye, had decreed that no one should ever refer directly to the death of any Asantehene. The message was understood without a single word passing.

As soon as the messenger had deposited the two heads in a basket, he laid his neck upon the Chief Executioner's stool. In a moment the heads were three. The headless bodies were dragged away leaving trails of blood. The Chief Executioner, still spattered with his own first victim's blood, went at once to inspect the late King's body. Then he summoned his cohorts to prepare for their work by dancing that fearsome dance which they alone were entitled to perform.

"Tonight, let the knives speak: let no other tongue be heard," they sang.

The male relations, brothers, sons, nephews, gathered in the room of the dead King. Prince Owusu Ansa opened the cupboard where he knew his late father kept his private hoard of imported liquor. They drank quickly to fortify themselves for the task at hand.

"Our father, Nana Osei Kwadwo, is on his way to the next world. The ancestors will know his greatness by the size of the entourage which accompanies him," said Owusu Ansa. "Drink up, collect your weapons and let us get to work."

The Chief Executioner had an escort ready for them. A death drummer, beating his fateful message, led the way out of the palace. A party of sober professional executioners followed the drunken family amateurs. Last came the apprentices bearing empty baskets.

"Wait, let me collect my musket," said the Prince as they came by his wife's courtyard.

Then he had a drunken idea. The two pretty young girls who served his wife and looked after her baby would join his father's escort. Konadu Yaadom might be Queen Mother, but she was also now his wife. He would teach her who was master in the house.

"Esi," he called, "Ama."

He knew their names, though he had never spoken to them.

"Where are you, slaves? Come out and meet your honourable fate! My father must not go on his journey alone!"

Through their peepholes, Esi and Ama could see sword and knife blades glinting in the flickering light of the torches. Both were bathed in sweat and conscious of the rapid beating of their hearts.

The royal prince fired his musket into the air. In spite of herself, Ama cried out. Esi clapped her hand over her companion's mouth.

"Prince, come. Let's get going, there is no one here," someone said.

*****

Back at the royal quarters, Osei Kwadwo's favourite wives were carrying out their last earthly duties, preparing their common consort's body for burial.

They were surrounded by the most senior of the late King's 'souls.' Bound and gagged, their red, white and black faces were turned away from the corpse and the indignities to which it was being subjected.

It was Konadu Yaadom's shriek which had awakened Ama. She had been sitting by Osei Kwadwo's bed, dozing fitfully. She had opened her eyes and seen at once that the King had stopped breathing. She had felt his pulse and then put her ear to his heart. It was then that, against all custom, the involuntary scream had escaped her lips.

"Amma Sewaa," she said, shaking her niece to awaken her. The baby slept on peacefully.

"Where are Esi and Ama?"

Amma Sewaa sat up, rubbed her eyes and looked around.

"Nana, please, I don't know. I was sleeping."

"Give me my boy."

She would keep the baby securely strapped to her own back for the next few hours at least.

Koranten Péte came through the gate.

"Wofa, where were you? I was worried," said Konadu Yaadom.

"I was detained," he said, looking around and observing the activity in the courtyard. "Is it over?"

Konadu Yaadom nodded. Koranten Péte quickly assessed the situation. He thought he discerned the first glimmer in the eastern sky.

"It's too late to bury him before dawn. It will have to be next midnight. Everything is ready. All I need to do is to send Nana Mamponhene a message. I shall do that at once. Atakora's forces will leave Mampon as soon as it is dark. They will be in a secure position on the outskirts of the city before dawn tomorrow. Then let Ntoo Boroko do his worst: we shall be ready for him. Now let me go upstairs and pay my last respects. I am sorry I was not here to bid him farewell."

*****

Osei Kwadwo's male relations had done their customary duty and were returning to the royal quarters.

"Wait," said Owusu Ansa when they came to his wife's courtyard. "This work has tired me out. Let's rest a while."

Ama and Esi peered through their peepholes. Their mistress's husband, like his companions, was smirched with blood. The professional executioners helped their apprentices to take down the loads from their heads. The lads, too, were covered with the blood which had seeped from their baskets. Ama and Esi gripped each other in fear. Every basket they could see was full of severed human heads.

"Wife," they heard Owusu Ansa call, using an address of unusual familiarity. He was pissing against the wall of the courtyard. Konadu Yaadom might be Queen Mother. She might be several years older than he. But he would show everyone that he was her master.

"Wife," he called again, "bring drink for my guests. Their work has made them thirsty."

"Husband," replied Konadu Yaadom, appearing suddenly, "your noble task is not yet complete. Deliver the results of your work. Then bath in your own quarters. When you have slept off the effects of what you have drunk, then, and only then, you may bring me your condolences on the death of our father. And never let me find you pissing against the wall of this courtyard. There is a proper place for that and you well know it."

Owusu Ansa thought better of replying.

"And another thing," she said, "I hope that the heads of my slaves Esi and Ama are not in one of those baskets."

"How can you think to accuse me of such a thing?" he replied sulkily as he led his companions away.

*****

All morning the death drums sounded in Kumase.

Only the executioners, the licensed assassins, roamed the streets, using muskets and swords, clubs and knives to kill whomsoever they found, without discrimination.

The wise had fled the city or had locked themselves securely in their compounds. It was not that they had not loved their late King; it was not that they doubted that he should arrive in the land of the ancestors at the head of large army of servants and retainers; it was just that they were themselves not quite ready to join that army at this time.

No one cooked, for smoke rising from a fire would warrant forcible entry and guarantee summary execution. The adults drank palm wine and chewed kola and the children drank water and cried silently.

In their hideout, Ama and Esi's shit began to smell in the heat of the day. They would have to endure the discomfort at least until after dark but they were nervous that the smell would rise through the stairs and lead Konadu Yaadom to investigate and find them.

"How long do you think we shall have to remain cooped up here?" Ama whispered, not for the first time.

Esi replied sharply, "Now how would I know? But if you want to stay alive, be patient. The worst of the slaughter must be over but we shall not be safe until after the burial. If we are lucky that will be tonight. Now shhh!"

She could hear approaching footsteps.

In the other cities of the confederation, Mampon and Kokofu amongst them, similar events were in progress. Each city was expected to provide a hundred corpses and twenty barrels of gunpowder for the burial and its aftermath.

At Bantama, the royal burial ground, the 'souls' of the dead King were digging his grave, and their own. Their faces and their bare torsos were covered with the lines of white and red clay and charcoal which marked them off as sacrificial victims. By noon the huge hole was ready and the headless corpses began to arrive. They laid them shoulder to shoulder, head to toe, covering the bottom of the hole. The King's corpse must not be allowed to touch the earth. When the bottom was covered they began to build up interlocking walls of corpses, leaving only a space in the centre for the body of their ruler. The executioners guarded the site from foolhardy curious eyes and stood by with whips and swords in case of trouble. But there was none. Ever since Osei Kwadwo had so honoured him, each 'soul' had lived with the certain knowledge that he was destined to accompany his master to the next world.

*****

That night the royal horn blowers did not disturb the deathly silence which hung over the city.

The pallbearers manhandled the pallet with Osei Kwadwo's shrouded body down the narrow stairs. Without a word, lit by a single torch, they carried it to a place in the back wall of the palace where a hole had been cut. They passed the pallet through the hole. A single death drummer led the small cortege. No other sound was heard as they passed through the dark streets and then along the road to Bantama. The Chief Executioner supervised the placing of the royal body in the recess which had been left for it amongst the headless corpses. When dawn broke, there was nothing to be seen but a large mound of earth beneath the sacred Kumnini tree which gave the city its name, and a simple stake to mark the position of the mortal remains of the late king. Some time in the future the next Asantehene would order the exhumation of Osei Kwadwo's skeleton, also at dead of night. It would be taken to the Royal Mausoleum. The bones would be sewn together with gold thread and the assembled skeleton would be installed in a furnished room, supplied with food and drink. Each year the current holder of the office would pay homage to his royal ancestors in a secret ceremony, this way nurturing the bonds which tie the living to the spirits of their dead ancestors and to those of the as-yet-unborn.

*****

When Konadu Yaadom returned shortly before dawn, Esi and Ama had cleaned out their refuge and bathed.

They had hot water on the boil for their mistress's ablutions.

"Where have you two been?" she asked and then continued at once, "Wake Opoku Fofie and bring him to me. While I am feeding him, get my bath ready. And prepare yourselves too. We shall be going out. Now get a move on: I'm in a hurry."

Konadu Yaadom was clearly nervous. She found it difficult to decide how to split the forces at her command. Some must remain at home to guard her children: who could know what mischief Ntoo Boroko and his henchmen might get up to? At the same time she might herself be in great physical danger should the meeting turn nasty.

The Asanteman-hyiamu, the highest assembly of the Asante nation, was already in session when they arrived. Konadu Yaadom noticed the gross discourtesy done her by starting the meeting in her absence. At least, she thought, they had left a seat for her.

"Ama and Esi, go and sit where I can keep my eye on you. You, guards, keep close by, in case I need you. Amma Sewaa, bring a stool and sit just behind me. Listen well to what is said. Today history will be made."

Ntoo Boroko was in full flight. As Konadu Yaadom took her seat he paused briefly and grudgingly acknowledged her arrival. Then he proceeded. He was setting out his view of Asante law.

Carefully disguising her unease, Konadu Yaadom looked around for Koranten Péte.

Ntoo Boroko drew attention to the absence of some person whose name had been expunged from the nation's history.

"He is talking about Akyaamah," Esi whispered.

It was Ntoo Boroko's considered opinion that the offence that person had committed automatically debarred her children from any right to the succession.

Koranten Péte crept up behind Konadu Yaadom and whispered in her ear.

"Everything is in order. The Mamponhene will be here any moment now," he told her.

"I have heard," she replied.

"This debarment," Ntoo Boroko was saying, "must include all descendants of the mother of the person whose name we may not . . ."

He paused without completing his sentence. Atakora Mensah, with the young Kwame Panin by his side, was leading in the ranks of his heavily armed Bron striking force. Immediately behind the Mamponhene, strode the tallest man Ama had ever seen.

"Konkonti," Esi nudged Ama. "See his insignia: the Chief Executioner of Mampon."

Ntoo Boroko retired to his seat without a word. Atakora Mensah, satisfied with the disposition of his forces, put his arm around Kwame Panin's shoulder and led him to the centre of the Council. The Mamponhene's seat was waiting for him and another was hurriedly provided for Kwame Panin. The man and the boy sat down without a word.

"Hasn't he grown?" whispered Amma Sewaa into Konadu Yaadom's ear. "He looks like a man."

"Hush," replied her aunt, secretly amused and pleased by her niece's pride in her brother.

"He looks just like a man," Ama whispered to Esi, "so handsome in his kente and sandals. And so haughty!"

Ntoo Boroko was bamboozled. He had been outflanked.

"Nana Bremanhene . . . " said Atakora Mensah quietly, indicating with a wave of his hand that his adversary should continue his speech.

Ntoo Boroko decided that his only course of action was to brazen it out and mobilise, by skilful oratory, the support in the Council which he had long been so assiduously courting.

"Nananom, my fellow Kings and Queen Mothers," he said, "this is unheard of. It seems that we are faced with a coup d'etat. Any decisions we make in the presence of these forces will be made under duress. I propose that we suspend immediately our discussion on the selection of the successor to our dearly beloved Osei Kwadwo. I propose that we discuss instead this invasion of our constitutional rights by Nana Mamponhene."

Atakora Mensah sprang to his feet.

"Nananom," he said, "we deeply mourn the passing of our revered and beloved Osei Kwadwo. By law and custom established since the time of Nana Osei Tutu and Okomfo Anokye of blessed memory, responsibility for the designation of the successor to Nana Osei Kwadwo lies with our beloved Asantehemaa Nana Konadu Yaadom. It is for us only to approve or dispute her nomination. The Asantehemaa has authorised me to announce that she nominates her son Kwame Panin as the next occupant of the Golden Stool. I propose that her nomination receive our unanimous approval."

Konadu Yaadom sat impassively. She would intervene if she had to, but for the present she chose to permit the Mamponhene to act as her spokesman.

Before Atakora Mensah had finished, Ntoo Boroko was on his feet shouting, "I protest, I protest . . . "

Ama did not fully understand the cause of the excitement but she could feel the tension in the air. She saw the Mamponhene make an almost imperceptible signal. Searching for its target, Ama saw Konkonti, the tall Chief Executioner of Mampon, dart away behind the seated Councillors. As she watched him, he came up behind Ntoo Boroko, immobilised his victim's arms with his own left arm and with his right hand drew a sharp knife across the Bremanhene's throat. There was a sudden spurt of crimson blood. Ama clutched Esi in alarm and muffled a scream. Then she covered her eyes with her hands.

Esi's attention had been diverted by the baby Opoku Fofie and she had not witnessed the assassination. She looked up in time to see Konkonti release his victim. Ntoo Boroko's partly severed head fell backwards as his body fell forwards. As the body hit the ground the head bounced forward again. Then she heard the sound of retching. Ama was down on her knees and Esi went to her. A man tripped over her foot and almost fell. He swore at her as he rushed away. She thought she recognised the Kokofuhene, Kyei Kwame, preferred candidate of the assassinated Ntoo Boroko.

For a moment there was utter silence in the assembly; then uproar. In the confusion, Konkonti's assistants dragged away the corpse of their master's victim. Konadu Yaadom sat immobile, dumbfounded by the murder which had taken place not a stride away from where she sat. This was not what she had intended, not what she had discussed with Koranten Péte. She would have to take charge of the situation. That was her constitutional duty. But how?

Koranten Péte saved the day for her. He strode across and took Kwame Panin by the hand. The boy was confused, uncertain what he should do.

"Wofa?" he queried Koranten Péte. His voice was breaking.

"Kwame," said the boy's hero, "just do exactly what I say. Now stand here by your mother. Keep cool. Show a straight face, as if nothing has happened."

"Nana," he said to Konadu Yaadom, "you must act at once. Otherwise things might get out of hand."

"Yes, but how?" she asked him.

"Disassociate yourself from this cold-blooded murder. State your determination that whosoever proves to be responsible, not only the one who carried out the act, but also whoever gave him his orders, will face the full force of Asante law. Say that the confederacy is in danger. Tell them that the only way to avoid widespread fratricidal strife is to elect Kwame Panin as Asantehene immediately. Demand a vote at once. When you win, and you cannot lose, insist that the Golden Stool be brought out and that Kwame be enstooled without further delay. Do all this in the name of Osei Tutu, Opoku Ware, Kusi Obodum and Osei Kwadwo."

He turned to Kwame.

"My boy," he said, "it is time for you to become a man. Are you ready? Then stand by your mother as she speaks. Stand straight and tall. Remember all you have been taught. You are about to be called to a great office."

CHAPTER 11

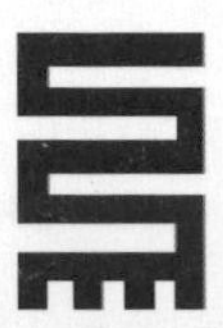

Pity the adolescent King! Kwame Panin was plain Kwame no more.

Even his aunt, Konadu Yaadom, whom Osei Kwadwo's royal edict had made his mother, could no longer address him as 'Kwame', at least not in public. Now he was Nana Osei Kwame, fifth Asantehene, successor of four illustrious forebears, whose feats in war and peace he was bound by duty and tradition to emulate. He was no longer free to wrestle and tumble and roam the palace with his cronies; to speak his mind to commoners and slaves; to jest with fools; to throw a tantrum.

He strained at the leash, impatient at the restrictions placed upon the freedoms he had so recently enjoyed. He was bored by the lessons in history, language and custom, law and public administration which aged men with grey stubbly beards imparted to him each day in Osei Kwadwo's old quarters. They taught him that as ruler of the Asante empire he might wage war but yet must never strike another human being; nor must he allow himself to be struck, for that would be an abomination. Neither must he ever walk barefooted, not even in the privacy of his own bedchamber. Like it or not his person was now sacred. He must spend his life in frequent communion with the spirits of Osei Tutu, of Opoku Ware, of Kusi Obodum and of his beloved Osei Kwadwo; and in return the heroic ancestral spirits would guide him in the exercise of the heavy responsibilities he now bore.

He invented a nickname for each of the old fogies who were his teachers: the one who was forever scratching his balls; and the other who picked his nose in public. But now there was no one to share an innocent malicious chuckle with him. He much preferred the Muslim clerics to whom he gave weekly audience. They told him gripping stories from their Holy Book and the Tales of a Thousand and One Nights, preparing the ground for ambitious future projects which they discussed amongst themselves only in whispers.

He appointed Koranten Péte to act as chairman of the Regency Council. This was one man he could admire and respect, a welcome substitute for his natural father, Mamponhene Safo Kantanka, whom he had hardly known. Koranten Péte called on him every day to brief him fully on the affairs of state and the decisions which had been taken in his name. He heard in this way of the removal of his erstwhile sponsor, Atakora Mensah, from the stool of Mampon and learned that at times high office demands the renunciation of such qualities as loyalty and gratitude, prized by men of humbler origin.

He was eager to prove himself in war. Koranten Péte had great difficulty in persuading him that he was not yet ready to lead his forces in person. On his Regent's advice he appointed Osei Kwadwo's young protégé, Opoku Frede-Frede, Opoku the Swift, to lead an Asante force which he sent to chastise the Asens for their impudent rebellion against his ailing predecessor. He celebrated Opoku's resounding victory with generous gifts and a lavish public celebration over which he presided in person.

Koranten Péte and Konadu Yaadom advised him to court popularity amongst the common people as a counterweight to the schemes of ambitious enemies who might seek to take advantage of his youth. So he decreed that only convicted criminals would henceforth be killed at public executions; and that only once a year, on the occasion of the Great Adae.

For a while he shunned female company. He hardly noticed Esi and Ama, who had helped to raise him and had sometimes joined his boisterous childhood games. When he did deign to acknowledge their respectful greetings, he did so with haughty indifference. He stopped bullying his elder sister Amma Sewaa and now ignored her completely. He kept his distance, too, from Konadu Yaadom. The Queen Mother was the only person with the constitutional right to scold him in public, and although she wisely held this privilege in reserve, he feared her zeal and her acid tongue.

He continued to live in Konadu Yaadom's quarters but he now had a bedroom of his own.

It was one of Esi's duties to tidy his room each day, but whenever she was menstruating, Ama took over this task. Esi generally waited until he had left the courtyard before she entered his room, so that he hardly knew who it was that cleaned up the mess he often left in his wake.

One day Ama, it being her turn and thinking him absent, entered Osei Kwame's bedroom, humming to herself, thinking of her little brother Nowu and how big he must now be. She was already halfway across the room when she realised that Osei Kwame was there. He was lying on his bed, face down, and sobbing. Ama stopped dead in her tracks. Becoming aware of a presence in his room, Osei Kwame turned. Before she averted her eyes, Ama saw the tear stains on his cheeks.

"What do you want," he snapped at her.

She fell to her knees.

"Please, Nana, I didn't know Nana was here. I only came to tidy Nana's room."

He stared at her but said nothing so she rose and started to back out of the room.

"Wait," he said.

Then, "Latch the door."

She was not sure if she had heard right.

"Latch the door, I said."

He was sitting on the edge of the bed.

"Come," he said.

She approached him slowly, hardly knowing what to expect, until she stood before him.

He wiped his eyes. Then he looked up at her. Ama wondered if it were not improper for the King to be raising his eyes to a slave and whether she should not perhaps sink to her knees before him. But this was only Kwame Panin, whom she had known as a boy, who had patiently taught her the rules of *oware*. And he was still a boy, she saw.

"Ama," he said, "Ama."

And then the flood burst. Sobbing uncontrollably, he sank his face into her breast. Suddenly she remembered Suba and how they had cried together after he had helped her to bury Itsho. She held the boy's head to her and caressed him.

"I don't want to be Asantehene," he said through the sobs.

"There now, don't talk," she said, holding him tight and comforting him, though unsure how she should address him.

After a while the sobbing subsided. He kept holding her though, his head between her breasts, afraid to show his face. Then she became aware of the pressure of his erect penis. All of a sudden her mind was in a turmoil. She was consumed by a deep, almost maternal, compassion for the boy. She was sure he had never before been with a woman. Then she struggled to impose her will upon her own rising desire. What would be the consequences? Was she condemning herself to a wasted life in the royal harems like the old women she had heard talk of? What if Konadu Yaadom or Koranten Péte should come to the door?

Itsho. She tried desperately to conjure up Itsho's presence, but he did not respond.

Since Abdulai had raped her, she had never felt any desire for a man. Now she was overwhelmed. She pushed him gently from her.

"Lie down," she said.

She pulled his cloth away from under him. He lay naked; she was aware of his rigid organ, but, knowing that he would be shy, she did not look at it. Instead she stroked his cheek with the back of her hand and looked straight into his eyes. He returned her look, his mind confused by strange emotions. She let her cloth drop to the floor and unfastened her beads. Then she climbed onto the bed and, taking him in her hand, lowered herself onto him.

She played him like a *sanko*. She let him move a while and then she pinned him down, holding him immobile.

"Ama, Ama," he begged her.

When she felt he could hold it no more, she held him tight to her and rolled them both over so that he could ride her to the finish like a man.

When they had rested, he said, "Ama, you will be my first wife."

"No, Nana, no," she replied, suddenly terrified at what she had done.

"Why 'no'?" he asked. "I will command you. It is my right."

"Nana," she said, "I beg you. I will make love to you whenever you desire it, but please do not force me to be your wife."

"You should be honoured," he said, sulking, "It is not every woman who gets to marry the King of Asante."

She looked at him, wondering whether she might risk a cheeky reply.

"Only three thousand, three hundred and thirty three," she said.

"Oh, that's what it is, is it? Anyway, there is no hurry."

She rose.

"Nana," she said, "I must go. My absence will be noticed. Nana Asantehemaa will be calling for me."

He pulled her back and put his moist lips to a nipple. She saw another erection coming and pulled away.

"Where did you learn that?" she said and then, "Not now. Keep it for another time."

"When?" he said. "Tonight?"

"No," Ama replied, "I will tell you when."

She went out and busied herself in the courtyard. Soon he followed and called his personal bodyguard. He paid no attention to her but she noticed a new jauntiness in his step as he passed through the gate.

*****

Osei Kwame soon found an excuse to quarrel with Esi.

He demanded that she should no longer clean his room. Ama alone was now to do so and she was to do so only in his presence, before he left for his classes each morning. She was to report to him every day at dawn.

The boy's lust for Ama was insatiable. Sometimes he would have her twice in quick succession, before he took his breakfast. He was barely willing to abstain during her periods. She could only hold him off by threatening him with the wrath of his ancestors for breaking the customary taboo.

And then he would pester her every day: "Haven't you stopped bleeding yet?"

It was only his fear of Konadu Yaadom's anger and unpredictable response that dissuaded him from boasting about their relationship.

Ama cursed herself for falling into a trap of her own making. She seemed destined either to life-long imprisonment as a rejected royal wife or to early execution for her temerity in introducing the young King to the mysteries of sex without the prior permission of the Queen Mother. She had no illusions about the boy's fidelity to her. Once the novelty had worn off, he would look around for a substitute or substitutes. On the other hand if Konadu Yaadom were to get wind of what was going on, she would have no compunction about handing her over to the Chief Executioner. She could see no way out, except a desperate attempt to escape from Kumase, an attempt that she knew was doomed to failure.

Ama found it difficult to fall asleep at night and when she did, she was disturbed by frequent nightmares. She could no longer concentrate on her work. Esi sometimes found her crying, but Ama refused to take her into her confidence, fearing that, with the best of intentions, her friend would not be able to keep such a secret. Most dangerous, she found that she most often had to feign pleasure for Osei Kwame. If he should begin to suspect, that would be the end of her.

Then, one day in the market, she caught sight of Minjendo. They ran to meet, fell about each others' necks and cried.

"Minjendo," said Ama, "I had given up hope of ever seeing you again; and now you tell me that you have been working in a house I pass each time I am sent to the market."

"Nandzi," said Minjendo, "how are you? Tell me everything, everything that has happened since we were parted."

They found a quiet spot and Ama began. In the joy of speaking in her own mother tongue, her resolution failed. She felt she would go mad if she could not tell her troubles to someone. When she came to talk of her relationship with Osei

Kwame, Minjendo's eyes opened wider and wider in astonishment.

"You mean the King, the Asantehene himself?"

Ama nodded ruefully. Then she went on to talk about her fears, her insomnia, her nightmares.

"It sounds to me as if a spirit of the bush is afflicting you," said Minjendo.

Ama looked at her. She had heard talk of Benekpib, spirits of the bush, evil ghosts of criminals, or of those who had not been buried with the proper ceremonies which would guarantee their spirits entry into the domains of the ancestors. The Benekpib, she knew, selected one poor person to persecute. Sometimes, they would harry their victim until he died. The only escape was treatment by a skilled diviner, who would capture the errant spirit, tame it and force it into the service of its former victim.

"There is a diviner, one of our own people, in our house. He is called Dzimwa. He might be able to help you. He works in the kitchen. I am sure he could find the time. Would you like me to speak to him?"

*****

"I have thought deeply and at length about your case," the diviner told her. "I do not believe that the ancestors are punishing you for failing to observe our customs. The ancestors are aware that we are no longer our own masters. And I do not believe that it is some unattached malevolent spirit of the bush which is attacking you. No, I believe that the key to your problem lies with the spirit of Itsho. Spirits are not that different from us. After all they were once also human beings. Indeed some sages say that they are destined to become human again in another form. They like us to make a fuss over them. It is clear from what you have told me that in the months immediately after Itsho's death, his spirit was watching over you intently. I suspect that since then you have neglected to speak to him regularly and to give him food and drink. So he feels abandoned and as a result he has withdrawn his protection from you. Does that sound plausible?"

Ama pondered.

"Sometimes I try to speak to him, but he doesn't hear me," she said.

"I will teach you how to reach out to him and what to say to him. It will not be easy and you must not expect immediate results. He may wish to test your patience and dedication. Are you prepared to try?"

Ama nodded.

"Then next time you come you must bring me a white cockerel. I know that, like me, you are only a poor slave without resources, but I also know that you will find some way, because this is important to you."

*****

"Ama," said Konadu Yaadom, "I am going on a trip.

The baby will come with me and you will come too, to look after him. Esi, you will stay behind to keep an eye on the older children."

"Please, Nana, what of Nana Asantehene's room? " asked Ama.

"Nana Asantehene will just have to make his peace with Esi," replied the Queen Mother.

"Please, Nana, when do we leave?"

"Tomorrow at dawn," replied Konadu Yaadom.

Ama thought, *I'll be glad to get away. I hope the boy won't take it too badly. Perhaps he will find some one else in my absence.*

Maybe Esi, she speculated and smiled to herself.

To Esi she said, "Where do you think we are going?"

"You are going, my dear sister," replied Esi, who, unobserved, had been watching Ama's reaction to the news, "you are going on the great annual inspection of Nana Asantehemaa's kola estates and gold mines."

*****

Each village vied to outdo its neighbours in welcoming the Asantehemaa; so their progress was slow.

While Konadu Yaadom sat patiently listening to the views of the elders, Ama would wander around with Opoku Fofie on her back. He was growing quickly and was now quite heavy. Soon it would be time to wean him. Then Konadu Yaadom would allow her new husband, Owusu Ansa, into her bed and then she would become pregnant again. Ama wondered why she had never become pregnant, not with the seed of Itsho, nor that of the rapists Abdulai and Akwasi Anoma, nor, most surprisingly, with the child of Osei Kwame. Perhaps she was barren. Or perhaps Itsho was preventing her from conceiving.

"Do you see why we have to have slaves?" Konadu Yaadom asked Ama as they made their way out of Konadu-krom. "You people of the north like kola too much and we Asante are the only ones who have it. It takes much labour to collect it and send it to Kafaba. Since there are not enough native born Asante to do this work, we need slaves. It is the same with gold mining, as you will soon see. That is why we have to bring your people to help us. We treat you well. No man will point at your children and call them the children of a slave. In just one generation, you will all be Asante yourselves. As for you, Ama, you already speak our language like a native. When we get back to Kumase I shall start looking for a good Asante husband for you. Then you will marry and have children and your children will be Asante."

Ama looked up at Konadu Yaadom, sitting in relative comfort in her hammock. The Queen Mother was in a good mood. Ama considered exposing the flaws in her argument. No, that would not do. She knew her mistress too well to trust her. She was too proud, too arrogant, too fixed in her way of thinking, too intolerant of the views of anyone not of her own station, to listen to the opinions of a slave.

So she dissembled and replied, "Yes, Nana. Thank you Nana. Nana is very kind."

Maybe that would solve her problems, she thought: an Asante husband. But that did not take account of the precocious sexual passion of the Asantehene. Until he tired of her, he would not willingly give her up to another man. And, young as he was, he was the King. There could be nothing but trouble ahead. *The longer this excursion lasts,* she thought, *the better.*

*****

Konadu Yaadom's temporary home was one of the few with walls, though they were only of woven grass matting.

It was divided into four, a bathroom, a reception room, a bedroom for the

Queen Mother and another where Ama slept with the baby.

One day Ama was feeding Opoku Fofie a fine pulp which she had mashed from the food in her own bowl. He was a slow eater, but Ama had plenty of time. It had been her job to wean Nowu, so she was not without experience.

It was midday. Konadu Yaadom had spent the morning on an inspection of some distant mine workings. She was unused to walking long distances and had returned exhausted and soon fallen asleep in the next room, on the other side of a wall of matting.

Ama heard a whispered conversation outside but she could not make out the words.

Then a male voice called out, "Àgòo!"

Ama thought she recognised the voice but before she could react, Konadu Yaadom replied irritably, "Who is it?"

"Please Nana, my name is Mensa. Nana Koranten Péte has sent me with a message."

The baby had fallen asleep. Ama laid him down on the mat and then lay down beside him. There was nothing for her to do until Opoku Fofie woke up. She could hear the sounds of Konadu Yaadom preparing to receive the messenger in the next room. Nana would call her if she was needed. She wondered idly what could have brought the musketeer. Her eyelids were heavy. She was about to doze off.

"You may enter," Ama heard Konadu Yaadom call.

She heard Mensa make the customary greetings.

"Nana there is no bad news. Nana Asantehene is well. Nana's children are all well. No one has died. No one is ill. None of the tributary states has rebelled. There is peace in all the land," said Mensa.

"Nana Koranten Péte has not sent you all this way to tell me this," replied Konadu Yaadom.

If he had come straight to the point she would have been outraged at his crassness; yet she was impatient with the niceties of custom.

"Nana is right," said Mensa, "I have learned Nana Koranten Péte's message by heart and with Nana's permission I will now recite it."

Konadu Yaadom must have nodded, for he continued, "Firstly I am to convey to Nana, Nana Koranten Péte's respectful greetings. Secondly I am to say that Nana Koranten Péte has received certain intelligence that makes it essential that Nana return to Kumase with the utmost haste."

Ama pricked up her ears. She raised herself on one elbow, no longer drowsy. Suddenly it struck her that the Queen Mother was almost certainly unaware of her presence. It was too late now to slip away: she would be heard. She decided that it would be best to feign sleep.

"Thirdly," continued Mensa, "I am to say that the details of the matter are so confidential, that they cannot be entrusted to any messenger. Fourthly, Nana is respectfully requested to advise Nana Koranten Péte of her approach to Kumase so that he can meet Nana and brief Nana fully concerning the matter, before Nana enters the city. Fifthly, Nana is respectfully requested to ensure that the slave girl, Ama, returns with Nana."

In spite of the heat, Ama felt suddenly cold when she heard her name. *What can all this mean?* she wondered. She had done nothing wrong. She shivered.

Could it be . . . Osei Kwame? She dismissed the thought. No one knew of their relationship except Minjendo and Dzimwa. Both were aware of the seriousness of her predicament. She felt sure that neither would have betrayed her secret.

"Finally," concluded Mensa, "I was instructed to make sure that this message should fall on no one's ears but Nana's."

Ama's heart was pounding. She lay down, taking care to make no sound. She screwed up her eyes, willing herself to fall asleep.

"I have heard," replied Konadu Yaadom. "Is that all you know? You have no idea of the meaning of the message?"

"Nana, please, that is all I know."

"Repeat your message, then. Say it slowly, one sentence at a time."

Mensa repeated the message, using precisely the same words. Koranten Péte had put his faith in him, Mensa knew. Success in this mission, he knew too, would be generously rewarded: he had been told as much. On the other hand, he had no illusions: if he got one word wrong, he might well be handed over to the Chief Executioner.

"How long did it take you to get here?" asked Konadu Yaadom when he had finished.

"Please, Nana, three days. Nana, I beg your pardon, three and a half days, including today. I ran all the way."

"You will rest this afternoon and tonight. Have you eaten?"

"Please, Nana, not since last night," replied Mensa.

"Amaaa!" called Konadu Yaadom.

In his sleep, Opoku Fofie, heard his mother's voice and whimpered. Ama's heart pounded even faster. She said nothing and kept her eyes shut.

"Where is that girl?" she heard the Queen Mother mutter.

Then she heard the sound of the matting being pushed aside.

"Ama," said Konadu Yaadom sharply, shaking her shoulder.

"Nana?" asked Ama, rubbing her eyes, acting as if she had suddenly awoken from a deep sleep.

"Sleeping? At this time of the day? Have you no work to do? Didn't you hear the messenger come in?"

"Please, Nana. I beg you. I fed the baby and then I just fell asleep."

"This is . . . what did you say your name was? Yes, Mensa. See that he gets something to eat. And then find him somewhere to sleep tonight. He will be returning to Kumase before dawn tomorrow. Give him some food to take with him. Understood?"

Ama's heart skipped a beat. Her subterfuge had succeeded. She took care not to look at Mensa.

"Please, Nana, yes," she replied humbly.

"And, Ama. Get everything ready. We shall also be leaving early tomorrow."

*****

"Ama," said Mensa, as she served him, "How are you?"

"Please, sir, I am fine," she replied meekly.

"Are you sure? What have you been up to?"

"Up to? What do you mean?"

He gripped her lower arm and held it tight while he spoke.

"Promise to forget at once that I ever told you this."

"Told me what? You are talking in riddles."

"What I am going to tell you now. But first you must promise."

"If you say so. I promise."

He relaxed his grip and looked around to make sure that no one was within hearing distance. He looked her in the eye. She dropped her gaze, apprehensive, wondering what this was all about.

"Ama. I have no idea what mischief you have been up to, but I must warn you: you are in deep trouble. That is all I know. Now forget that I ever told you this. You promised, remember?"

She nodded.

"Now bring me another bowl of palm wine. Or rather bring me the whole calabash. I will serve myself. I am thirsty. This afternoon I am going to get drunk."

*****

Ama pushed her way through the undergrowth at the edge of the settlement.

Soon she was inside the high forest and she could move more easily. She stopped and looked back through the dim light to make sure she had not been followed.

"Ama," she told herself, "take your bearings. You have not come here to spend the night with the forest dwarfs."

The sound of distant voices drifted up from the mine camp. All else was still and silent. She moved on and the dry leaves crackled under her bare feet. Around her the trunks of great trees rose up towards the dark green canopy above. She dropped down between two buttresses of a silk cotton tree and tried to think. The thoughts refused to come. Her mind was a confusion of fear and misery. She lay on her back and looked up. The sun was overhead. Its light fell on the roof of the canopy and was absorbed. Dust particles danced in a beam of light. She closed her eyes and tried to think.

When she awoke, the sun had sunk towards the horizon. For a moment she panicked: Opoku Fofie might have woken in her absence. Then she remembered: Konadu Yaadom had said she would look after him this afternoon while Ama made preparations for the journey back to Kumase.

She sat on her knees, her back upright. Taking up the small calabash of palm wine which she had brought with her, she spoke aloud.

"Itsho. Spirit of my dearly beloved Itsho. It is I, Nandzi, whom they now call Ama. Itsho, you gave your life trying to save mine. Itsho, if you are there in the world of the spirits, hear me, I beg you. Dzimwa says I have been neglecting to bring you food and drink. He is right. I beg your forgiveness. Only, it is difficult. I have nothing of my own. Even this palm wine which I bring you now, I had to steal.

"Itsho, I am in trouble. I know it is so. What Mensa told me has only confirmed it. I know it is my fault. I should never have started this thing with the boy. But I was tempted. I pitied him. I had no intention. He is just a boy. It is true that I am fond of him, but I cannot love him, even though he is the King. My love is reserved for you, Itsho. All my life I will never forget you."

She saw him. For the first time in many months she saw his face. He was smiling; there was laughter in his eyes. Ama began to sob. She sobbed with joy.

"Oh, Itsho. You have heard me. I knew you would not forsake me. You know everything. I know you will help me in my trouble. Tell me what to do."

She wiped the tears from her eyes and he was gone. But she was at peace now.

*****

Koranten Péte was waiting for them at the first village beyond the city gate.

The bearers lowered Konadu Yaadom's hammock. She stood up and stretched. The Queen Mother and the Regent exchanged greetings. Then they went into the house of the village chief.

Ama played hide and seek with Opoku Fofie, who shrieked with joy when he discovered her behind her fingers. She was calm. The fear of death, of cruel torture, had left her. Whatever was in store for her she knew that Itsho would be by her side.

She had considered trying to escape, but the logistical problems had defeated her. Which way would she go? How would she avoid capture? Where would she get food? Where would she sleep? It would be better, she had decided, just to take things as they came.

She picked the little boy up and swung him gently round and round.

Konadu Yaadom came out of the house. She neither looked at Ama nor spoke to her. She mounted her hammock and the party moved on into the city and to the palace.

*****

Esi was the only person in Konadu Yaadom's courtyard. She took the baby from Ama. The child babbled away at her.

"Esi, I want you to go to the market. Put Opoku Fofie on your back and take him with you."

Konadu Yaadom gave her her instructions.

"Nana, please, shall I go too?" Ama asked.

"No. Stay here," was the abrupt reply.

Ama went to her room. She was washing away the dust of the journey when she heard voices in the courtyard.

"Ama," she heard Konadu Yaadom call.

"Nana, please I am bathing. I will come in a minute," she called back.

The High Sheriff was waiting for her.

"You are called Ama?" he asked her.

"Yes, please," she replied.

"I have orders to search you and your room. Nana, with your permission."

Let them search, thought Ama as she waited. *What could they find amongst our paltry possessions?*

The High Sheriff stood chatting politely to Konadu Yaadom as his men conducted the search.

"What is this all about?" Konadu Yaadom asked him, knowing that Ama would hear.

"Nana, we have information that a quantity of gold has been stolen."

The policemen emerged, one of them triumphantly holding a small leather bag in the air. He gave it to his master, who handed it to Ama.

"Open it," the Chief said to her.

"I have never seen this bag before. It is not mine," protested Ama.

"Open it," he ordered again.

She untied the leather thong.

"Look inside," he told her.

"Please, it is full of gold dust," she said.

"You are under arrest. My orders are to take you straight to the Asantehene's court. You had better take your things with you. You may be away for a long time. Nana, with your permission?"

Konadu Yaadom nodded. Ama tried to catch her eye, but she looked away.

"Do as the man says," was all she said.

*****

The Great Court lay at the end of a broad colonnaded passageway in the innermost depths of the Palace.

It was surrounded on all sides by a gallery of plastered columns with shining ornamented bases.

Koranten Péte, Regent of Asante during the minority of the Asantehene Osei Kwame, sat on a raised platform. His wood and leather armchair was studded with brass and decorated with gold. It was shaded by the multicoloured royal umbrella. The ceremonial gold sword of war hung on the right of the chair, the sword of peace on the left.

Ama was hustled to a corner to await trial. Apart from her guards, no one paid any attention to her.

Koranten Péte was flanked, left and right, by nobles, important officials, generals, linguists, chiefs. Each of these was supported by retainers and each had his own umbrella, surmounted by a different gilded carving: a bird, a lion, a baboon. Before Koranten Péte sat court criers, every one of them deformed or maimed in some way and each wearing a monkey skin cap with a gold plate attached to the front and the tail hanging down behind. They created a constant buzz of noise with their cries of 'Silence in the Court! Pray hear! Be quiet.' Alongside them sat a squad of long-haired, bearded policemen, colleagues of Ama's guards. From time to time they would add to the general hubbub by calling the praises of the young (and absent) King.

A new law was being proclaimed as Ama entered. The Chief Linguist recited it several times, once to each member of the royal family who was present and then to the whole assembly.

"It shall henceforth be illegal for any ambassador or messenger of the King, in any country of the realm, including tributary states, to demand food from the inhabitants, without first offering to pay a fair price."

As the assembly was applauding the sense of justice and fairness of the young King, the Queen Mother entered, with her attendants. All, including the Regent, rose and remained standing until she had taken her seat. Esi, with Opoku Fofie on her back, took up a position within call. Ama waved to her friend, but one of the guards slapped her arm down.

The law was recited again for Konadu Yaadom to hear. There was fresh applause.

Then Ama was brought before Koranten Péte.

"The slave girl, Ama Donko," said the prosecutor, "is accused of stealing a bag of gold dust worth two peredwans, the property of her mistress, our esteemed and beloved Asantehemaa, Nana Konadu Yaadom, who is the owner of the girl. She returned only today from accompanying her mistress on a tour of her gold mines. It is thought that she might have acquired the gold there in return for certain favours to persons unknown. On receipt of information by the High Sheriff, her room was searched and the bag of gold was found."

"Has the accused anything to say in her defence?" asked Koranten Péte.

Ama turned to look at her judge. She looked him straight in the eye. He returned her look without flinching. *He knows I am innocent*, she thought. *He set this thing up this morning with Konadu Yaadom. It has nothing to do with this gold. It is about the boy, Kwame Panin, King Osei Kwame. He knows. That is why he sent Mensa to call Konadu Yaadom back to Kumase.*

For a moment she was tempted to turn her back to him, face the assembly and tell them the truth.

"This case has nothing to do with a bag of gold," she would say. "I am here because I am the lover of your King and because the Regent and the Queen Mother do not approve of our relationship."

She wondered where the boy was, whether he was aware of these proceedings, whether he had done anything to try to save her. *Probably not*, she thought. *Men are such cowards.*

She thought, *if I tell them all the truth, what will I achieve? They will surely find an excuse then to torture me as well as kill me. And the boy might also be made to suffer in some way.*

She was still looking into the depths of Koranten Péte's eyes. *It is you who brought me to Kumase*, she thought, *and now I am an embarrassment to you.*

"I have nothing to say," she replied.

"In that case, since you have stolen the property of Nana Asantehemaa, which is the property of the Asante state, the law requires that I sentence you to death," said Koranten Péte.

"No, no!"

A cry rent the air. It was Esi. She stepped forward. Opoku Fofie started to bawl. Esi stopped as she reached Konadu Yaadom's chair and loosened the cloth which bound the child to her back, allowing him to slip gently onto his mother's lap.

Then she was standing beside Ama.

"It is not possible," she said.

She spoke without waiting for permission, "I know Ama better than I know my own sister. It is impossible that she should steal. If the gold was found in our room, it must have been put there in our absence by some one who wants to be rid of Ama."

Koranten Péte gave a sign to the High Sheriff. One of the police pinned Esi's arms behind her back while another put a gag in her mouth and tied it behind her neck.

"The court is adjourned for a short time," Koranten Péte announced.

He rose and led the way to a private room behind the podium. Konadu Yaadom followed him. So too did the members of the Inner Council, the Minister of War, the Commander-in-Chief, the Minister of Finance and the Chief Executioner. As each rose, an attendant turned his chair or stool on its side.

There was a buzz of conversation in the court. Everyone present was clearly puzzled by this case. On the surface it seemed to be a trivial matter. Yet it was clearly of sufficient importance to merit a special private session of the inner cabinet.

"Esi, you fool!" Ama hissed. "Why did you have to get yourself embroiled in this thing?"

"Do you also want to be gagged?" a guard demanded of her.

Ama and Esi looked at each other silently. There was both love and sadness in that wordless exchange.

The councillors returned and the chairs were hurriedly set upright

"The pawn known as Esi, who took it upon herself to interrupt the proceedings of this court, is also sentenced to death," announced Koranten Péte. "However, at the specific request of Nana Asantehemaa, who is to be commended for her compassion, both sentences are commuted to transportation. There is no place in Asante for these women. They will be sent to the coast and sold to the white men at Elmina."

*****

The guard took Ama by the elbow.

He pushed her roughly through the doorway and left her in the dark room. She stood quite still. As her eyes adjusted to the dim light, she saw that she was not alone.

"Ama," said a voice she recognised, "Sit down. I want to talk to you."

It was Koranten Péte. He was sitting in an armchair. The only other furniture in the room was a stool. She did as he had directed.

Koranten Péte cleared his throat. Ama thought he sounded nervous.

"I know you did not steal that gold," he said. "I had it planted in your room; and it was I who told the High Sheriff to have you searched."

Ama said nothing. This was not news to her: she had already guessed as much.

"I am truly sorry that I have had to do this to you. I believe that you are not at fault, that you have simply been the victim of circumstances. In a sense, I am to blame. If I had not given you to Konadu Yaadom, this might never have happened.

"You must understand that Asante is more important than any single person. It is more important than me. It is also more important than you. Ama, you are being transported to the coast for reasons of state. I hope you will understand that."

Ama did not reply. She was not really interested in what he had to say. She had already moved into the next chapter of her life.

"While you were away with Konadu Yaadom, Nana Asantehene came to speak to me. He had not been told that you would be leaving Kumase and he was distraught. He told me that he had seduced you. He said that he loved you and that he wished to make you his wife, not even his first wife, he said, but his only wife. I understand your position. Even though he is still a boy, he is the King and you are only a slave. I realise that you would have been afraid to resist his demands."

In spite of herself, Ama was amused at Kwame Panin's brazen male impudence. *So he seduced me! Ha! The boy was a virgin! If there was any seducing, it was I who did it.*

"This is a critical period in our history," continued Koranten Péte. "Osei Kwame is our King and at the same time he is not yet our King. He is much too young, ignorant and inexperienced to take on the heavy responsibilities of state. What we are doing, Konadu Yaadom and I, and others too, is to prepare him, to train and educate him. We all agreed that we could not allow you to supplant us as the major influence on him at this time. Some of the councillors would have had you summarily executed. Both the Queen Mother and I argued that that would make it extremely difficult for us to exercise any influence over the boy."

So that is why you commuted my sentence, thought Ama. But still she said nothing.

"These matters are, perhaps, beyond your comprehension. However there is one simple matter which I have to make you understand. You must never talk to anyone of what passed between you and Osei Kwame. If you do, and if it should come to our ears, I have to warn you that your life would not be safe. Let me repeat what I have just said. Never speak of your relationship with Osei Kwame to anyone. If you do, you will be sealing your own death sentence. Do you understand?

"Ama, you will never see my face again. I would not like you to take your leave on such a harsh note. I cannot foresee what future awaits you. The white men will no doubt send you across the great water. I do not know what lies on the other side, but whatever it is, I wish you well."

He rose and she followed suit.

"Will you shake my hand?" he asked as they came to the door.

CHAPTER 12

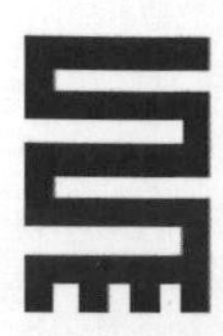

"In the beginning," said the storyteller, "Onyame, creator of all things, made three black men and three whites. To each of these he gave a woman of the same colour. The six blacks were our first ancestors and the others were the ancestors of the whites.

"Onyame set before them two things: a large clay pot and a piece of paper, folded and sealed. Then he made them draw lots and, the black men winning, he gave them the first choice. They discussed the matter amongst themselves.

"The first said, 'Of what use is a piece of paper?'

"The second replied, 'None, and the pot is large; in it we shall surely find everything we need.'

"The third said, 'Let us take the pot.'

"So they took the pot. But when they broke it open all they found was a piece of gold and a piece of iron."

The story-teller paused to wet his throat.

"Now it was the turn of the white men. When they opened the paper and examined it they found it told them everything there was to know.

"Then Onyame gave this country to the blacks. Leaving them in the bush, he took the whites to the mouth of the great water and taught them to cut down trees and build a ship. When the ship was ready they boarded it and sailed away to a far country which Onyame had prepared for those who would select the paper.

"Many years later the descendants of the first whites returned to this country with goods to exchange for gold and slaves. It is from that paper that they had learned to make the goods.

"That is the end of my story."

There was silence around the camp fire as the slaves and their guards reflected upon the significance of the tale.

"These white men," Ama asked a guard who had become her friend and who sat nearby, "What are they like?"

"They are very tall, twice as tall as we are, and very ugly. They are so ugly that it hurts ones eyes to look at them. Indeed, if you look at them for too long, you are sure to become blind."

Ama shuddered.

"What do they eat?"

"They eat all the things that we eat. Like us, they like meat best. But their favourite is human flesh."

Ama started. She had heard this once before.

"I don't believe it," she said.

"Well," he replied, "When we reach Elmina you will see. And another thing: they like woman flesh pass man."

Ama decided that he was having her on; but a small doubt remained in her mind.

"When will we reach Elmina?" she asked.

*****

Kwadwo Akyeampong, the Asantehene's ambassador, trade representative and rent-collector in Elmina, was waiting for them at Manso.

The town reminded Ama of Kafaba. The slave market was subdivided into fenced compounds, each with a few rickety sheds to provide a modicum of shelter from the elements. The slaves sat around, immobilised by chains and shackles, depressed, uncertain of what future awaited them. Traders from the coastal states would come and buy them. They would then take them south either for resale to the resident Europeans, who kept stocks in their dungeons, or to wait for a passing ship whose captain might come ashore looking for bargains.

Ambassador Akyeampong received no salary from his King but, provided that he met his obligations to Asante, he was free to enrich himself as he saw fit. So he also worked for the Dutch, collecting a commission on all purchases which he arranged for the Governor. When the demand was heavy, he would travel to Manso himself to meet a caravan.

He addressed the slaves, "You have already been sold to the Dutch governor, my friend De Bruyn. When you reach Elmina you will see the great stone castle there. None of you has ever seen a building of such size. On the coast, the strength of the Dutch is like that of their castle. In the whole country it is only Asante which is more powerful. The Dutch are our friends. Governor De Bruyn has asked me to tell you that if you behave well he will be your friend too and treat you well. If you are disobedient and rebellious, he will see to it that you experience the might of the Dutch King - on your backs."

He flicked his wrist, miming the use of a whip, in case they did not understand.

"We leave at dawn tomorrow. We shall be in Elmina in three days."

*****

Kwadwo Akyeampong called a halt in the early afternoon.

They camped near a small village in the hills behind Elmina. The slaves were given soap and sent to bathe and wash their cloths in a stream and their heads were shaved.

"Why are you doing this to us?" Ama asked the woman who was shaving Esi's head.

"It is for the white man," came the enigmatic reply.

Early next morning Akyeampong checked the inventory. Then they set off.

"Ama, look!" Esi exclaimed as they topped the crest of a hill.

A scene of the utmost strangeness and beauty presented itself to them. In the middle distance, row upon row of coconut palms; beyond the palms a strip of white sandy beach; beyond the beach, the great white-flecked expanse of the Atlantic bounded only by the curve of the horizon; above the horizon the paler blue tropical sky decorated with brilliant white fluffy clouds. The breakers rolled in upon the shore with a distant roar. Beyond the breakers, stretching far into the distance were canoes, some moved by sails, some stationary. In the canoes, they saw tiny figures.

"Is that the . . . ?" Ama asked the guard, her eyes and mouth open with wonder at the scale of it all.

Even on the open savannah in the dry season, one could not see so far into the distance. And out there there were no hills and trees to block the view. She had imagined that the great water would be like the Volta River, only wider.

The guard laughed, amused at the astonishment of this simple country girl, as he always was at the slaves' first sight of the Ocean.

"That, my sister, is indeed the sea, the same sea of which we have spoken."

"And you say that that is all water?"

"I do. But it is salt water, indeed so salty that if you try to drink from it, it will make you vomit."

She looked at him. Not for the first time she suspected that this man was pulling her leg.

"Why would anyone want to put salt in it? There must be a lot of water there. Where would they get so much salt? Next you will be telling me that it is blue because someone has poured accassie into it."

"No one put the salt into it. It has always been there. As for the colour, it is not caused by dye. That is just its colour, like green is the colour of plants. Except that in the rainy season, when there are storms, its colour can change to a kind of green, too."

Ama thought, *there is much here that I do not understand.* The guard looked at her curiously. He thought, *this is a strange girl, with all her questions.*

The path took them through a broad grassy swamp and up onto the low sandy hill where the coconut palms grew.

A gang of small boys stood around the base of one of these trees, peering upwards. They paid little attention to the passing slaves: the sight was not unusual. Suddenly, as Ama passed, a heavy object fell from the tree and the boys scattered. She looked up and there, at the top of the slender stem, sitting amongst the fronds, sat another boy. How on earth, she wondered, had he got up there?

But there was no time for further speculation. They were now on the beach itself. Here nothing grew. The sand was a blinding white in the bright sun. Ama screwed up her eyes. The hot sand burned the soles of her bare feet so that she had to keep moving. More small boys played in the surf. She flinched as a wave bore down on one of them. He disappeared. She was about to call out to a guard when there he was again. She wondered at his bravery. But why was he in the water? It was not like swimming in a river. *River* made her think of crocodiles and she scanned the shoreline.

"What is that?" she asked, grabbing the guard's arm.

At the end of the curve of the bay there rose a great white edifice, sparkling in the sunlight, dominating everything else in sight.

"That is the house of the white man, the Dutch governor," he replied with a twinkle in his eye. "Did I not tell you that the whites are twice as tall as normal human beings? It is because they are so tall that they need such big houses. It is called Elmina Castle. That is where we are going. Do you see the smaller castle up on the hill? That is called Fort St. Iago."

They passed two imposing houses, each surrounded by beautiful gardens with trees laid out in straight rows.

"Do you see those trees? The white man, again. He orders the trees: 'grow in straight lines,' and they obey him."

That was too far-fetched. *I am not such a fool,* thought Ama. *Everything this man is telling me must be lies. But then, whom should I believe; and what?*

Their way was barred and they turned right along the bank of the stone-lined channel which connected the Benya Lagoon to the sea. Ahead of them was a curious bridge and beyond it Ama could see what looked liked a small forest of dead trees, without leaves but with a network of ropes hanging from them. As they climbed from the beach to the road, she saw the brig, floating in the lagoon, but she could make nothing of the masts and rigging. *There are just too many mysteries in this place,* she thought. *But give me time and I will sort them out.*

They crossed the bridge and climbed the short hill beyond. On their right was a large town.

"Women and children slaves this side," cried Akyeampong. "Set down your loads over here."

Two men came out of the castle. One was black. Though the skin of the other was light in colour he was of normal size. Like his fellow, he a wore peculiar red garment, somewhat the worse for wear; but apart from that he looked just like a bleached version of a normal man. Ama thought to ask her friend the guard if this was a white man, but he had been called away. These two also seemed to be guards, judging from their long whips.

Ama was at the head of the line of women with Esi beside her.

"This way," called the white in a sort of broken Asante. He was looking in her direction but she assumed that he was speaking to someone behind her.

She looked back and saw the shackles being removed from the first of the male slaves. Then the guard grabbed her arm roughly and manhandled her across two short wooden bridges which crossed a deep channel filled with water. Esi tried to follow her, but the other guard restrained her. They called out to each other plaintively. Who could tell if they would ever see each other again? Perhaps Ama was being taken away to be eaten?

The guard stopped in a dark portico. She saw shadowy figures and heard a voice speak in a language she had never heard before. She thought she recognised Akyeampong's voice, too, but she could not understand what he said. Before her eyes had time to adjust, the guard pulled her again so that she almost fell. Then they passed out of the darkness and into the bright light again. She was aware of a great courtyard with white walls as high as the highest forest trees rising up on all sides. She caught a glimpse of many people, as in a dream. Then she was pulled down a dark narrow passage into another courtyard, with walls as high but smaller and quite empty. The guard took a key from his belt and unlocked a narrow iron gate. He thrust her through the opening, banged the gate closed and relocked it.

Ama was bewildered. She had heard and seen so many strange things that morning. She gripped the iron bars and looked out at the courtyard. The sun was overhead and the stone floor was drenched in sunlight. Then she heard a sound behind her. Startled, she turned quickly. In the darkness all she could see was the whites of many pairs of eyes. They all seemed to be staring at her. She pressed her back against the gate. Then she heard quiet sobbing. It sounded like the crying of a child. Now she could see that there were women sitting shoulder to shoulder with their backs to the walls of the room. Others sat and lay on the damp stone floor. Apart from the gate where she stood, there were no other openings for light or air. She took a step forward and breathed deeply. The air she inhaled was pervaded with a foul smell of unwashed bodies and old shit and piss.

There was a noise from the courtyard. The gate was flung open and Esi was pushed inside.

"Esi, it is me, Ama."

Ama put her arm around Esi's shoulder and hugged her. Esi was rigid with shock and fear.

"Come, let us see if we can find some place to sit."

*****

When Ama woke, there was not a single glimmer of light in the dungeon.

The smell struck her and she wanted to vomit. The air was unpleasantly hot and humid, yet the floor she lay on was cold and damp. She was thirsty and she wanted to piss. She screwed up her eyes but she could see nothing. She could hear the sleep sounds of many women and children.

She tried to think. That very morning she had been walking along the beach, watching the naked boys playing in the waves, breathing deeply in the salt air. Now she was in a place worse than death. *Or, is this death?* she wondered. The dungeon had already been crowded when she arrived. All the other women in the caravan had followed her, one by one. The women who had already spent some time in the dungeon - *how long*? she wondered - had resented the new arrivals and there had been squabbles and abuse in several languages, her own, Asante and others she did not understand at all. They were all victims of the same unseen oppressor and yet they fought amongst themselves.

She tried to pray to Itsho, but the words would not come. She needed peace, a quiet place on her own, before she could communicate with him. She would pollute the world of the ancestors if she tried to call him from this place of damnation.

She heard a sound from the courtyard. Keys turned in the lock. Esi was sleeping next to her, nearer to the gate. She shook her gently and whispered her name in her ear.

The gate opened. Esi sat up.

"What is it?" she asked. "Where am I?"

A man entered, carrying an oil lamp, keeping it low, looking at the faces. His own face remained in the shadows. He brought the lamp up close to Esi's face. Then he said something, just one or two words, in a strange language. He grabbed Esi's arm and pulled her upright. She gasped and stretched for Ama, but it was too late. The man dragged her through the gate and banged it shut. Some women woke and spoke.

"Ama," Esi cried but her voice was muffled as if a hand had been placed over it.

Silence settled over the dungeon. Ama lay awake, not knowing what to do, what to think.

Time passed. Then there was the sound of the key turning in the lock again. The gate opened and Esi was pushed inside. She was sobbing deliriously. Ama stepped over bodies in the dark, guiding her to her place. She tried to comfort her.

"What happened?" she asked, but Esi could not speak.

EUROPEANS

Both thy bondmen, and thy bondmaids, which thou shalt have shall be of the heathen that are round about you; of them shall ye buy bondmen and bondmaids. Moreover, of the children of the strangers that do sojourn among you, of them shall ye buy, and of their families that are with you, which they begat in your land: and they shall be your possession. And ye shall take them as an inheritance for your children after you, to inherit them for a possession; they shall be your bondmen for ever.

Leviticus 25, 44 - 46

When Dom Diego de Azambuja, the agent of the Portuguese king, built the Castle of São Jorge da Mina in 1482, he established the first long-standing European presence in West Africa. In 1637, after several abortive attempts, a Dutch force expelled and supplanted the Portuguese. The Dutch were to keep the Castle for 235 years, until the British bought them out in 1872.

CHAPTER 13

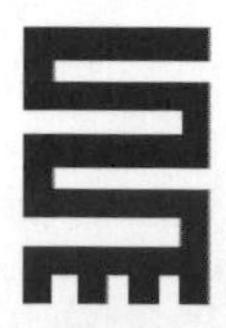

Director-General Pieter De Bruyn stood in the shadow, leaning against one of the plastered arches which framed the second floor balcony.

It was Sunday afternoon. He had spent the morning in church, eaten to excess in the company of his officers and drunk enough wine to make him drowsy. He unbuttoned his high collar and fanned himself ineffectively with his left hand. The air was still within the high enclosing walls of the courtyard. On the roof a row of white-breasted black crows cried their raucous cry. It was hot. The moisture in the air was almost palpable. Drops of perspiration trickled from his balding pate, down over his wrinkled forehead, onto his thick grey eyebrows and into his eyes. He felt the sting of the saltiness of his sweat and wiped his eyes with the handkerchief which he kept clasped in his right hand.

Sven Jensen, the young Chief Merchant, stood leaning over the balcony a few paces away. Jensen was immaculate. His white uniform was perfectly pressed. His shock of blonde hair shone in the midday sun. The gold braid on his epaulets sparkled as he turned to speak. Jensen seemed immune to the climate. Indeed he seemed to thrive on it. De Bruyn sighed.

"They are coming now, sir", said Jensen.

Remaining in the shade, De Bruyn peered down into the courtyard below. He heard the grinding of the hinges as the iron door was opened.

"I hope you have a better selection for me than last week," he said. "Emaciated, ugly bitches. I took the best of a bad lot but she turned me off. I sent her back to her hole unused. Must be old age creeping up on me. When I was younger I would have just covered her face and got on with it."

"This is the batch which Akyeampong brought in on Thursday," replied Jensen. "There are some with a bit more flesh on them."

He knew: he had already tested a sample.

Impotent bugger, the DG, thought Jensen, *I cannot live without a fuck practically every day and yet it seems that De Bruyn can manage a stand only on Sundays. And two weeks without a woman. The old boy must either be pulling himself off or he is impotent.*

"I hope you will find a candidate more to your taste today, sir," he said.

The Company's Board in Amsterdam had its rules. Company servants were not permitted to take concubines. The lower ranks were forbidden from so much as spending a night in Edina and they were locked into the Castle before dark every evening. They were certainly not permitted to bring women to their quarters nor even to handle the slaves. Offenders were flogged till the blood ran. But the officers, including the Director General, flouted the rules with impunity. All that was required of them was that they exercise reasonable discretion.

Two guards, Kobina and Vroom, lounged against the wall in a corner of the courtyard. They were dressed in ragged scarlet trousers, inherited from deceased Dutch soldiers. They were barefooted and stripped to the waist. Idly, they flicked their rawhide whips at one another. The third guard, Kofi Kakraba, was somewhere in the dungeon, shouting at the seated women, kicking those who did not understand him, cracking his whip in the dark, to force them onto their feet and out.

The women blinked and rubbed their eyes. At this time of the afternoon, the sun lit up the wall opposite De Bruyn and half of the stone floor below. Vroom shouted at them in broken Dutch, careless of whether they understood or not. Kobina clapped his hands and gesticulated, herding them into a corner. More women came streaming past the iron gate. The guards divided them into two lots and lined the first up against the sunlit wall. They stood there, confused and uncertain, flexing their limbs and looking around. One yawned and stretched her arms. Some began to chatter. One woman began to sing a dirge in a high-pitched voice. Coming out of the dungeon behind them, Kofi Kakraba silenced them with a harsh command and a crack of his whip. They cowered against the wall.

Ama stood in the shade and hugged herself. She thought she recognised Vroom.

What now? she wondered.

She looked around the courtyard. The floor was of stone flags, their surface worn smooth, if she had only known it, by nearly three hundred years of traffic of the bare feet of female slaves. Near the far corner there was a raised platform covered with wooden boards. Above it stood an iron frame supporting a wheel of the same metal, from which there hung a chain, coiled alongside. A wooden bucket stood on the platform. Ama raised her eyes and examined the whitewashed walls. The sunlight reflected from the white surface made her blink. She looked away to avoid the glare. High above her, she caught a glimpse of a head of golden hair.

Vroom prodded the women with the butt of his whip, urging them to stand upright and look ahead. They murmured in sullen confusion and resistance.

De Bruyn put the telescope to his eye and focused on the first female slave. Satisfied that the women would give them no trouble today, the guards relaxed; but kept their eyes on Jensen. They could not see De Bruyn, who was concealed in the gloom, but they knew he was there. De Bruyn did not fancy the first woman: she was scrawny and ugly. He examined each female slave in turn. Most of them were dressed in torn and ragged cotton wrappers, wound around the waist or under the arms, with the loose end tucked in to hold it in position. Their heads had been shaved. De Bruyn waved the back of his hand dismissively to Jensen who conveyed the message with a sign to the guards.

The guards moved the first group of women away and motioned to the other set to replace them. Ama was fifth. By her side stood Esi, short, fat Esi, her eyes meekly on her feet. Ama looked up and, with a start, again caught sight of Jensen. The golden-haired red-faced god in his spotless white uniform astonished her. *That must be a real white man*, she thought. She nudged Esi and, with a nod of her head, directed her gaze up at Jensen. Esi stared, her mouth open. She recognised him; she was sure of it. It was Jensen who had had her the night before, in the dark courtyard, against the wall, from behind, without ceremony. She could still feel the pain in her loins and the humiliation and degradation of being taken like a dog.

"That is the pig," she muttered to Ama. "I am sure: that is the pig that raped me last night."

De Bruyn raised the telescope again. He was looking for youth, a smooth ebony complexion, a full face, a well rounded torso and a clean body-cloth. But above all he searched the slaves' unseeing eyes, seeking . . . He could not put a word to whatever it was he was seeking, perhaps some sign of humanity, some sign of the human warmth he craved, the warmth only a woman could give. Invariably what met his eye was pain, humiliation and despair

He stopped at Ama. Wide-eyed, forgetful of her condition, Ama was trying to make sense of the divine apparition above, the golden pig-god, the essential white man.

Without lowering the telescope, De Bruyn brought his thumb and index finger together.

"Fifth from the left," he said.

Jensen raised the five fingers of his right hand and then moved the index finger from left to right. Kofi Kakraba placed a hand on Ama's shoulder. She flinched, but he held her firmly. The guard looked up at Jensen, who nodded. Seeing this silent exchange of body language, Ama guessed what lay in store for her.

"Mama, the pig wants to eat me," she shrieked in her mother tongue.

"The pig wants to eat her," echoed another woman, following Ama's line of sight.

A third woman took up the refrain. Soon they all raised their voices, in a babel of languages and in a mixture of fear, anger, sympathy for Ama and relief that she had been chosen rather than themselves.

De Bruyn put the telescope down and covered his ears with his hands. The threats of the guards and the crack of their whips rose above the women's voices. Kofi Kakraba walked across to a corner of the courtyard and returned with a wooden chair which he placed in the sunlight in view of the watchers above. Then he dragged Ama across and signalled to her to stand on the seat. She was confused. *What do they want of me? Perhaps the pig-god up there is a cannibal.* She shuddered at the thought. Stubbornly she stood her ground, staring at the guard with narrowed eyes, hating him. Kofi Kakraba was a big man. His shoulders were broad and paddling a canoe through the breakers had given him huge biceps. In Kumase, Ama thought, he would have been an executioner. He took three steps; then stopped just behind her, bent his knees and suddenly wrapped his arms around her waist. Ama screamed, but before she knew what had happened, she was standing on the chair. Then her tormentor reached up and grabbed her cloth where it was tucked in above her left breast and pulled it down. Without giving her time to react, he ripped off the beads which hung around her waist. Kobina applauded; Vroom shouted an obscenity.

Ama now stood stark naked. She noticed Jensen looking down at her and covered her pubis with her hands. For a moment the other women were silent.

Then they took up their wailing again. From behind, Kofi Kakraba grabbed hold of Ama's wrists and, moving one foot back to maintain his balance, pinned her arms behind her back. She cried out in pain but he held her immobile and exposed. Vroom looked up and Jensen nodded. Vroom was light skinned. The Dutch called him "Yellow," avoiding giving him the name of his Dutch father. He forced Ama's legs apart so that he could better see her private parts. He was looking for signs of the clap. He stuck his index finger into her vagina making a lewd comment to Kobina, who stood by his side. Ama struggled to free herself from Kofi Kakraba's grip and screamed abuse at Vroom. He withdrew his finger and raised it to the light to examine it. Then he put it under his nostrils. Satisfied, he stood aside and showed the finger to Jensen and shook it once, signalling a clean bill of health.

All this time, De Bruyn's telescope had been focused on Ama, her eyes, then her breasts. Her chest was pressed forward by Kofi Kakraba who still gripped her arms behind her back. Her breasts were small but they stood high and firm. Anticipating future pleasure, De Bruyn felt his rising penis straining against the tight trousers of his dress uniform. Now that Vroom had moved aside, he dropped his sight. Within the circle of his view he saw the mound of her pubic hair.

"Dear God", he prayed silently, "forgive your humble servant for his carnal desires," and forced himself to think of chess. At his age, he knew, too much forethought and he might not be able to manage an erection when the time came.

"That one will do," he said to Jensen.

Jensen gave his final signal of approval. Their whips cracking, the guards herded the women though the gate, forcing them back into the dungeon. Kofi Kakraba had released his grip. Ama now stood silent and alone on the chair, attempting to pull herself together, to muster her spirit to face the next ordeal.

The guards came back. Kobina returned Ama's cloth to her and told her, not unkindly, to get down from the chair.

"Send me a bucket of warm water," De Bruyn said to Jensen as he turned to open the door to his bedroom.

Jensen clapped his hands.

"Water, warm water," he called.

De Bruyn unbuttoned his coat as he walked across to the tall south-west window. He opened the shutters and lent out to hook the clips to the iron hoops. He scanned the distant curve of the horizon for sails but there were none. He stretched and yawned. The air was still; it was too early for the afternoon's sea breeze. He took a deep breath and turned to study his image in the standing mirror.

There was a knock at the door.

"Enter," he called.

It was the guard Kofi Kakraba, carrying a large copper basin on his head.

"Bring it here," said De Bruyn and helped him to lower it to the floor, a few feet before the mirror. He dipped a finger into the water to test the temperature.

"You may go," he said, turning again to the window, "but wait outside the door."

Barefooted, Kofi strode silently across to the door and closed it just as silently behind him.

Ama had been given a bowl of rice and palm soup. It was the first real meal she had had since her arrival. She was hungry and she ate quickly. As soon as she had finished, Kobina told her to get up.

"Where are you sending me?" she asked him.

"Oh, so you hear Fanti?" he asked.

"Where are you sending me?" she repeated, scowling at him.

"Never you mind," he said, taking her by the hand.

"Come," he said, but she resisted.

"My little sister," he said, turning to her. "Let me give you some friendly advice. In this place you will find life easier if you co-operate. Do you understand? Now come with me. The Director is not going to eat you, he is only going to fuck you."

He laughed as he pushed her gently before him. It was a pun that always amused him.

Ama did not understand. For one thing Fanti sounded different from Asante, it was full of 'z' sounds. And then Kobina had used the same Fanti word for 'eat' as he had for 'fuck' and she could neither fathom his meaning nor understand his play on words.

What she thought she heard was, "He is not going to eat you; he is only going to eat you."

In her fear, Ama remained silent. Kobina directed her to a long, steep flight of black and white stone stairs, keeping close behind her. She was startled by the first of three strokes of a bell close by. There was a landing and then they turned to climb the second flight, this time of wood. The stairs creaked as they climbed, reminding Ama of Konadu Yaadom's staircase in Kumase. How happy she had been there, in spite of her captivity, and how stupid to have got herself into this pickle. Two polished brass guns, *pattereroes*, protected the top of the stairs. Now she thought that they had reached the level of the balcony from which she had seen Jensen looking down into the courtyard. She looked down over the balustrade. The courtyard was empty. The 'pig-god', as she thought of him now, was nowhere to be seen. They turned a corner. At the end of a wainscoted corridor their way was blocked by a solid white door, covered with ornate mouldings. Kofi Kakraba was on guard, squatting on his haunches with his back against the wall. Silently, he withdrew the clay pipe from his mouth, acknowledged their presence and with a sideways gesture of his head, indicated to Kobina that he should knock on the door.

"Enter," called De Bruyn from within.

Kobina opened the door and gently propelled Ama into the room.

"Yessir," he said, poking his head through so that he could be seen.

De Bruyn, gazing out at the Atlantic, did not turn. Receiving no reply, Kobina gently closed the door. Then he squatted against the wall opposite Kofi Kakraba.

"Got a light?" he asked.

When he heard the door close, De Bruyn turned. Ama was standing where Kobina had left her. De Bruyn walked across and stood before her. He looked her straight in the eye. Confused, afraid, shy, modest, Ama dropped her eyes to the ground. *This is not the 'pig-god,'* she thought. *This is an old man. Or perhaps they can change their appearance at will?*

She shuddered.

De Bruyn took a step back and ran his eye over her body.

"You are very young, my child," he said, "and very nervous."

He spoke in Dutch and Ama did not understand.

She remained silent, her eyes still averted from his gaze, thinking, *how harsh and unpleasant their language is.*

De Bruyn took her hand. Again she was afraid and she trembled. No white man had touched her before. She wanted to look at him, to see what was wrong with his skin that made him such an ugly colour. She was curious, too, about his hair, but she was scared to look at him. His unwashed body smell mingled with that of the civet perfume with which he had anointed himself. Ama was conscious that she smelled of the dungeon. She wondered whether he would notice.

De Bruyn led her to the mirror and stood her before it, facing it. The copper basin was just behind her.

"Look," he said, lifting her chin with his hand.

Ama had seen small hand mirrors before in Kumase. Her mistress had had one and she had often stolen a secret moment to study her own face, trying to puzzle out the meaning of the image, as she once had with Itsho. But she had never stood before a full length looking glass. Forgetting De Bruyn, she gazed at her reflection with wide eyes. She moved a hand to stroke her shaven scalp and, seeing the movement copied in the glass, dropped it to look at the original. De Bruyn watched her with a smile, pleased with himself. This trick never failed to amuse him.

"There was never yet fair woman but she made mouths in a glass. . ." he said in English.

Then, without warning, he grabbed the end of her cloth and pulled it from her, quickly crushing it into a bundle and throwing it to a far corner of the room. For the second time within an hour, Ama stood stark naked. The beads which Kofi Kakraba had torn from her earlier had not been returned to her. Instinctively, she covered her nakedness with her hands. Her feet, she felt, were stuck to the floor. She turned her head to look at De Bruyn and then as quickly dropped her eyes. Again she was afraid. As for rape, it would not be the first time. She would fight. But Kobina had said this man would eat her. She stared at her eyes in the mirror, a deep penetrating stare. The eyes stared back at her. She saw the anguish in her own expression and her fear was compounded. Then, for the first time she noticed the image of her own naked body, her round arms, the swell of her breasts, the dark areolas about the nipples, her full hips, her slender legs, her little feet. Her eyes widened. She moved her hands away and saw the mound and her private hairs.

All this time De Bruyn was talking to her in his language, but Ama understood no word of what he was saying and paid no attention to him.

"Now my little princess," he said, "you are really very beautiful. You must surely be of royal blood? Most definitely a princess. And that is what I shall call you, Princess. No, no, on second thoughts I shall call you Pamela."

"Now Pamela," he continued, "I am going to give you a bath."

In anticipation of the pleasure of cupping Ama's breasts in his soapy hands, lathering her cunt hairs, massaging her lips, inserting a soapy index finger into her pussy, De Bruyn felt his penis struggling against his tight trousers. Quickly, he pulled off his boots and socks, stripped off his coat, shirt and trousers and threw them onto the bed. Now he was wearing only his drawers. Pausing for no more than a moment, he let them drop to his feet. Now they were equal in their nakedness. *As God made us*, he thought. Ama saw his erect penis reflected in the mirror and braced herself for what was to come.

De Bruyn took a cake of soap and washed and lathered his hands. Standing behind Ama, he placed his left hand on her left shoulder and took her right breast in his soapy hand. Ama panicked. Twice before she had been taken by force. Instinctively she swung round. Thrown off balance, De Bruyn took a step back, placing his foot on the edge of the basin, tipping it over and flooding the floor boards. At the same time Ama's outstretched arm swung round and her clenched fist struck him. Already off balance, De Bruyn toppled over backwards. As he fell, the back of his head hit the corner of a table, drawing blood and causing him to cry out in surprise and pain.

Outside the door, the guards, hearing his cry, stood up, uncertain what to do. A moment later, they heard De Bruyn calling, "Guards, guards!"

No sooner had the words escaped his lips than De Bruyn became aware of the ludicrous nature of his situation. He lay there stark naked, the black woman, equally naked, standing there immobile staring at him. The blood had left his engorged penis and it had shrivelled to its normal size. He stretched out to grab his drawers and threw the garment over his organ.

The guards opened the door.

"Wait," called De Bruyn, but it was too late. Pausing only for a moment to assess the situation, Kobina rushed to De Bruyn, lifted him to his feet and helped him to a chair, De Bruyn all the time clutching his shame cloth.

"Oh my God," cried De Bruyn.

Kofi Kakraba spun Ama around and for the second time that day grabbed her wrists and pinned her arms behind her back. He began to run her out of the room.

"Wait!" commanded De Bruyn.

He had lifted a hand to the wound in his scalp. Now he lowered it to look at the blood.

"Pass me that towel," he said to Kobina. "Now dip it in the water."

There was a little water left in the basin.

"Now pass it to me. Pass it to me," he repeated.

Keeping his drawers in position with one hand, he wiped the wound on his scalp with the wet towel. It stung a little, but he realised that the damage was superficial.

"Now get out! Both of you, get out," he screamed at the two guards.

They scurried for the door and closed it noisily behind them.

Ama remained standing where Kofi Kakraba had released her. She had struck this old white man who seemed to be the chief of the castle. Surely now he would kill her. She wanted to run. But where to? The guards were outside the door. There appeared to be no escape. And how far could she get in her nakedness?

Ama got down on her knees and, cupping her right hand in her left, blurted out hysterically,

"Nana, grandfather. My lord, my master. Forgive me. It was a mistake. I didn't mean to harm you. You startled me and it was in my surprise that I swung round.

Do not kill me, I beg you. It was a mistake. It was a mistake. I didn't do it on purpose."

Her words were swallowed by her crying. She sank her head upon her knees and sat there, unable to decide what to do next and unable to control her sobbing.

De Bruyn, guessing the general import of her plea, pulled on his drawers and rose gingerly to his feet.

"Get up, you stupid baggage," he said as he picked up the basin and took it to the door.

"More water," he ordered as he passed it to the guards. "And mind, if one single word about this incident gets abroad, you will both be on the next ship leaving for Guyana. Do you savvy? Not a single word," and he drew a finger across his throat.

When Kobina returned with the basin, De Bruyn had donned a gown and had persuaded Ama to get up and wrap her cloth around her. He directed the basin to the alcove he used for his weekly bath.

"I suppose you know how to bath yourself?" he said to Ama wryly and handed her the cake of soap, a loofah and a towel and pushed her gently into the alcove. Then he drew the curtain to allow her to bath in privacy.

Ama's mind was still in a turmoil but she didn't need a second invitation to scrub off the filth of the dungeon. As she lathered herself, she slowly recovered her self-control. She concentrated her mind on Itsho and when she succeeded in summoning up an image of his face, he was laughing. Then she began to see the ridiculous side of what had happened and smiled involuntarily to herself. The soap was mildly perfumed and the water was warm. Enjoying the luxury and in no hurry for whatever was to come next, she took her time.

"What are you doing in there woman? Hurry up, I also want to take my bath," called De Bruyn.

"Here, take this and put it on," he continued and hung upon the curtain rail a piece of Ijebu cloth which he had taken from his wooden chest.

They had no single word in common but were somehow managing to communicate. Ama dried herself and wrapped the blue cloth around her. She drew the curtain and came out, not quite sure whether that is what he had intended.

"Yes, very pretty," he said in response to her questioning look.

"Come now, Pamela," he continued, taking her hand firmly in his.

"This is our marriage bed," he said, chuckling at his own joke. "Lie on it and I will join you shortly."

All her life, Ama had slept on a mat on the floor. She had seen Konadu Yaadom's ornately carved bed in Kumase, indeed Nana had taught her how to arrange the bedclothes. But this massive four-poster was something different. She climbed onto the white cotton sheets and lay there stiffly, unable to relax. De Bruyn went to take his bath, delicately drawing the curtain behind him.

Ama had only a short time to consider her next move. The man would reappear soon and there was no doubt he would try to climb on her. What should she do? She thought of Tabitsha, her mother. Tears came to her eyes and she began to sob quietly, considering her predicament. She had seen De Bruyn's penis. It seemed to be no different from any other she had seen, in spite of its peculiar pink colour. There was no doubt what he wanted of her. But what then?

Surely when he had squirted his semen into her and had his little sleep, he would send her back to the dungeon of the female slaves, to the darkness, the fetid smell of stale piss and septic shit, the damp, the shared misery of a hundred women without hope. What if she were to resist him, to fight? She knew that she could not succeed. She could not match his strength and anyway, the guards were at his beck and call. He seemed to have forgiven her for what she had done to him, but would he do so a second time? What if she were to succumb to his wishes? She knew how to please a man and, unless white men's sex was very different from that of blacks, she was confident she could persuade him of her own excitement, even though she felt only repugnance and pain. She propped herself up on one elbow and looking through the open window saw the broad blue expanse of the ocean. She recalled the walk along the beach on the way to the castle. How she would like to go and touch it. She had no doubt that it was water, but it looked so different from the rivers and lakes she knew. Perhaps she could swim in it as she had learned to do as a child in the flood lakes of the Oti and seen the little naked boys doing not three days ago?

De Bruyn's call from behind the curtain, "Well, are you ready for me?" brought her back to reality. Then she knew what she would do. She would not resist, but neither would she co-operate. She would lie there limp and let him do what he had to do, but she would not help him and she would not encourage him. If he wanted her to give him real pleasure, he would have to earn it. And even if he sent her away in disgust, back to the dungeon, at least she would have kept her self-respect.

"Ah, Pamela, " said De Bruyn, as he drew the curtain. "There you are. Now we shall see," and he licked his dry lips.

CHAPTER 14

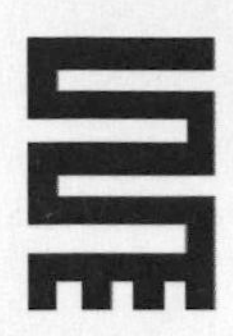

Ama was startled by the sound of a cannon.

"Oh, shit," said De Bruyn and went to the window.

"Pamela," he said, starting to put on his uniform, "please accept my most abject apologies. That cannon shot signals the arrival of a ship. I shall have to go and meet the captain. I would much prefer to spend an afternoon of pleasure with you. However, young Jensen has caused me enough trouble already with our noble Assembly of Ten, and I cannot afford to give him another opportunity to undermine me. Mr. Jensen, I must tell you, my dear Pamela, is after my job."

Ama wondered what he was jabbering about. She lay where she was on the bed. De Bruyn leant over her, looked into her eyes for a moment and then kissed her on her forehead.

"Until this evening then."

"I shall look forward to it," he called back as he left the room.

Ama heard the key turn in the lock. She rose from the bed and went to the window. All was quiet now. The ship had rounded the outcrop on which the castle was built and was out of sight. Wisps of smoke rose from Edina. She thought she heard voices drifting up from the thatched roofs which lay amongst the coconut palms but she could see no sign of human life.

She wandered around the room, examining the furniture. Four old elm armchairs stood in one corner. She ran her fingers over the brass buttons which secured the elaborately brocaded upholstery. Then she knelt to feel the carved hooves at the ends of the cabriole legs. *Strange*, she thought, *chairs with feet like those of a deer*.

Suddenly she felt overcome by exhaustion. The stress of the past three days in the female dungeon and of the afternoon's events had drained her. She went back to the bed and within moments she was asleep.

It was dark when she awoke but the room was lit by candles. A small dining table had been laid. De Bruyn had ordered a light meal for two. He had shared a brandy with the captain of the Dutch ship and, making his excuses, had delegated Jensen to entertain the visitor.

He took Ama by the hand and drew her to the table.

"I am sorry that I had to abandon you, my dear Pamela." he said. "However, business before pleasure, as they say. I have left our guest in the capable hands of that young scoundrel, Jensen."

Ama let him ramble on. *What can he be talking about?* she wondered, rubbing the sleep from her eyes. De Bruyn pulled a chair for her and guided her into position.

"When a gentleman pulls a chair for you, my lady Pamela," he said, "You must move in front of it, so, and as he slides the chair forward, you sit your pretty rump on the seat, like this. Are you comfortable? A little further forward, perhaps?"

Mellowed by the brandy and anticipating the pleasures of the night ahead, De Bruyn was in a genial mood, amused at the pantomime he had set up.

"Now, my love," he continued, knowing full well that Ama did not understand a single word, "you must learn to use a knife and fork like a Dutch lady."

The words *Dutch lady* reminded him of his late wife, Elizabeth De Bruyn, but he resolutely erased the image. Elizabeth would certainly not have approved of this tête-à-tête. He carved the duck and served a portion onto Ama's plate, humming tunelessly as he did so. Then he tasted the warm Rhenish wine and poured a full glass for Ama.

"That will relax you, my darling," he said.

Ama watched him use his knife and fork.

"Eat, eat," he told her, his mouth full, noticing her hesitation. He rose and moved to stand behind her and taking her hands, showed her how to hold the implements and cut the breast of duck which he had served her. The contact with her bare arms and shoulders excited him but he controlled himself and returned to his seat.

Ama cut a piece of the duck, impaled it on her fork and, watching De Bruyn for approval, put it in her mouth.

"Excellent," he said. "And now," raising his glass and indicating to her that she should do the same, "A toast."

Looking her straight in the eyes and touching his glass against hers, he said, "To a long and *intimate* friendship."

Ama returned his gaze for a brief moment and then, puzzled, dropped her eyes.

"Drink, drink," he urged her as he put the glass to his lips and sipped the wine.

Ama was thirsty and drained her glass as if it were water. De Bruyn was amused.

"Slowly," he said, chuckling and chucking her chin. "A lady drinks her wine like this," and he demonstrated.

Relaxed by De Bruyn's evident good humour, Ama smiled.

"Oh, that is beautiful," he said. "Please smile like that again, for me."

He bared his ugly stained teeth at her and, feeling the glow of the wine, Ama could not help laughing at his expression.

"This conversation is too one-sided," said De Bruyn. "You haven't opened your mouth once to speak. And, come to think of it, we have not been properly introduced. My name is Pieter. Pieter De Bruyn. But it wouldn't do for people to hear you calling me by my name. You should call me *Mijn Heer*."

He pointed to his chest and repeated, "Mijn Heer."

Then he pointed to her and said, "Pamela."

Ama pointed to herself and said, "Ama."

Her name had already been changed once and once was enough for her.

But De Bruyn insisted, "No, I am *Mijn Heer* and you are *Pamela*. Say your name, say *Pamela*."

Ama decided to humour him.

"Pamela," she tried.

"Excellent." said De Bruyn, "Now again. *Pamela, Pamela, Pamela*."

"Pamela, Pamela, Pamela," echoed Ama.

"You have a sweet, melodious voice. Now try *Mijn Heer*. *Mijn Heer, Mijn Heer, Mijn Heer*," he said, pointing to himself again.

"Mijn Heer, Mijn Heer, Mijn Heer," sang Ama, beginning to enjoy the game and pointing boldly at De Bruyn.

"What is my name?" he asked her, pointing at himself.

"Mijn Heer," replied Ama.

"And yours?" pointing at her.

"Pamela?" Ama tried.

"Splendid. You are a clever girl."

Sensing the approbation in his voice, Ama glanced up. For a moment De Bruyn appeared lost in his thoughts and Ama was able to observe him unnoticed. Thin wisps of grey hair swept untidily across a bald red crown. He had enormous, untidy, grey eyebrows. His light blue eyes seemed to vanish into his head. Ama had never seen blue eyes before. She stared at them, fascinated.

"But one thing you must know and remember very well at all times," said De Bruyn, as if continuing his unspoken thoughts, "is that I am the Director-General of this great castle of Elmina, which we took from the Portuguese in the year of our Lord 1637. I represent the Assembly of Ten who control the United Dutch West India Company from our headquarters in Amsterdam. I have to maintain the dignity of my office. You must treat me with respect. If you fail, if you dally with any other man, I shall send you straight back to where you came from this afternoon. Do you understand?"

What with the brandy and the wine he had taken, De Bruyn's speech was beginning to be slurred. He rambled on as if talking to some one who understood his every word. Then he rang a small bell. *What next?* Ama wondered. A servant came to clear the table.

"No, no. Leave the wine and the glasses," he said. "And tell the chef I say the duck was very good and the yam pudding, too."

"Now, my dear, it is time for bed," he told Ama after the man had left.

He put his hands on her bare shoulders and looked into her eyes. She dropped her gaze. He lifted her chin and forced her to look at him, as one might do with a pet dog. With his fingers still under her chin, he leant forward and kissed her gently on the lips. Then he looking into her eyes again and holding her gaze, he loosened her cloth. Instinctively, Ama grabbed it, but it was too late and it fell to the floor. She felt doubly naked without her beads.

This man may be ugly and his breath may smell of drink, she thought, *but at least he seems quite gentle.*

De Bruyn feasted his eyes on her body. Then he began to remove his clothing. As he took off each piece, he handed it to her, indicating that she should lay it on an armchair. When only his drawers remained, he beckoned to her to remove them for him.

What choice do I have? she thought. *My fate cannot be worse than Esi's.*

"Mijn Heer," she asked him as she pulled his drawers down over his erect organ, "who is the pig-god and what does he do here?"

"I beg your pardon?" replied De Bruyn, wondering what she was saying. "Do you want to piss?"

He showed her the chamber pot and went to wait for her. Ama took her time. On the bed she found him snoring quietly. She covered him with a sheet and lay down by his side.

De Bruyn woke in the middle of the night with his bladder bursting. After relieving himself, he returned to the bed and woke Ama from a deep sleep. His foreplay aroused him but drowsy as she was, Ama was barely aware of the man's caresses.

As he entered her, she saw a vision of Abdulai. By an act of sheer will she wiped it clear.

De Bruyn moved in her. At first she felt nothing. Then she thought of Itsho. She saw his crushed skull. She buried him again in his shallow grave. De Bruyn was losing control and he stopped his plunging to prolong the coupling. He sought her lips. She struggled to free her mouth.

"Itsho," she called out, "Itsho, Itsho."

Itsho was inside her. Again she called his name. Fiercely, she drew him to her.

De Bruyn could no longer control himself. As he moved in her again, she responded and they drove each other on.

"Itsho," she called again, "Itsho," and together they came to a climax.

"Pamela," said De Bruyn. Then he forced her mouth open and sought her tongue.

"Pamela, thank you," he said when he had kissed her.

A moment later he had rolled away. Soon he was snoring again.

Ama lay on her back, thinking. It was strange. Itsho was dead. She had buried him herself. Yet she had felt his presence, felt him making love to her as if he were still alive. Perhaps he had sent his spirit from the place of the ancestors into the body of this strange white man. She tried to reach out to him, whispering his name but he had come to her call once and he would not come again.

Her thoughts drifted. She forced herself to concentrate and consider her options. *I am a slave. This Mijn Heer has bought me, along with so many others. I am his property. He is the master of this great castle and my master too. He will send me back to the female dungeon at sunrise if he so chooses. Apart from Esi, trapped down there (and there on my account too) I know no one in this place. I have no friend, no one I could speak to, no one to advise me, no one to speak for me. Mijn Heer seems no different from other men: a little childish; lonely, perhaps; needing to be cuddled and loved; and with his sex's animal need to penetrate a woman. True, he is ugly and he is old. But he seems reasonably kind.* She smiled as she recalled how she had knocked him down. Now it seemed funny. *I was so scared. He could have had me killed. What if I had done such a thing to the Asantehene, or to any free Asante man for that matter? Why did Mijn Heer spare me? And why did he make me sit with him to eat?* Never before in her life had she sat at a table to eat and never had she eaten with a man. *Except, just once,* she thought, *with Itsho.* They had arranged to meet in the corn fields and she had grilled a chicken and taken it for him. Itsho had insisted that they share it. *Yet he was usually such a stickler for custom. Itsho is dead. Itsho tried to save me. The Bedagbam killed him. I shall never see him again, until, one day, I join the ancestors myself.*

Is there really another world where the ancestors live? she wondered. *Where? Under the ground or in the sky? Or are their spirits all around us, but somehow invisible? When Mijn Heer was inside me just now, I really felt it was Itsho. Could it be so? If his spirit could come into Mijn Heer's body like that, is Itsho trying to tell me something, to advise me, to help me?* How she longed to hold him to her, to caress him, to take his head upon her chest. She looked across at De Bruyn. He had stopped snoring. *Men look so defenceless and innocent when they sleep, especially after they have spent their energy.* She wiped a strand of hair from De Bruyn's forehead and then wondered at her nerve. Her thoughts returned to Itsho. *What could his message be? Could his spirit influence Mijn Heer to help me, to look after me?* She had heard their guards say that they would be sold to other white men and sent far across the sea. *How could that be? Will they send us in canoes, like the ones I saw in the sea? The sea seems so huge and I could see no land on the other side. Even when the Oti is in flood, you can see the far shore. Maybe the sea is in flood now? Maybe in the dry season it will shrink to a trickle as the Oti does when the rains fail?*

De Bruyn was snoring again. Ama gathered her cloth and went to the window. The sky was clear and full of stars. The light of a full moon was reflected on a calm sea. She could see the white surf breaking on the shore and she heard its gentle roar. Edina lay below the castle walls, enveloped in dark mysterious shadows. She sat on the broad window cill with her back against the Dutch bricks in the jamb. She hugged her knees. *What is the moon*, she wondered, *and the stars*? She knew some of their names, but what they were, that was a puzzle. *Could each star be a dead ancestor? Which one is Itsho then? And are the ancestors of the Bedagbam and the Asante and the white men there too? How can one know? So many things in the world are so difficult to understand.* When they had first fallen in love, Itsho had been amused at her outrageous inquiries and this had encouraged her to search for more questions to ask. Soon it had become a habit and she had begun to look at the world in a new way. But Itsho had become scared. She was trespassing upon the territory of the earth priests. If she was not careful, he had warned her, she would be accused of witchcraft. Noticing the subtle change in his attitude (she knew Itsho much better than he knew himself) she had stopped sharing her inquiries with him. But her secret habit of speculation and reflection had acquired a life of its own and was not easily denied.

Itsho or no Itsho, I have no choice. I am lucky this man selected me for his pleasure. I have had two good meals and a bath; he has given me a fine new clean cloth to wear; I have slept in his bed. It is true that he has used me, that he did not ask my consent, that I am his chattel to deal with as he chooses; but he did not take me by force, he did not hurt me. If I am honest with myself, I have to admit that I have missed having a man all this time. Kwame Panin didn't really count, for all his boyish passion. Old and ugly as he is, this scrawny man is surely my only chance of survival. If I could only make him love me and need me, perhaps one day he would even let me go back home.

She concentrated her mind on those she loved best. *Tabitsha, my mother, how you must have mourned the kidnapping of your first born. You cannot even know that your daughter Nandzi is now called Ama. Tigen, my father, wise old greybeard, so stern, but with a twinkle in your eye. How you loved and cherished me when I was small.* Her first memories were of Tigen grasping her hands and swinging her through the air, round and round and round, up and down, and then, when he had put her down on her feet again, the two of them stumbling around dizzily as if they had taken too much pito. *I must have been as old then as Nowu was when I was taken. Poor Nowu, he was so ill and he must have had such a shock. And baby Kwadi, he must be quite a big boy now.*

They could not even imagine a small part of what she had been through. *And here I am now, sitting at the window of this great castle, with its master, a white man, sleeping there in his bed.*

The sea reminded her of the savannah, it was vast, open, you could see far into the distance. Except there were no baobab and silk cotton trees growing in the sea!

De Bruyn spoke in his sleep.

"Elizabeth," he said, "I will be home soon."

For a moment, Ama was startled; then she chuckled to herself. She yawned and stretched her arms. Then she went back to bed and fell into a deep, dreamless sleep.

*****

When De Bruyn awoke, it was already light.

He was late for his morning inspection. He rose and dressed quickly and quietly, without waking Ama. He leant over her and gazed at her sleeping form. Such a beautiful child, he thought, surprised at the tenderness he felt for her. Then the bell for seven o'clock brought him back to the real world of duties and responsibilities, trade and correspondence, and he turned to go.

As he left the room, Augusta was waddling down the corridor, chewing on a *tweápeá* stick. Following her at a respectful distance, a bare-footed slave girl bore a bucket and broom and ostrich feather duster.

"Good morning, Augusta," De Bruyn said hurriedly as they shook hands.

Barely allowing her time to remove the chewing stick and return the greeting he continued, "I am late. I overslept. You will see the reason."

He indicated the door behind him with a cock of his head.

"I like this one. She is beautiful; and clever, too. I think I will keep her for a while."

He squeezed Augusta's hand and continued in a confidential whisper, "Speak to her and tell me what you think."

"I am late for my inspection," said De Bruyn. "We will talk later."

The young slave curtsied to De Bruyn as he passed and he nodded to her absent-mindedly.

Augusta watched him until he turned the corner.

Not for the first time she thought, *As the years pass, you look more and more like a swamp reed dried in the sun and,* looking down at her own corpulent frame, *I look more and more like a ball of fufu.*

"*Àgòo*," she called, announcing her entry, as she opened the door to the De Bruyn's bedroom.

She was surprised to hear the customary reply, "*Amêê.*"

"So, young woman, you understand Fanti?" she asked as she entered, looking to see whom it was that she was addressing.

Ama had been feigning sleep as De Bruyn dressed, uncertain as to how she should behave, but she had risen from the bed as soon as he had closed the door.

She had washed her face in the brass basin of water she found on the dresser and was drying it with the towel as Augusta entered.

"Please, yes, Madam," she said.

"I mean, no, Madam," she continued in some confusion, curtsying as she spoke, "but I do hear Asante small."

"Oh, Edinas and Fantis and Asantes, we are all the same family, " replied Augusta, settling her considerable bulk into one of Mijn Heer's comfortable arm chairs. "We are all Akans. We fight amongst ourselves, of course, but it is the fighting of brothers."

"Where do you come from?" she continued, signalling to her assistant to get on with the work.

"Please, they brought me from Kumase," replied Ama, thinking it best to avoid the complication of trying to explain the location of Tigen's hamlet.

"Ah, Kumase, I hear it is a great city," said Augusta. "Some time you must tell me about it. What is your name?"

"Please, they call me Ama."

"Ama. That is a good name. My name is Augusta, alias Efua Kakrabaa. I am one of the most important traders in this town."

She nodded towards the open window, beyond which lay the grass and matting roofs, the winding narrow streets and whitewashed swish walls of Edina. She gestured impatiently to the young girl who was holding the brass chamber pots mutely requesting her approval to take them out of the room.

"I deal in cloth," she continued. "Bombay, broad cloth, calicoes, ginghams, guinea cloths, sattins, seersuckers, silks, taffaties, worsted damasks, fringes and all kinds of cotton stuffs. Every kind of cloth the Dutch bring in their ships, from all over the world, from India and Batavia and from Europe. Linens from Germany. And the new cotton prints from Manchester, in England. Have you heard of these places? No? Well I do not know them either. The Director General tells me they are far away, many months journey on the sea. As for me, I have been once to Axim and many times to Manso and to Cape Coast, but that is as far as I have travelled."

Augusta was fond of talking, especially about herself.

"I am best known for my cloth, but I also sell beads. Amber, crystal, coral, glass: I have them all. Jewellery too, earrings, chains, necklaces, bangles. And aggrey beads of course. I sell them all. You can find my store in the market in Edina. Just ask for Augusta. Everybody knows Augusta."

It struck her suddenly that she was talking to a slave woman, a chattel, without property, without money, but the thought gave her only slight pause. *If Mijn Heer keeps her for a while,* she thought, *he is sure to want to buy her presents. And Mijn Heer pays cash, in unadulterated gold dust.*

All this time Ama had been standing respectfully before her. She had picked up the general trend of what Augusta had said but there were many words she did not understand.

"Sit down, sit down," said Augusta, indicating a chair. "I have something to tell you. Mijn Heer has asked me to talk to you."

"Tell me first, how long have you been with him? Oh, no need to answer," she continued. "You were not here when I came on Saturday, so he must have taken you yesterday. Were you in the dungeon? It is not very pleasant, is it? So you are a very lucky girl to be selected by the Director-General. If you are clever, he might marry you. He might even set you free one day. But I must warn you. You are not the first slave girl he has taken. Sometimes they last only one night and he sends them back to the dungeon. A week later, perhaps, a ship will come and collect them away over the sea. Sometimes he keeps them for a week or a month. So you must behave well and you must be very careful to keep him happy. You are lucky he has asked me to advise you, because I know Director-General Pieter De Bruyn better than any black woman in this country, or any black man for that matter."

Ama listened to all this in amazement, straining to catch Augusta's meaning and to keep up with the torrent of words.

"I am the best person to advise you, because I, Augusta, alias Efua Kakrabaa, was the first wife of your Mijn Heer."

Ama's eyes opened a little wider. Augusta noticed.

"You do not believe me? It is true. You can ask anybody in Edina. Ask Mijn Heer himself.

"Many years ago, when he was young and handsome (as white men go) and new to this castle, my father (of blessed memory) who was one of the leading *caboceers* in Edina, took a liking to him. So he sent me to serve him as his wife. I was young and beautiful then, like you. I was a virgin. Mijn Heer was my first man. It was he who gave me my name, Augusta. I stayed with him for two years but I failed to bring forth. A pity. I would have liked to have had a European child. But it was not my fault, I have had eight children since and five are still living. And Mijn Heer has had only one, and that one none of us has ever seen.

"Then, when we had been married two years, the company transferred him to a distant place they call the Cape. I asked him to take me with him but he said it was too far, though it is also in this our Africa, not in Europe where the whites come from. In the Cape he married a white woman. Many years later, when he was already quite old, they sent him back to Elmina as Director-General and he brought this wife with him."

Ama was lost in the romance of Augusta's story. She loved a good story and this one was very different from those of her childhood and the Anansesem she had learnt in Kumase.

"By the time he came back here, I had already born six children. I had buried my second husband and taken a third, but still De Bruyn had only one issue. To this day he has had only one, a son he left behind at the Cape.

"His wife was called Elizabeth De Bruyn. She was a good-for-nothing woman. About your size but without colour. She was already sick when she came to Elmina Castle and she was sickly all the time she was here. She did nothing with her time but sleep and read books. Do you know what books are? No? Effibaa, bring me a book."

Effibaa was just then dusting the books in the glass-fronted cabinet. She brought a book. Augusta signed to her to give it to Ama. Ama took it.

"Open it," Augusta told her, holding her palms together and then opening them as if they were pages in a book. Ama did so. She could make nothing of the marks on the paper, but she found a picture of European men in wigs and ladies in hooped skirts and studied it with interest.

"Can you imagine? The woman spent the whole day, every day, looking into books like that. Mijn Heer is the same but he does not waste as much time on it as she did. I cannot think what they make of all those little marks. I have asked Mijn Heer, but he always makes fun of me with his answer. He says that there are stories in those books. Can you believe that?"

"Anyway, when Madam Elizabeth was not reading books she was lying on her bed and fanning herself or sitting at the window looking at the sea. The only time I ever saw her go out of these rooms all the time she stayed here, was when she went to chapel."

Augusta saw Ama's blank look.

"Chapel. You don't know what chapel is? That is their room where they go to worship their gods. It is in the charge of the chaplain, who is like a fetish priest for them, an *Okomfo* you know, except that he does not know how to dance. When I was married to Mijn Heer, I had to go there with him every Sunday. Sometimes the chaplain tells them stories which he says comes out of a special book. That book is one of their main fetishes. Mijn Heer tried to tell me some of the stories when we were married. Some were not bad, but most were rubbish. I told him he should listen rather to our Ananse stories, they are much more entertaining and there is always a lesson to be learned from them."

Once she had started it was difficult to stop Augusta and while she watched constantly for the response of her captive audience, she gave little opportunity for questions or interjections. This suited Ama. Feeling her way in this relationship, she was too shy to attempt to turn the monologue into a discussion.

"Now where was I? Oh, Madam Elizabeth. The lady, she complained all the time. Once Madam Blunt came to visit her. Madam Blunt was the wife of that Cape Coast Fanti man who is the priest of the English at Cape Coast Castle. But our Madam Elizabeth could speak no English and Madam Blunt (or Quaque, for that is her husband's name) could speak no Dutch. Moreover our Madam Elizabeth would not countenance the other white woman because she was married to a black man. So Madam Blunt never came to visit her again. That is the only time that I ever saw two white women together. And now they are both dead.

"Oh, poor Madam Elizabeth. Either the weather was too hot or she didn't like the food; Mijn Heer didn't pay her enough attention; the European men were bush; there were no other respectable white women here for her to talk to: complaints, complaints, complaints. She wanted to go back to the Cape, she wanted to go to Holland on the next ship. She complained to me and she complained to her husband about me. She never knew that we had once been married. He could not tell her, and why should I? She was too lazy or sickly to supervise the domestic chores and Mijn Heer asked me to help. So I came every day to do the cleaning and washing. I saw the woman every day while she lived here, but I never got to understand her. I guess that white women are not like us. White men, I know them well. But the women?"

She shook her head.

"After one year Madam became very ill from fever. I nursed her day and night for a week. I sponged her, I fed her, I gave her herbs to drink. I slept here in this room on a mat on the floor. But in the end she died. I don't think Mijn Heer De Bruyn was too sad. He never complained, but I think that the woman had become a burden on him.

"Mijn Heer asked me to continue with the work. That was five years ago and

I have done it ever since. It is not for the money that I do it, you understand? He was my first husband and he is getting old now. He needs a woman to look after him. All men are children, you know."

Ama nodded her head sagely in agreement.

"Now Miss Ama. You strike me as a sensible young woman. You have seen what it is like in the dungeons. I can tell you, from the stories we hear, it is many times worse on the ships. Mijn Heer is your life line. Treat him well and he may save you from an early return to the ancestors. Treat him always with respect. Humour him. Soothe him when he is tired or angry. Conquer your own desires. Be his servant always and you may have a small chance of escaping from being a slave. I know the business and it is a small chance, I tell you, but it is a chance. Tomorrow, if you are still here, I shall begin to teach you to do the work that this child has been doing this morning."

"Effibaa," she called. The child had finished her work and made a bundle of Mijn Heer's laundry.

"Let us go now," she said as she drew her bulk laboriously up from the comfort of the armchair.

"Maame Augusta," Ama spoke quietly and with humility.

"Yes my child," the older woman replied.

"Maame. I thank you for what you have told me."

Augusta nodded.

"Maame, I beg you, my sister is in the dungeon. Already she has been raped once. They will kill her. Maame, I beg you to save her. Speak to Mijn Heer for me. Otherwise they will kill her."

For a moment, Augusta was taken aback by the girl's presumption.

"My child, you are a slave. You are nobody here. I have given you good advice and at once you show how headstrong you are. Never, never think of asking such a thing of Mijn Heer. This Castle belongs to a mighty European nation. Their nation is ruled by ten kings, each of them a giant. Mijn Heer is the master of this castle but he is the servant of the ten kings. Their business is to buy slaves from us. If Mijn Heer were to listen to every slave who says *my sister this, my sister that*, he would lose his job at once and maybe his head too. Ask him such a favour and you will join your sister back in the dungeon as quickly as you can blink your eye."

She turned to go. Ama was suddenly struck by the enormity of Esi's danger and of her own. Her limbs seemed to lose their solidity. She collapsed on the floor like a heap of old bones and began to sob.

Augusta bent down and grabbed her under the armpit.

"Stand up. Stand up. And stop crying at once. If Mijn Heer were to walk in now, it would be the end of you."

She thought for a moment.

"I like you, child," she said, "and I admire your love for your sister. What I will do is this. I will tell Mijn Heer that you have told me of your sister and praised her so highly that I wish to buy her myself. What is your sister's name?"

Ama stared at her, wide-eyed.

"Oh, Maame, I thank you, I thank you. She is called Esi," she said and sank down on her knees, embracing Augusta's own. "I thank you. I thank you. I thank you."

CHAPTER 15

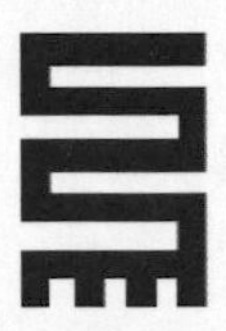

De Bruyn could not concentrate.

Again and again his thoughts turned to Pamela. Sometimes he thought of her with a tenderness which was almost paternal, sometimes with pure carnal lust.

"You're crazy," he told himself. "You are driving yourself silly over an ignorant, savage slave girl. Take a grip on yourself, Pieter De Bruyn. You are behaving like an adolescent boy in the first discovery of the other sex."

An image of Ama, naked, black, smooth, voluptuous, came into his mind. Self-indulgently, he considered it. He day-dreamed. He kissed her all over, her mouth, her nipples, her thighs. He was aware, not for the first time this morning, of his erection. He felt an ache in his balls.

His reverie was interrupted by a knock on the door. It was Jensen.

"How was the girl?" he asked.

"The girl? Oh, good, quite good," De Bruyn replied. "I shall keep her for a while."

Then he changed the subject.

Jensen, always on the lookout for something which might be of benefit to himself, was not entirely taken in.

Now why did my question disturb the old bastard so? he wondered. De Bruyn's accident the previous afternoon was common knowledge amongst the officers and had been the occasion of much bawdy mirth in their mess. He put the senior man's reaction down to embarrassment at the incident and stowed the thought away for future reference.

They discussed the conduct of the afternoon's business with the captain of the Dutch ship. The dungeons were full of slaves and, with the road to Kumase open, supplies were coming in more regularly than either of them could remember.

"Our turnover will be so great this year," said Jensen, "that we can afford to reduce our margins. Any more overcrowding of the accommodation and we might have an epidemic on our hands."

"Oh, Jensen," called De Bruyn as the Chief Merchant was leaving the room. "I am feeling a little under the weather. I think I shall take the afternoon off. Be a good chap and hold the fort for me. Let me have a full report tomorrow morning on this afternoon's palaver, will you?"

Jensen stopped and turned.

"I hope it's nothing serious," he said.

You bloody hypocrite, thought De Bruyn. *If I were afflicted with a mortal ailment your fondest hopes would be realised.*

"No, no, just a slight touch of fever," he said aloud. "I shall try to sweat it off. Not to be disturbed, please," he said, adding, as an afterthought, "but you might remind Van Schalkwyk to come in as usual in the evening."

*****

De Bruyn locked the door. He intended to devote the afternoon to the undisturbed fleshing out of his morning's fantasies.

He made Ama lie naked on the four-poster bed. Keeping his eyes averted, he covered her from head to toe with a clean white sheet, as if she were a corpse. Just as she was beginning to become concerned, he drew the top of the sheet back, exposing only her eyes and her small, broad, slightly upturned nose. He met her look of surprise with amusement. Guessing that this was some sort of game, she responded with a smile. He spoke to her quietly in Dutch, words of praise for her beauty and of his devotion to her, words that he would never have had the courage to speak if he had thought she understood him, words he had never spoken before, not to Augusta in their youth, never to holy Elizabeth. He devoured her with his eyes, her shaven head, her small ears with the modest gold earrings which Konadu Yaadom had allowed her to keep, the sweep of her dark eyebrows, the upward curve of her eyelashes. He bent to kiss her eyelashes, first one eye and then the other, gently, controlling his passion, suppressing the consciousness of the weathered naked body beneath the night-gown he had put on. He stroked her cheeks, tickling her with the hairs which grew luxuriantly on the back of his hand. All the time he spoke to her. He called her *Princess Pamela*; he repeated the name he had given her again and again; he would have sung to her if he had had any confidence in his croaky voice.

He exposed one small part of her at a time, a shoulder, a hand, examining it, exploring it. He hardly touched her and when he did it was with the gentlest of contact, sometimes with his fingers, sometimes with his lips. Ama began to bask in his adoration, watching his eyes as they surveyed the contours of her body, meeting them with wonder as he returned from each excursion.

When he uncovered a nipple, she moved, with instinctive modesty, to cover it. He took her hands away and kissed her palms. When he reached her most private parts, he did the same.

Ama was astonished at this performance. No man had ever treated her like this before. Even Itsho, kind, gentle, passionate as he had been, had never worshipped her as this peculiar white man was doing. She was afraid.

When De Bruyn had completed his mapping of her thighs, her legs, her feet and toes (hardened these, by a life time of walking barefooted), he rolled her over and began his exploration of the other hemisphere. He was completely possessed. His entire consciousness was concentrated on this fragile creature.

Ama turned her head on the pillow to watch him. She felt desire rising in her. She was his slave, his property, but, for the moment, she had lost her will to be free. She wanted him to possess her.

As he ran the surface of his finger nails down along her vertebrae, she spoke for the first time.

"Mijn Heer, Mijn Heer," she whispered.

*****

When they had spent their passion, De Bruyn looked into her eyes again and they laughed together.

He brought a basin and wiped their parts. Then he sponged the sweat from her body and wiped her with a clean towel. They lay naked together under the sheet, her head on his chest, and spoke to one another, neither understanding a word of the other's language and laughing at their mutual incomprehension.

When they awoke, he took her again, astonished at a capacity he thought he had long lost.

The sun, setting far along the line of the coast, sent slivers of orange light through the jalousies, making patterns on the far wall. They bathed and dried one another. Ama replaced her beads and wrapped her cloth around her.

De Bruyn dressed in a casual shirt and trousers. Then he went to the cabinet which held the books. Opening a drawer, took out a brass key. With it, he unlocked a wooden cabin trunk, elaborately carved with scenes of Dutch landscape.

"Pamela, come," he called her as he raised the lid. There was a smell of naphtha and a hint of stale perfume. He drew out a lady's dress in the European style, shook it, and held it up for her to see. Then he took her to the standing mirror which had been the scene of their battle the previous afternoon and, standing again behind her, held the dress up against her front. Ama recalled the picture she had seen in the book which Augusta had shown her. She was about to tell him and to fetch the book; but then she wondered how she would explain and whether Augusta had not perhaps exceeded her authority in showing her Mijn Heer's possessions.

"Try it on," said De Bruyn.

Ama feared the strange garment. But before she could react, De Bruyn had lifted the skirt over her head. He pulled her arms through the sleeves. There was no turning back. She looked at the mirror and was flabbergasted at the transformation in her appearance. The hem fell almost to the floor and the skirt was wide enough to conceal her bare feet. The waist was a little loose, but otherwise the fit was perfect. She was still wearing her cloth underneath and it showed at the low cut neck.

"Remove it, remove it," said De Bruyn and when she didn't understand, lifted the skirt and tugged the cloth until it fell around her feet.

"Ah that is better," said De Bruyn, admiring the swell of her breasts which was now visible in the décolletage.

"Not too loose?" he asked, squeezing her waist, and buttoning her up. "If it is, we shall just have to fatten you up. You *are* a bit lean. Now let me have a good look."

"Amazing," he said as he took her hand and turned her round. "But your bald head!"

He rubbed the stubble which was beginning to emerge upon her scalp.

"I am sorry we had to shave you like this, my love. If only I had known. What cruelties you have suffered at my hands."

These thoughts were uncomfortable and unwelcome to him so he changed the subject of his conversation.

"Let me see if Elizabeth has a bonnet which would fit you," he said and bent to search the contents of the trunk.

Speaking his late wife's name aloud set his thoughts off on another disturbing track, but they had not travelled far when they were interrupted by a knock on the door. It was the steward to take the order for dinner.

*****

An hour later, there was another knock. When Hendrik Van Schalkwyk, Minister of the Dutch Reformed Church, Preacher and Chaplain of Elmina Castle, entered, the candles had been lit and the table had been laid for three.

Ama was sitting in a high backed armchair near a window, looking out over Edina and the ocean. The moon had risen early and over the shoulder of the massive castle it shone on the town.

"You have another guest this evening, Director?" Van Schalkwyk asked, pointing to the table and raising his eyebrows just a little.

"What, has the Castle Intelligence failed?" De Bruyn asked with a chuckle.

There wasn't much that happened in the small European male society of Elmina Castle that did not come to the Chaplain's attention. Besides rehashing old sermons for the twice weekly compulsory church services he had little else to do but collect idle gossip.

"Well, I must admit I have heard rumours. Unconfirmed, mind you," Van Schalkwyk replied with mild embarrassment, "but they certainly did not lead me to expect . . .?"

"Expect what, my good Minister?"

Apart from Jensen, De Bruyn and Van Schalkwyk were the only educated men in the Castle. For years the two of them had been meeting every Monday evening to dine, drink, smoke and indulge in the civilised pleasure of conversation. They invariably spoke their native Dutch but their talk was liberally laced with Latin, French, German and English. They had heard each other's stock of anecdotes and witticisms time without number but, since neither had any alternative, they exercised a mutual tolerance of repetition. When the conversation ran dry, as it usually did after some time, they would suck their pipes and settle down to a leisurely game of chess.

"Ah, Director, you have me in a corner," replied Van Schalkwyk. "I concede defeat."

"What will you drink, Hennie?" asked De Bruyn, knowing well what the answer would be, but asking all the same. In private, he called the Minister by his first name. Since his childhood, no one, except Elizabeth, had called De Bruyn Pieter. He had considered extending that privilege to Van Schalkwyk but had never got round to making the suggestion. After all these years, it would be a little strange.

When they were comfortably settled, with drinks and pipes lit, Van Schalkwyk returned to the subject.

"Where . . . ?"

He hesitated and made another attempt.

"Where is the . . .?" but was again unable to complete his sentence.

"You are singularly inarticulate this evening, Hendrik," said De Bruyn. "What was the word you were looking for: wench? woman? lady? Wife, perhaps?"

Without waiting for a reply, he indicated the back of Ama's chair with a nod of his head.

"Miss Pamela," he said, "is contemplating the beauty of the African moonlight shining on the noble city of Edina and on the Atlantic Ocean beyond."

Ama heard her name, the name De Bruyn had given her. They must be discussing her. *How am I going to manage this meal?* she wondered. Eating alone with one white man had been difficult enough; eating with two promised to be infinitely more complicated. They would surely talk about her in her presence and she would not understand a word. She would guess what they were saying, of course. But what *would* they say? Would Mijn Heer describe their afternoon's lovemaking to his friend? Or would they just ignore her presence? She wished she could eat apart, but De Bruyn had made it quite clear, with the assistance of the Fanti steward who had laid the table, that he insisted on her presence.

She looked out. Cooking fires twinkled dimly in the town. Flickering shadows played on the mud walls. Dark figures went about their business. A woman sang. Another shouted an admonition to a child. Indistinct conversations floated up over the roar of the surf. All over the land black people were preparing and eating their evening meals in similar manner. So it had been in Yendi and Kafaba and Kumase and in all the small villages where she had spent a night on her long journey to the coast. So it was in her father Tigen's hamlet and all over the Bekpokpam country.

She had been thinking in Asante but when she thought of Tabitsha, she began to think in her mother tongue. *I will forget my own language,* she thought. *It will die in my mind from disuse.*

"Pamela," called De Bruyn, "will you not come and join us?"

Ama rose slowly. She had rejected the bonnet which De Bruyn had offered her and instead tied a silk *doek* which they had found in the trunk to cover her shaven scalp. The dead woman's dress (for such she took it to be) smelled slightly of mould and naphtha, but the smell was obscured by the civet he had sprinkled on her. Several visits to the looking glass had left her feeling more at ease with her new appearance. De Bruyn had tried to fit her feet into a pair of his late wife's shoes, but the foot of a female slave who has walked many weary miles on her own tough soles is very different from that of the idle lady wife of a Director General of the Westindische Compagnie; and so, under her spreading skirt, Ama's feet remained unshod.

Sensing her diffidence, De Bruyn approached her and presented his elbow for her to grasp. However, he had not yet taught her that particular trick and he had to show her how to take his arm. The Minister watched with some amusement,

"May I present," De Bruyn said to her, "Mijn Heer Hendrik Van Schalkwyk, Minister of Religion in the Dutch Reformed Church and Chaplain to the European residents of this Castle?"

Van Schalkwyk wondered whether his part in this charade required him to kiss the hand of this slave girl. He decided against and merely bowed slightly from his ample waist. The girl's appearance was undoubtedly striking, he thought. *De Bruyn, you lucky old lecher, how did you find such a jewel in amongst all the dross and dregs of dark humanity which enters these walls?*

"Hendrik, this is Miss Pamela," De Bruyn continued with the introduction.

Van Schalkwyk bowed again. For a moment they were at a loss for conversation.

"Please be seated," said De Bruyn and drew a chair for Ama, indicating with a movement of his head that she should sit.

They were beginning to understand each other's body language, he noted with satisfaction.

When the first course had been served and the wine had been poured, he said, "As yet, the wench neither speaks nor understands a word of Dutch, nor, so far as I can judge, any other civilised tongue. You need not, therefore, inhibit you sparkling conversation in any way."

He turned to Ama.

"Pamela, I am telling the reverend Minister that we do not share a common language and that he may speak without fear of embarrassing you."

Ama sensed that they were playing a little game and that the game was being played at her expense. She caught his eye with a look that mixed appeal and mild reproof. They had made love together that afternoon, she told him. Twice indeed. In their passion they had been equals. He should not mock her now before a third party. De Bruyn read her message and dropped his eyes. She was right, he had betrayed her. He looked up and apologised. She read his silent message and nodded her head ever so slightly in acknowledgement. De Bruyn felt profoundly excited. They needed no words to communicate. He wanted to be alone with her, to embrace her, to kiss her on the lips.

Van Schalkwyk busied himself with his food and wine, attempting to convey that he had observed nothing of this. In fact he had witnessed the confidential eye contact and was attempting to fathom its meaning. His dissemblance was unnecessary for his two dinner partners had for a brief moment been unaware of his existence.

"Pamela?" he asked. "That is not a common Dutch name. Presumably she did not bring it with her? You gave it to her?"

He stole a glance at the girl. She had dropped her eyes. *She is indeed pretty*, he thought, seeing her through De Bruyn's eyes and feeling suddenly very lonely. Van Schalkwyk had a reputation in the Castle as something of a dirty old man. His penchant for making accidental body contact with female slaves and, believing no one else to be watching, for grabbing their buttocks or their breasts, had not gone unobserved. He was inhibited, however, from taking a concubine by fear of the consequences of breaching Company rules, by fear moreover that his status in the Castle would be undermined and by the certainty that eternal damnation would be his reward for fornication. Minister Van Schalkwyk led a secret life of unconsummated sexual fantasy.

"English," said De Bruyn. "Surely I have told you of the book of that name I have been reading? Samuel Richardson the author. It is one that Captain Williams brought me."

"Ah, yes, I do recall." replied Van Schalkwyk. "Pamela is a maid-servant, not so? And she sets out to marry her employer?"

"Not exactly, but that is the book," said De Bruyn, looking at Ama and hoping that she would not misconstrue the continuing use of her name. Van Schalkwyk understood his host's tone of voice to discourage further discussion on the matter.

The two white men continued to talk in a desultory way about matters of no great consequence, washing down the five course meal with healthy draughts of Rhenish wine. Ama had eaten greedily the day before but the gnawing hunger had now passed and she left food on her plate in spite of De Bruyn's urging. She had also learned the effect of the wine and gave him no chance to recharge her glass.

"She doesn't like our chef's cooking," said Van Schalkwyk, but De Bruyn again changed the subject.

The table was cleared and Ama had time to observe the two men as they re-lit their pipes. Her Mijn Heer was long and thin, scrawny even. In the flickering candlelight, his features appeared even more gaunt than they did by day. He seemed depressed. She had put him down and she was sorry. Yet, she told herself, if she were to consolidate her hold on him, and to do that seemed essential if she were to survive, she had to obtain his regard for her dignity. His carnal desire for her might not last long and he had the power to discard her without ceremony in much the same way as he had had her plucked from the dungeon. It was risky but she must insist on his respect. She must keep something back, so that he never felt that he had fully possessed her. He was old but he could be good to her. She could see in his eyes his passion for her. She might even grow to love him. Not like she had loved Itsho, never like that. She wondered again whether Itsho had sent his spirit to possess the man and make him love her. She would show Mijn Heer some of the things she and Itsho had done together. She smiled at the thought and De Bruyn saw the smile and, not knowing about Itsho, smiled back. A white man! What would Tabitsha say if she knew her daughter had a white man as a lover! And her father! They had never even seen a white man.

The other man was short and fat. Indeed he was obese, almost obscenely corpulent. He reminded her of one of the eunuchs at the Asantehene's court. She wondered if his balls, too, had been cut off; if there were perhaps some causal relationship between castration and obesity. His chin cascaded down in fold upon fold of fat. Even his eyes were surrounded by fatty tissue, so that they seemed to look out through a tunnel. She was sure that when he stood up straight he would not be able to see his own feet. His skin was sallow, almost translucent. He did not look unkind but she could not be sure whether he would be her friend or her enemy. If he was Mijn Heer's friend it was important that he should be hers too. What was his name? She had forgotten.

De Bruyn got up to go and piss, leaving the two of them alone together.

Ama pointed to herself and said, "Pamela."

Then she pointed at the fat man's chest and, with a coquettish smile, inquired what he was called.

The Minister was successively astonished, amused at her boldness, and entranced by her smile.

"My name?" he replied with a chuckle. "Well since you are so charming, you may call me *Henk*. But only in privacy, mind you. In public you must call me *Minister*."

He pointed at the wall and then described a circle with his index finger. Then he pointed at the floor and then to himself.

"Henk," he said.

Though she was not quite sure what it meant, Ama reproduced his sign language and then pointed again at him.

"Henk," she repeated.

Van Schalkwyk's heart fluttered at hearing his name on her lips and he chuckled again.

"Young lady, you are not only beautiful, you clearly also have brains," he said. "Now see if you can understand this."

He pointed again, outside the room, far away.

"In public," he said, repeating the gesture, and then pointing again to himself, "you must call me *Minister*. In public, *Minister*. Do you understand?"

Again Ama did not quite understand but she mimicked his gesture and repeated the second name he had given himself. *If I have three names*, she thought, *it must be all right for him to have two.*

"What's all this now?" asked De Bruyn, reappearing at the end of this conversation.

"Never you mind," said Van Schalkwyk, enjoying his little conspiracy with Ama, "that is between the two of us."

*****

"Pamela," said De Bruyn, "would you be so kind as to fetch us the chess board?"

He had laid it on the writing cabinet before dinner and he now pointed it out to her. She sent him an inquiring glance as she picked up the folded board.

"And the box too, please," he told her.

"That's a clever girl," he praised her. "Now pull up your chair and watch us."

The board was just like that the Asante used for playing draughts, she noted, but with only eight squares along each side, rather than ten.

"Your turn with the whites tonight, Hennie," said De Bruyn as he tumbled the pieces onto the board, "I'll take the Africans."

Ama had expected to see a game of draughts, but these tokens were unlike any draughts she had seen.

"Now, Pamela, watch this," he told her as he laid out the black pieces. "First the two castles: we also call them rooks. Then the knights, looking like horses - do you know what a real horse looks like? Not many of those in this part of Africa, eh Hennie?"

Bedagbam, thought Ama, taking a knight and examining it. *Abdulai*. She put it down and clenched her fists, her finger nails cutting into her palms, at the recollection of the man who had raped her.

"Next the bishops. Priests if you like, but not Hennie's kind, eh? Now watch closely. This is the king. Like me at Elmina."

He puffed himself up in jest and beat his chest, to demonstrate his importance.

"*Ohene*," said Van Schalkwyk, using one of his few Fanti words.

Ama nodded vigorously. The pieces had been made in Batavia. De Bruyn had acquired them during his tenure at the Cape. She was fascinated by the intricate carving.

"Always on the right," continued De Bruyn, showing her first the correct disposition of the king and queen, then exchanging them and indicating his displeasure; and finally placing them back in their correct positions.

Van Schalkwyk repeated the demonstration.

"I wonder if she knows her left from her right," he ventured.

"And these are the pawns, the foot soldiers, the slaves if you like. There to take orders, one step at a time."

Then they demonstrated to her the various moves which the pieces might make. Ama screwed up her face in concentration. She had become quite skilful at oware and draughts while she was in Kumase, but this game was quite different, each piece had its own rules.

De Bruyn got to his feet and demonstrated the knight's legal moves.

"Two steps forward and one to the right. Or to the left."

He was already quite tipsy and staggered and almost fell.

"It is quite complicated when you try to explain it, not so, Henk? I doubt if she will pick it up," he said as he recovered his seat.

"Director, before we start to play, there is something which I have to say to you," said Van Schalkwyk.

"Yes, I know. Fornication. The consequence of which is eternal damnation. Not to speak of the regulations of the noble Company regarding the taking of concubines. I have been waiting for you to summon up the courage to tackle the subject. Let us just take it all as said, shall we? I have heard it all before. I promise to pray to God to forgive me for my weakness. Now play," replied De Bruyn.

Relieved of any obligation to say more on the subject, Van Schalkwyk made his opening move. As the game progressed, Ama watched, transfixed. Flattered and amused by her interest, each player explained each move to her as he made it, confident that he was giving away nothing that his opponent did not already know.

Where games are concerned, the rules of chess may be quite complicated; but, considered as a language, chess is easier to learn than Dutch. Ama watched each player as he deliberated on the next move and screwed up her eyes in concentration as the move was explained to her. The spoken words were superfluous: a finger pointed out a threatened line of attack by a bishop, or the alternative possibilities open to a knight. Only when the Minister castled, exchanging the white king and its rook, was she confused, but she set that move aside in her mind for future study. As pieces were taken, they gave them to her to keep in the box. *Itsho,* she thought, as a black pawn was taken by a white knight, *poor Itsho.* When there were only a few pieces left on the board, they explained the developing end game to her. Her mind reeled with complications as she tried to see the consequences of each possible move. She left her chair and kneeled on the floor beside De Bruyn.

His king was under attack. Ama perceived the threat. It was De Bruyn's move.

"Mijn Heer," she said to him and showed him with her outstretched finger how his queen could take off a threatening white knight.

"Pamela," he replied, his eyes wide in astonishment, and suddenly took her face in his hands and kissed her on the lips.

He had forgotten Van Schalkwyk's presence. Now he covered his embarrassment by demonstrating to Ama that the move she had suggested was not quite as clever as she had thought and would certainly lead to the loss of his queen. His position was indeed irrecoverable. Soon the Minister was calling *Check!* at every move and finally *Checkmate!*

"Check," said Ama, "Checkmate!" looking at De Bruyn with sympathy and the two men laughed.

In the excitement of the game she had lost all her reserve. Now she was shy again.

"Another?" suggested Van Schalkwyk.

De Bruyn yawned and stretched his arms.

"No thank you," he replied. "That's enough for one session. But let's have a night-cap."

He poured the two cognacs as Ama put the chess things back in their place. When she came back he offered her a sip from his glass. The liquor was too strong for her and she screwed up her face and shook her head when she had tasted it. They laughed. The couple's obvious intimacy increased Van Schalkwyk's loneliness. He gulped down the brandy which he had been swilling round his mouth.

"Director-General," he said, "you have discovered a young woman of astonishing intelligence. I have never before come across such a clever black, let alone a female."

"Well, you don't have much to do with the natives," said De Bruyn. "And what about Augusta? You know Augusta, don't you?"

"Of course I know Augusta," replied Van Schalkwyk, "and I admit that she is clever, and especially quick, so I am told, when it comes to business. But Augusta is an older woman with a lifetime of contact with Europeans and their ways. She speaks some Dutch, but can she read or write? She can reckon, no doubt, but has she learnt to keep books of account? And can you imagine Augusta mastering chess, as Pamela seems to have done, by watching a single game?"

"Well, no, I must admit that chess is not Augusta's style. What exactly are you suggesting, though?"

Van Schalkwyk had suggested nothing but De Bruyn had read his mind.

"Well, no doubt Miss Pamela will soon pick up Dutch from you. Indeed, probably more quickly than we whites seem to be able to pick up Fanti. However, I think you might consider also teaching her to read, perhaps even to write and figure arithmetic."

"What would be the benefit of that?" asked De Bruyn.

"Well," replied Van Schalkwyk, improvising, since he had not yet considered the implications of his suggestion, "it would be an interesting experiment. I mean, to see just how much she can absorb and how quickly. She could read to you. And in the course of time, she might be brought to receive the grace and salvation of Our Lord."

"No," said De Bruyn, "I am no schoolmaster and I would not have the time."

Jensen, he thought, would waste little time in getting back to the Ten a message that Director-General De Bruyn was spending several hours a day teaching a slave girl to read and write. He could imagine the consequences. Then he had a brain-wave.

"*You* would have to teach her. It would do you good. You have plenty of time on your hands. But if she is to read to me, you would have to teach her English, not Dutch. All I read in Dutch is correspondence from Amsterdam. For relaxation I read only English and a little French. De Foe, Richardson, Fielding and of course Shakespeare and Milton; there is nothing in Dutch to match them. We can teach our neighbours across the Channel a thing or two when it comes to painting pictures and, of course, trade, but you have to admit it, we have not produced a single writer in Dutch who can match the English."

He had a pleasant mental picture of Pamela reading to him each afternoon while he sat back, relaxed, and smoked his pipe. Then they would talk about the book. In spite of his education, Van Schalkwyk was not much of a reader. *What use is a good book,* De Bruyn thought, *if you cannot share your pleasure in it with another?*

Van Schalkwyk needed no convincing. He anticipated with secret joy the prospect of spending several hours each day with Pamela. The arrangements were quickly made. Augusta would call each morning to train the girl to perform her domestic duties. In mid-morning, the Minister would take over and teach her spoken English, reading and writing. If that proved successful he would teach her also to count and do simple arithmetic. De Bruyn would speak to her henceforth only in English. The Minister would pay a visit the very next day to Cape Coast, there to solicit from the Rev. Philip Quaque, who conducted lessons for a small group of mulatto children in his rooms in Cape Coast Castle, an English primer and simple reading materials.

"Just tell Jensen to fix you up with a hammock and bearers," said De Bruyn, "and don't forget to convey my greetings to the English governor."

Ama could make nothing of this conversation, though she realised that it concerned her. She was suffused with the excitement and stimulation of her first encounter with chess. After Van Schalkwyk had left, they quickly undressed and went to bed. She hugged De Bruyn tightly and kissed his lips in innocent gratitude.

CHAPTER 16

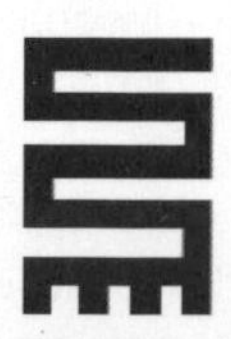

One morning, while Van Schalkwyk was still in Cape Coast, De Bruyn sent for Augusta.

They shook hands formally and exchanged greetings. He asked after her health and that of her husband and her children. For a while, they talked business, about cloth and the glut of slaves. Then De Bruyn reached for his pipe. Augusta shifted her weight on the narrow wooden chair.

"Well," he asked, "what do you think?"

"Think about what, Mijn Heer?" she asked innocently.

"About the girl, Pamela," he replied.

"Oh," said Augusta. "The girl. Well, she is quite pretty; a bit bush, but all the *donkos* are like that. On the other hand she learns quickly and she is polite and obedient. A good girl, I would say. But why do you ask?"

"Oh, Augusta, you know how I value your opinion and how I rely on your advice. Were we not once man and wife?"

"How is she . . .?" Augusta asked, looking him in the eye and screwing up her face in an attempt at a wink.

De Bruyn coloured. It amused Augusta to make him blush.

"Oh, that," he replied. "Augusta, no woman has been so good for me."

"Not since you, of course," he hastened to add. "You know, Elizabeth was like a stone in bed."

Are all white women like that? Augusta wondered. *If they had some of their own women here, would they still chase after our girls as much as they do?*

"Ah, Elizabeth," she replied.

Elizabeth was the only white woman she had ever got to know at close quarters and she had not been impressed. As for herself, she had been fifteen when her father had sent her to live with the young De Bruyn and eighteen when he had left for the Cape. She had given him the years of her prime. But that was long ago.

"Augusta, I am going to get Rev. Van Schalkwyk to teach her to read and write. What do you think?"

Augusta was surprised.

"I am not a fit one to answer that question, Mijn Heer. Teach her to understand Dutch, by all means. But what good will it do a *donko* girl like that to read and write? When you have finished with her, you will sell her like the rest and send her over the sea."

"No, Augusta. This girl is different. She may be a slave, but I really love her. If she learns to read and write and becomes a Christian, I might even marry her. What would you say to that?"

"Let me tell you a story, Mijn Heer. After you left me, all those years ago, and went to the Cape, there came a young black man by name of Capitein, Jacobus Capitein. One of your people had bought him when he was a child and taken him home with him. When he was grown the Company sent him here as chaplain. He set up a school for some children in this very castle. The new Director then, de Pettersen, had brought his wife with him, and he put his own two small daughters in the school. The rest were mainly castle offspring. Poor Capitein. He tried to teach them reading and writing and Christian matters, but the children preferred to play on the beach. My father wanted me to go to the school, but I refused. I said I was already a married woman."

And she thought, *even though you, my husband, had abandoned me.*

"Capitein? I have seen the name in the old files. When I first arrived here, the chaplain was a man called Ketelanus. Do you remember him? He was a bad influence. On Sundays he would preach the word of our Lord in the church and the rest of the week he would spend fornicating with the female slaves. Like Jensen. The company had to sack him. He was bad for discipline. Then there was no chaplain at all. Not until I left.

"Capitein, eh? What happened to him in the end?"

"Trouble, trouble; poor man. He wanted to marry my sister, Ekua Amankwaa, the second daughter of my mother's brother. My uncle was willing, but Capitein said he must first send the girl to Holland to learn to be a Christian. Ekua was her mother's only daughter and the mother would not let her go. So the Company sent him a white girl from Holland instead, Antonia she was called. Not that that did him much good. Some of the whites did not like having a black man preaching to them about fornication with black women. They said he was sending reports about them to Holland. No doubt they were jealous that the Company had sent him a wife, and a white woman at that, while they were not even allowed to go into the town at night. You know what I mean? Especially one Hubert van Rijk. He was another scum, like your Jensen. He used to get drunk and then he would abuse Capitein. Capitein wanted to leave the work, but the Company wouldn't agree. He was an unhappy man. He did not hear Fanti well and our people treated him as if he were a white man. But the whites, except for the Director himself, treated him like a black.

"Then he started trading; but he was a bad businessman and he soon got into debt. Next thing he fell ill and died and that was the end of Capitein. His grave is in your cemetery. I think they sent the wife back to Holland."

"What happened to his school?"

"It died with him. Some of his pupils are still in the town. Sister Ekua is there too. They have forgotten everything he taught them, except a few Dutch words. Christianity is good for you whites. As for us, we already have Tweneboa, the spirit of the Benya and seventy six other gods in our town and that is enough."

"But what do you think might go wrong if I taught Pamela to read and write?"

"I am not saying that anything would go wrong. It might even keep her out of mischief. Mijn Heer, you know you are not as young as you once were. She is a pretty girl. I wouldn't let Jensen get anywhere near her."

"Ag, Jensen, never mind him. Anyway I shall let her stay in my room for the time being. By the way, we have decided to teach her English, not Dutch. Then she will be able to read my books to me. Will you try to explain all this to her, please?"

Augusta thought, *he will spoil this girl, teaching her to read books, putting ideas into her head and then throwing her out when he is tired of her. As for men, they are like children; and we women are their playthings.*

But she left these thoughts unspoken and took her leave.

She had completely forgotten her promise to talk to De Bruyn about Esi. By the time Ama summoned up her courage to remind her, Esi had been sold and shipped to God knows where.

*****

"Ah, Hendrik, back from your travels?" De Bruyn greeted Van Schalkwyk on Monday evening.

"I missed you at Church yesterday, Director," replied the Minister.

"Ah, Church, yes," De Bruyn dissembled. "I was a little, um, indisposed.

"What will you drink, Hennie?" he continued, closing the discussion on that subject and busying himself with the decanters.

As he poured the drinks, he recalled the lazy Sunday morning spent with his Pamela.

"Well, what have you brought from our English friends?" asked the Governor.

"Greetings. The English Governor expressly asked me to convey his warmest respects to you."

"The hypocrite!" interjected De Bruyn.

"And also from Philip Quaque. A charming young man and most hospitable, I must say. Highly educated too. He had an English wife, you know, Madam Catherine, they called her."

"Ah, yes. She came to visit Elizabeth once, but they didn't get on."

"She was an educated woman, it seems, and helped him with his school, but she died after only a year on the Coast. A lonely woman, I gather. She had no friends of her own sex, indeed no friends at all besides her husband. And he has few enough. He mourns her still, though he has remarried. A lonely man, Quaque, too. He despises his own people for the heathens that they are. He is really a kind of black Englishman. He says the English tongue was sent by heaven as a medium for religion and civilisation. On that account he will not use his native Fanti and indeed he claims that he can no longer speak it or understand it.

"Now the English . . . Well the English are an uncouth lot if you ask me. The Governor is an irreligious man. Quaque tells me that he loses no chance to undermine his position as chaplain and will suspend divine service on a Sunday on the slimmest of pretences. He certainly did not attend last Sunday. But," and Van Schalkwyk paused, "then neither did you, Director, yesterday!"

"I know the English governor," said De Bruyn, ignoring the last comment, "and I cannot say that I like him. But what about our little project? Was Quaque able to help?"

"Aha!" he exclaimed as Van Schalkwyk opened the buckle of a leather satchel he had brought with him and began to extract a small hoard of books.

"The late Madam Catherine," said Van Schalkwyk, "purchased a large number of children's books in London. Her intention was to use them in the school. However, Quaque regards most of them as frivolous and unsuitable for educational use. He says he prefers to use religious texts for his teaching. He agreed to let me take them all and added some more serious volumes of which he has several copies. Like all of us, he complains that he is short of money and I therefore took the liberty, on your behalf, and knowing your love of books of all descriptions, of purchasing them from him. Here is the bill."

De Bruyn raised his eyebrows.

"Let me see the books," he said, impatiently.

The Minister handed them to him one by one.

"*A New Playbook for Children,*" De Bruyn read aloud, "*Or an Easy and Natural Introduction to the Art of Reading, in which is Introduced a Great Variety of Providential and Proverbial Maxims with Several Little Moral Tales and Fables in Prose and Verse in order to Render their Little Lessons a Diversion rather than a Task.*"

He paused for breath and then continued, "*The Whole Embellished with a New Set of Initial Letters Containing the Whole Alphabet* - aha, that's what we need; and now here is a little poem:

"The Cynic Tutor fruitless lectures reads.

"He who gilds o'er his Precepts, best Succeeds.

"An excellent philosophy which, it would seem, your friend Quaque might well practice, and you too, if you please, Hennie. *Printed and sold by Thomas Harris, Bookseller and Stationer in Aldergate East, Seventeen Hundred and Forty Nine.* Well, not exactly the latest edition. *Price six pence.* In that case, we can hardly complain, can we?

"Now what is this? *Mr. Weston's New and Compendious Treatise of Arithmetic.* Well I suggest that you leave the arithmetic for a later date. Concentrate on the reading. But this is not frivolous stuff. By no stretch of the imagination. What can the man mean?"

Van Schalkwyk preferred to let that question pass.

"Look at this curious chapbook," he said, "published by one John Newbery. *The History of Goody Two Shoes; otherwise called Mrs. Margery Two-Shoes with the Means by which she Acquired her Learning and Wisdom, and in consequence thereof, her Estate.*"

"Well, now, *her estate*, you say?" asked De Bruyn. "That might be a somewhat premature ambition to plant in the breast of an illiterate slave girl, don't you think? Let me look at that, please. Ah, you missed something, Hennie, you old devil you. It says here *From the original manuscript in the Vatican at Rome, and the cuts by Michael Angelo.* What! Papist propaganda and at a price of just six pence? Now what is one to make of that? Let me see the rest, please.

"But this is a treasure trove, Hennie. You deserve a promotion. Do you know, I am going to sit down and read all of these myself? Yes, and I shall recommend to the Company that they create a new post of Archbishop of Elmina, especially for you."

"You should not make fun of the Reformed Church, Director. I have two books left. Look at this one."

"Hennie, Hennie. *A History of Pamela, or Virtue Rewarded. Abridged from the works of Samuel Richardson, Esq.*"

Ama, who had been busy ironing De Bruyn's linen, came up, hesitated when she thought she heard the name De Bruyn had given her, and then curtsied shyly to Van Schalkwyk.

"Well?" De Bruyn asked her.

"Good morning, sir," she stuttered the rehearsed reply and, giggling, covered her face with her hands.

"Excellent, excellent, my child," replied Van Schalkwyk, applauding.

"Good *evening*," De Bruyn frowned at her.

"Never mind, never mind. An excellent beginning. Morning or evening, what is the difference? The finer points will come with time. Show the girl the book."

"Pamela, this is your very own book. See your name on it, P-A-M-E-L-A," De Bruyn said to her.

Ama looked at the book, understood nothing, and looked at De Bruyn for enlightenment; but his attention was already engaged in the prize which Van Schalkwyk had kept for last.

"Look at this now: an English bible, *The Authorised Version of King James the First* it says on the frontispiece, bound in fine black leather and brand new by the look of it. See, the pages are still uncut. There is no charge for this: it is Quaque's personal gift. He has a considerable stock of these."

"Oh, I'll have that, if you please," said De Bruyn. "It will be some time before Pamela is ready to tackle the Holy Book. In fact, you keep the primer and the copy book and leave the rest with me. Minister, I congratulate you on a task completed with a success beyond my expectations."

He stood up and formally shook Van Schalkwyk's hand, while Ama looked on puzzled.

"I shall send Rev. Quaque his gold dust tomorrow morning."

Miming the action of ringing a bell, he said, "Pamela, will you ring for dinner, please?"

"What about the school at Cape Coast?" he asked,

"It is a hardly a school, Director. Quaque has six mulatto children come to his own rooms each morning and there they learn the elements of reading and a little writing for a few hours. He drills them in the catechism of course, but, determined as he is, he is also deeply pessimistic about the prospects of introducing Christianity to the Fantis. I have to say that I agree with him. Their heathenish beliefs and customs are so deeply ingrained that they are not easily shifted."

*****

"Good morning, sir," Ama greeted Augusta the following morning, practising the English which De Bruyn had been teaching her.

"What do you say, child?" the older woman asked her in Fanti.

"Ah yes," she continued when Ama had explained, "Mijn Heer told me that he planned to teach you English. But you are wasting it on me. I hear enough Dutch, but as for English: at all. English is for Cape Coast people, not for Edinas. I do not understand the way these whites' minds work. Why English, after all? He could tell you all you need to know with a few words of Dutch, surely?"

She shook her head and eased herself into an armchair.

"Sit," she said, and indicated to Ama that she should take the leather footstool.

"Young woman," she said, "Mijn Heer has spoken to me about you. I have been thinking about what he said. You are nothing to me, a stranger, do you hear? But I like you. You have made a good impression on me. You are young and can have had little experience of men; and none of white men. You are far from your family and you have no mother to advise you. So I have decided to speak to you of what is in my mind. You may listen to what I have to say, or you may close your ears to it. I know, that is the way of the young. Each generation must learn by making its own mistakes. But you are in a perilous situation which you might not recognise and it would be wise for you to hear me out. Do you understand?"

Attentive, but puzzled, Ama nodded her assent.

"Mijn Heer is not a young man. He is old enough to be your father, or even your grandfather. To live to such an age is quite unusual for a white man in Africa. This our climate does not suit them well. Many of those who come here die within months, sometimes weeks. I have heard them call Africa the white man's grave. It must be something in the air. Perhaps it is the fevers which they say rise from our swamps; or perhaps it is our gods and the spirits of our ancestors who strike them down. It is worse with their women and that is perhaps why they so seldom bring them to our country. Mijn Heer's Elizabeth lasted just a year."

Ama watched Augusta attentively, concentrating on making sense of the Fanti words which were strange to her.

"Be that as it may," continued the older woman, "I must tell you, if you do not already know, that the man is in love with you."

Ama lowered her eyes.

"Men are strange. Mijn Heer was like that with me too, many years ago. While their passion lasts, they are ruled by it; they will kill for it, even kill themselves.

"But that is today only. In a few years Mijn Heer will be too old for this work. He will go back to his own country. What will happen to you then? He says that if you learn to read and write, and become a Christian, he might marry you. I doubt if he has given any thought to how it would be for him to take a black wife back to his country. Or how it would be for the woman, all alone in strange surroundings, with none of her own kind to turn to for comfort and support when the man turns sour. Moreover, I have never heard of a white man who took his black wife home with him. When the time comes, I do not believe that Mijn Heer would decide to take you with him. And even if he did, what would happen to you? Mijn Heer is old. When he dies, what would happen to you, I ask you again, left alone in the country of the Dutch? Who would look after you then? Do not imagine that you could return to Africa, all alone. Holland is many months' journey across the sea."

Augusta paused. Ama's mind was in a turmoil. Augusta had put into words the vague concerns which already lay there, confused and suppressed. She was in no way the mistress of her fate. Augusta had forced her to face up to reality. It was a comfort, at least, to have someone to talk to about her worries.

"Maame Augusta, what should I do?" she asked in a low, troubled voice.

"You are a slave, my child. You are his property. He can do with you as he pleases. The only hold you have on him is this love that has grown in him for you. If he tires of you, you are lost. You must nurture that love. First in the physical sense. You understand what I mean? Mijn Heer, forgive me, is a fool. You have not told me what your feelings are for him, but whatever they are, I can say that to you. That is my privilege. He was my husband once. I say, Mijn Heer is a fool.

He imagines that he is young again. His love for you has made him think that. But he is no longer young. And when men get old they lose some of their powers, you understand?"

Ama thought for a moment of her dead lover, Itsho, and of Satila, the dried out old man who was to have been her husband. Mijn Heer was much older even than Satila.

"You must help him. You must hide his age from him. You must nurture his passion for you. You must pander to his every wish. You must flatter his male pride. You must be diligent in learning his language and his ways. You must never encourage the attention of any other man, especially a younger man. You must do all these things without revealing your motives. You may not love him, yet you must never let him doubt that you do. If you do grow to love him, which you may well do, for he is a kind and gentle man, if you do grow to love him, you must always keep something back. Never forget for one moment that he is a free man and you are his property, his slave. You must do all this to gain power over him, to make him feel that he cannot live without you. When you have achieved this, and only then, you must ask him to grant you your freedom. Manumission they call it. It is not enough for him to agree. He must make public announcements, in the castle and in the town, so that it is known to all. And he must give you the proper paper. This will be a dangerous time for you. Only you can judge the best time. You must not ask him too soon and you must not wait too long, until his passion for you begins to cool, or until another woman takes his fancy. He will want to know why you ask for your freedom. He will suspect that you want to leave him for another man. Somehow, you must reassure him.

"Once you have achieved this, you will be free to make your own decision, whether to go with him to Holland if he asks you, or whether to stay behind. If you decide to stay behind, I will help you. I have finished. Have you anything to say?"

Ama kneeled before Augusta and bowed her head.

"Maame, I bend my knee to you. I thank you. I shall try to do as you advise."

"Get up my child. Now get on with your work," replied the older woman.

"Maame . . ." Ama paused.

"Yes my child. Speak out."

Augusta felt suddenly tired.

"Maame. If I do all these things; if Mijn Heer were to give me my freedom," and she paused again.

"Yes, yes?"

Ama summoned the courage to speak what was in her heart.

"Would I then be able to return to my own home and family, to my own mother?"

Augusta laughed, but there was little joy in her laughter.

"Young woman, you cannot cross a river until you have reached its bank. What is the point of searching for a canoe when you are still so far away? But I will answer you. You yourself, you know how far you have come to reach this place. Could you find your own way back to Kumase, or wherever else you come from? Through the forests, across the mighty rivers. Who would protect you? And, travelling without protection, what chance would you have of arriving without being captured and sold into slavery once more? In Edina, with Mijn

Heer's paper and my word, your freedom would be guaranteed. But even half a day's journey from the sea, Mijn Heer's writ is worthless. And my word too. You must wipe that dream from your mind. You will never see your mother again.

"Don't cry my child. I know my words are cruel, but when you think on them, you will realise that they are true. Act on my advice. I have set you a difficult task. Work at it. Do not waste your energy on dreaming idle dreams."

CHAPTER 17

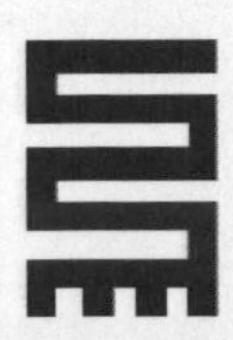

"A was an Archer, and shot at a Frog," said Van Schalkwyk, pointing to the picture in the primer.

Ama looked at the picture. It was nonsense. Who ever heard of shooting frogs with a bow and arrow?

"Say after me, 'A was an Archer'," he repeated.

"A was an Archer," said Ama.

"Good. Now again. 'A was an Archer'," he demanded, pointing at the picture again.

"A was an Archer," said Ama again.

"Now what is this?" he asked, pointing to the 'A'.

Ama looked at his face, searching for guidance in his narrow eyes.

"A was an Archer," she tried.

She had already learned to recite the alphabet by heart, but she had no idea what the sounds meant.

"No," said the Predikant. "This is 'A' and that," pointing to the picture, "is 'Archer' A. A. A. Archer. Archer. Archer. Now try again. What is this?"

Again Ama looked at his face.

"You will not find the answer in my face," he said. "Look at the book. What is this?"

Ama looked at his face again.

"A?" she asked doubtfully.

Augusta had told her that Van Schalkwyk would be teaching her to read. She had a vague and inchoate idea that he would in some unfathomable manner reveal to her the hidden mysteries of books, much as the elders had learned, she knew not how, to understand the arcane secrets of the spirits of the earth and of the ancestors. She thought the sounds she was being induced to make were some sort of magic incantation in the language of the whites, a prelude, perhaps, to future investiture into the priesthood of those privileged to interpret the enigmas of the papers that speak.

"Again," demanded Van Schalkwyk, pointing at the letter.

Ama pondered. Here was a new sound, not far removed from the other two. What should she reply, 'A' or 'Archer' or 'again'?

"A," she guessed.

"Good girl. Good girl. You are beginning to get the hang of it," said Van Schalkwyk. "Now again."

So the drill started and so it went on. *A was an Archer, and shot at a Frog; B was a Blind-man, and led by a Dog; C was a Cut-purse, and liv'd in Disgrace; D was a Drunkard, and had a Red Face.* Ama narrowed her eyes in concentration. First Van Schalkwyk drilled her on each letter and its picture. Then he chose each of the four letters consecutively, then one at a time at random. After an hour, they were both exhausted, but Ama had acquired a skill, somewhat akin to that of an 'arithmetical' dog at a Dutch fair, trained to respond by one or two or three or four barks when its owner pointed to a number on a blackboard.

"That is enough of letters for the time being. Now we will proceed to more serious work," said the Predikant. "We will start with the English version of the Lord's Prayer. Now recite after me 'Our Father, which art in Heaven.'"

She felt her head would burst.

*****

The following morning Ama had forgotten everything she had learned the previous day.

The Predikant was disappointed but patient and she soon recovered the lost ground.

Day in, day out, they laboured at it, teacher and pupil, until she had the whole alphabet fixed in her memory.

De Bruyn would come into the room in the late afternoon and find her standing at one of the high windows looking out at the sun setting far beyond Edina town and practising her recitation of the Lord's Prayer, of which she still understood not a single word.

Ama was a constant source of amazement and joy to him. When she had finished, he would cry out "Amen," take her in his arms and kiss her fiercely on the lips.

He would misquote Goldsmith, "And still they gazed and still the wonder grew, that one small head could carry all she knew," and then he would undress her and she would undress him and they would make love in the great four poster bed.

The alphabet and the Lord's Prayer of the daily lessons were still mystical incantations to Ama. She imbibed them with steadfast devotion to the goals which Augusta had set her. At the same time she was absorbing, from living with De Bruyn, a very different English vocabulary, more practical and down to earth. It began in bed. He asked her to call him Pieter, but only, he warned her, when they were alone together. She soon learned the names he gave to all their private parts: *cunt* and *tits* and *nipples*, *prick* and *balls*, *arse*. Such inhibitions as she had soon fell away before her indiscriminate eagerness to learn. Speaking to her in English, De Bruyn, too, felt liberated from the weight of Calvinist sin which each Dutch word seemed to carry. Soon too she learned: *hair*, *skin*, *ears* and *nose*, *tongue* and *teeth*, *lips* and *cheeks* and *neck*, *hands* and *fingers* and *palms*, *thighs* and *knees* and *toes*. The verbs: *kiss*, *suck*, *lick*, *taste*, *smell*, *feel*, *stroke*, *caress*, *tickle*, *bite*, *want*, *need* and *love*; *piss* and *shit* and *fart*; *wash* and *dry* and *iron*; *dress* and *undress*; *sleep* and *dream*; *eat* and *drink*; and the names of all they ate and drank. The adjectives: *smooth*, *sweet*, *beautiful*, *ebony*, *young* (and *old*), *moist*, *dry*, *clever*. And the pronouns: *I*, *you*, *we*. And *inside* and *together* and *thank you*.

At first she heard the words and learned to understand them. Then slowly, tentatively, she began to speak them herself. Though she was shy, she had no shame. Itsho had never used the words of love in her own language. There was no need. She assumed that the custom of the whites was different and, following Augusta's advice, she spoke as De Bruyn spoke in the privacy of his bedroom. Soon, she gained in confidence and the words began to run into sentences. He had only to teach her the words once for her to learn how, when she was ready, she could rouse him to a final frenzied movement within her by calling out, "Oh fuck me, Pieter, fuck me, fuck me, fuck me!"

Of course Van Schalkwyk knew nothing of all this.

In the evening, when they had eaten, they would sit at the table with the candles flickering in their long silver candlesticks and Ama would rehearse her lessons for the next day, expecting De Bruyn to test and correct her work; but the Governor would soon grow bored and weary of the repetitive exercises which Van Schalkwyk had set her. The chaplain's teaching methods were little different from those he had suffered in his own school days and it did not occur to him to question them. He sat back, sucked his pipe contentedly and sipped his brandy. Then one evening, searching his small library for a book to read, he came across the children's story books which the Predikant had put aside, believing that Ama needed to master the alphabet before learning to read.

"Pamela, look at this," he said, taking his pipe from his mouth.

Sitting down beside her, he put his arm around her shoulder and kissed her fondly on her cheek.

Then he put Goody Two-Shoes on the table and said, "Let's see if you can read this."

Ama could recognise and recite all the letters of the alphabet, in both upper and lower case, but Van Schalkwyk's pedagogics had not yet conferred on her the ability to read a single word. She triumphantly picked out all the A's and B's she could find. To her disappointment, De Bruyn was not impressed.

"All right," said De Bruyn. "One step at a time. I'll read the story to you and we'll see how much you understand."

He read slowly in the candlelight. The story told of how Margery's father, Meanwell, was ruined by the wicked farmer Graspall and Sir Timothy Gripe, who turned him out of his home. Meanwell died from a violent fever and his wife from a broken heart a few days later, leaving Margery and her brother Tommy orphaned, living in barns and from what they could pick from hedges. A kind gentleman found Tommy a job as a sailor and the good Rev. Smith gave Margery a pair of shoes. Judging that Mr. Smith's goodness and wisdom arose from his great learning, Margery decided to learn to read. Known now as Goody Two-Shoes she was soon teaching other children. Eventually Tommy returned rich and Margery married Sir Charles Jones. After which they all lived happily ever after.

When he had read the last page of the little book, De Bruyn asked Ama, "Did you understand the story?"

Ama nodded enthusiastically.

"Then tell it to me in your own words."

Ama hung her head in shame. Her affirmative had been a lie. Parish meetings, financial ruin, legal expenses, a proper settlement and hedges and barns meant nothing to her. She had really understood very little.

Van Schalkwyk had been teaching Pamela for weeks and there was little to show for it. De Bruyn wondered whether their experiment was doomed to failure. He decided to start from scratch.

"This girl is called Margery," he said, pointing to the picture. "The story is about her. What is her name? Right, 'Margery.' Now this is the word for Margery. See, M-A-R, mar, G-E, ger, R-Y, ree. Mar-ge-ry, Margery. It has a big M at the beginning because it is the girl's name. Spell it. Good. Now say it again. Excellent. Now see whether you can find the word 'Margery' somewhere else in the story."

Ama screwed up her face and searched. Triumphantly she put a finger on the next instance of 'Margery' and raised her eyes to De Bruyn's.

"Excellent. Clever girl," he said and rewarded her with a kiss. "Now find another 'Margery.'"

At his first attempt, De Bruyn had, almost by accident, succeeded in conveying to Ama the idea that each printed word was a symbol for a spoken word. Soon she could read the first sentence. Within a week she could read the first page. From that point on there was no holding her. Comprehension was another matter, but even a strange concept such as *parish meeting* presented few problems when interpreted as a gathering of village elders.

De Bruyn had cut the pages of the English bible, Rev. Quaque's gift. He was reading a few chapters each evening. Sometimes he would read to himself, sometimes aloud, savouring the beauty of the language. Ama would listen, straining to understand, but her vocabulary was still too small and Mijn Heer read too fast for her. She heard the words flying past and struggled to catch one which she thought she recognised, but even as she did, the torrent of new words continued and the one which she had captured was also lost, carried away in the turbulent stream, without meaning, its context destroyed.

De Bruyn noticed her frustration and when she had mastered the children's stories, he started her on the first chapter of Genesis, a few verses each evening. He tried to explain to her the meaning of the words she could not understand. Some he could not understand himself, for though his English was good, he was not a native speaker of the language. Then he would make a search in Dr. Johnson's dictionary. Soon Ama learned how to use her knowledge of the order of the alphabet to find a difficult word in that marvellous book.

Ama's domestic tasks were as nothing to her. All her life she had worked. Work was part of her life. Even as a little girl, the games she had played were an imitation of her mother's work: carrying firewood or water on her head, hoeing in the groundnut farm, washing, cooking, carrying a baby on her back. And as she had grown up, the games had changed imperceptibly into the real thing. She had never given it a thought. Life was work. Men had their work and women had theirs. Tabitsha's example had taught her to work with joy. Now she danced and sang through the dusting and polishing of Mijn Heer's room and the washing and ironing of his clothes. She had no need to cook or wash dishes: for that the Governor had his own kitchen whose staff served him and his senior officers.

Soon Augusta needed to instruct her no more, but still she came most mornings, out of habit partly, but also because De Bruyn expected it. She, in turn, needed to retain her connection with her former husband. And the young slave girl exerted a strange fascination upon the older woman. Ama treated Augusta like a mother. She trusted her absolutely and had few secrets from her. She told her about her childhood, about her mother Tabitsha and her father, Tigen; about her small brother, Nowu; about their home and how they lived; about her capture; about Yendi and Kafaba and Kumase; but she did not tell her that she had worked in the Asantehene's palace and she invented a lie to explain why she had been sent to Elmina.

Of Itsho, too, she said nothing. She could not share her memory of him with anyone, not even with Augusta. She knew Itsho was dead. Had she not buried him herself? But she knew too that his spirit lived on in the place of the ancestors. Often, he appeared to her in her dreams. Almost always his spirit was kind and benevolent. But, in trying to rescue her, Itsho had died a sudden, brutal death and sometimes, especially when it was time for her period, she would see the hooves of Abdulai's horse rise in the air and come crashing down on Itsho's head, cracking his skull, scattering blood and brains. She would hear his last agonised scream and her own scream too, fading as she woke from the nightmare. De Bruyn, his sleep disturbed, would comfort her, but she would hardly notice his presence. How could she tell Augusta of all this?

The other subject which she could not bring herself to speak of to Augusta was Esi, her much loved friend. For she remembered that when she had asked Augusta to intercede with Mijn Heer on Esi's behalf, she had forgotten. Ama wondered where Esi was now. She felt guilty that she had been saved to live in comfort while Esi, whose only fault was that she had spoken up for Ama in Kumase, had been consigned to an unknown fate. Sometimes, her mind spoke in two voices, one telling her that there was no way in which she could have saved her friend, that both Augusta and Mijn Heer had been strangers to her at that time and that she had had no language then with which she might have communicated with the powerful white man. Yet still she felt guilty and could not bring herself to talk to either of them about her lost friend. The subject was too painful.

*****

Van Schalkwyk was a methodical man. Ama could now recite her alphabet from A to Z and she could identify each letter, both lower case and upper, and the word in the primer which was the clue to its sound.

She could recite the Lord's Prayer by heart and he had started her memorising the Articles of Faith. As she made progress, so grew his ambition to save her soul for Jesus Christ.

Van Schalkwyk had forgotten his intention to start to teach her to read using the children's books; indeed, obsessed as he was with using education as a tool for spiritual progress, he had forgotten all about those books. He pictured himself demonstrating his success with her to Rev. Quaque. If he could succeed with Pamela, if he could make a Christian of her, perhaps he would open a school of his own for the little native girls of Edina.

The bible lay open where De Bruyn had left it the previous evening.

"Pamela," said Van Schalkwyk, "this morning we are going to start reading. We will start at the beginning of the Holy Book, that is to say with Genesis Chapter 1, Verse 1. This is such an important event that I think we should say a prayer first. Let us pray together to mark the occasion and to ask the blessing of our Heavenly Father for our enterprise."

Van Schalkwyk transferred his bulky frame stiffly from the chair to a kneeling position before the table. Ama had never seen him do this before and she watched bemused. He noticed that she was still sitting on her chair.

"Come, do as I do," he said, pointing to the floor.

Ama complied. She watched him place his palms together and close his eyes.

"Our Father," he began but when he reached "Heaven" he noticed that he was praying alone. He stopped and made her put her palms together and close her eyes.

"Now, together. One, two, three. Our Father . . ." and they recited the Lord's Prayer together.

When they had finished with "Amen", the Minister struggled to get to his feet and Ama had to help him. *You are really very fat,* she thought. *I have never seen any one as fat as you. Though Augusta comes a close second.*

Van Schalkwyk read the first verse, "In the beginning God created the heaven and the earth," he intoned.

Then, pointing to the passage, he said, "Now you try."

Ama was already familiar with the story of Creation. She repeated, with only an occasional stumble, the passage that Van Schalkwyk had just read to her.

"And the earth was without form, and void; and darkness was upon the face of the deep," he continued, reading one sentence at a time and letting her read it after him.

When she had read, "And the evening and the morning were the first day," he motioned to her to continue, without waiting for him to read each sentence first.

The fat Predikant was astonished. This was far beyond his expectations. She was reading intelligibly from the Good Book at her first attempt, her very first attempt. It was a miracle. He hardly had to prompt her.

The first time Ama had read this with De Bruyn, she had tackled one word at a time, understanding some but not enough to extract more than the vaguest meaning from the passage. But by now she had read it so many times that she knew it practically by heart. Mijn Heer had patiently explained the meaning to her. Now she read quite fluently and appeared to Van Schalkwyk to understand what she was reading.

"A miracle, a miracle," the Minister whispered to himself in Dutch as he listened, watching her with rapt attention.

Ama was wearing a simple calico cloth wrapped around her under her armpits with one end tucked in to hold it in position. It had come a little loose as she rose from her knees and now it threatened to unwrap itself, slipping down to expose the upper part of her breasts. She needed to stand up to rewrap the cloth but all her attention was concentrated on her reading and she merely tucked the loose end in as a temporary measure.

Van Schalkwyk watched her unobserved. He saw her profile, her round bare shoulders: he looked down the exposed cleavage between the swell of her breasts. He was moved. Astonished at her miraculous skill in reading, he felt the presence of the Holy Spirit. At the same time he was struck by the beauty of the girl's young body. He felt his penis come erect. He loved this black girl. He wanted to touch her, to stroke her, to hold her. Automatically he helped her over a word when she hesitated. Her concentration was intense. He looked down. She was sitting with her legs apart, her cloth hanging between them, outlining her thighs. Unable to control himself any longer, he placed his hand on the inside of her thigh near the crotch and squeezed.

Ama sprang to her feet in surprise. Her chair fell over backwards. The flesh had fled the Minister's hand, leaving it clutching a handful of cloth. The loose material unwrapped itself from Ama's body and fell to the ground, leaving her clad only in her beads. For a moment, Van Schalkwyk saw her naked body. It was a vision which would return to haunt his dreams. In an instant Ama had grabbed the cloth, wrapped it around her and tucked the end back in where it belonged. Her heart was thumping. She took a step back and stared at her teacher, old, ugly, obese and now contemptible. Van Schalkwyk stared back for a moment, hardly believing what he had done. Then he bowed his head, put his palms together in prayer and closed his eyes. *Oh, Father*, he whispered to himself in Dutch, *What have I done? Forgive me, forgive me this abominable sin*. A vision of the lake of fire and brimstone came to him. *What shall I do, what shall I say*? he prayed.

He opened his eyes. Ama had moved to the other side of the table and was watching him warily, ready to slip away should he pursue her.

"Pamela, forgive me, I beg you. I don't know what came over me. I lost control of myself. Forgive me, please. I promise you that that will never happen again. I beg you. Please tell Mijn Heer nothing of this. I promise you, in the name of God I promise you, it will never happen again. I will do anything you ask of me."

Keeping her eyes on the man, Ama retrieved her chair and carried it to the opposite side of the table from Van Schalkwyk. She sat down. She was feeling calmer. What had he meant to do, she wondered. To rape her? He could never have succeeded. As a man, she had never given him a thought. Now she saw him for what he was, a lonely, ugly, pitiable old priest, without wife or family, far away from his own country. She stretched out and took the book, turned it round to face her and began to read again from where she had left off.

"And it was so. And God saw everything that he had made, and behold, it was very good. And the evening and the morning were the sixth day."

CHAPTER 18

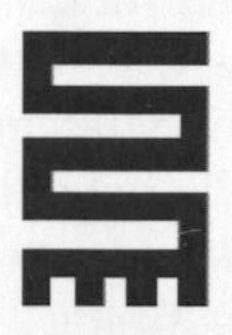

Although De Bruyn had been brought up within the narrow Calvinist conventions of the Dutch Reformed Church he was not a religious man.

He read the English Bible because he loved the poetry of the language, not in expectation of some revelation of divine intentions, nor indeed as a duty or a penance for his sins. So when he had finished Genesis and Exodus, he did no more than skim the boring passages of Leviticus and Numbers and Deuteronomy.

Then he started reading Genesis again, this time with Ama, his pleasure increased by her wide-eyed enjoyment of the magic of the stories: the Creation, the Fall, Cain and Abel, the Flood, the Tower of Babel, Abraham and Lot, Isaac and Rebecca, Jacob and Esau and Joseph and his brothers.

By the time they had finished Genesis together, Ama was reading fluently, even when she didn't understand all the words. De Bruyn's eyes were troubling him so he decided to rest them and let Ama read to him. He asked Van Schalkwyk to confine his lessons to writing and arithmetic; to which the chaplain insisted on adding the catechism.

So it was that the Director-General of Elmina Castle, Pieter De Bruyn, who had in his time bought and sold tens of thousands of slaves and even now had six hundred locked up in dark and filthy dungeons, which he never himself deigned to visit, this same Pieter De Bruyn sat down each evening and listened to his own private female slave reading to him the classic story of all times of delivery from slavery. If the irony of the situation had struck him, if he had had any inkling of it, he might have skipped the whole of Exodus. It did not strike him and he had no such inkling. The slaves of Elmina were one thing; the Children of Israel, slaves of Pharaoh, quite another.

*****

Ama had finished her domestic chores; no speck of dust was to be found upon the furniture; the bed was made; the laundry hung upon the line to dry; Augusta had sent a message to say that she could not come today; the fat Predikant had sent another: he was confined to his room with fever, nothing serious, but bad enough for him to cancel the day's lesson.

Ama hummed a tune she had learned in Kumase. She grabbed a damp handkerchief from the line and danced a few steps of *adowa*. She was free.

Nothing to do. She would choose a brand new volume from Mijn Heer's library and settle down to lose herself for a couple of hours in the doings of the curious and wonderful people who lived their lives in books.

She took up the telescope and glanced out of an east window. There was nothing new to see. She went over to a west window and sat herself on the broad cill. She aimed the instrument at the enormous canoe that was being carved on the far bank of the river and focused the lens. Progress was slow: the carvers had made several fires again, gradually burning away the heartwood of the log. Then she heard a noise, a great hubbub, shouting and laughter, the firing of muskets. Climbing down from her perch, she stretched out of the window and looked towards the hill of St. Iago and the Benya bridge.

Approaching the bridge from the north was a long procession. Slaves! In the lead were musicians, beating drums to the slow rhythm of the march, blowing horns, singing and chanting. They were followed by the merchants, responding in a condescending manner to the greetings of the townspeople who lined their route. The male slaves wore only loin cloths. Ama could see the dust-streaked sweat on their naked torsos. They walked in pairs, shackled, chained and heavily loaded, taking one deliberate, painful step at a time, driven by the beat of the drummers and the occasional flick of a manatee-skin whip. The female slaves followed, their condition much the same as the men's. Next were the children, boys and girls, stolen from their parents or forfeited by them, the unredeemed security for some trivial debt.

Ama closed her eyes. She went to the basin and washed her face and arms with cold water as if she was also covered with the dust and sweat and grime of the journey. She rubbed herself vigorously with a towel. Then she went back to the window and aimed the telescope at the procession.

Ignoring the musicians and their masters, she captured each slave in turn in the telescope's circular frame. Their necks were not bent, but it was only the need to support their head loads which kept them erect. She searched each face for some sign of dignity and courage, for some pride which had survived the suffering; but all she saw was sullen fear, despair and an infinite weariness; or, worse, a blank, devoid of expression, as if drained of all humanity. Face after face was the same.

Only once, in response to the flick of a whip on a naked back did she see a man turn his head towards the oppressor with a flash of hatred in his eyes. She tried not to think. She shivered as if she had fever. Perhaps she would recognise a face, a face from Kumase or from home. She started to look at the female slaves. Their expressions were no different from the men's.

Van Schalkwyk had painted for her a vivid picture of hell, the destination of all unreformed sinners when they died, he said. These slaves were clearly all in hell already; and yet they were still alive. *The living dead,* she thought.

Ama went to the tall mirror. She wiped the tears from her eyes and looked at her image. She kicked the soft leather sandals from her feet. She pulled the doek from her head and threw it to the floor. Staring at her own eyes, she unwrapped her body cloth folded it in two and wrapped it around her waist. Then she examined the image of her body, the round limbs, the full breasts, the healthy glistening black skin.

She went back to the window. The procession had reached the parade ground, but instead of swinging left to enter the castle, it bore right and headed towards the market square. She caught a last glimpse of each face as they turned.

She knew now what she had been searching for: it was her own face, hers and Esi's. They had come to Elmina in just such a procession as this and she had forgotten, she had buried the unpleasant memories. And yet she was a stranger to nothing she saw down there. *What have they done that their lives have been taken from them? What sin could merit such a punishment? The god of the white man must be without mercy, without compassion*, she thought. And yet that same god had led the Children of Israel out of their bondage in Egypt.

Then she wondered, *Why am I here, up here, and they down there?* She heard a noise at the door and thought it might be Mijn Heer, but it was nothing. *Mijn Heer is guilty*, she thought, *and Augusta too. Konadu Yaadom is guilty and Koranten Péte and all their people. Abdulai is guilty. And I am guilty, too, because I have been living a life of quiet comfort here, preoccupied with my lessons and my reading, and all this while my sisters and brothers have languished in the dungeons below my feet. Perhaps I am most guilty of all.* Then the thought came to her, *but what can I do? I am powerless*. She thought of the child in the bulrushes. *If I should become pregnant and bear Mijn Heer's son,* she thought, *I would call him Moses.*

She got down from the window, sank onto her haunches and, holding her head in her hands, dropped her forehead onto the wooden floor. Closing her eyes, she summoned Itsho.

"Itsho. Come to me. Tell me what I should do, what I can do, to stop this evil. Itsho come."

She remained there immobile for several minutes. When she rose, she was more at peace. She took up the telescope again and went to the window. The procession had wound its way into market square. Elephant teeth were lifted from the heads of the fettered slaves, who sank to the ground where they stood, rubbing their limbs. Young women of the town circulated amongst them, giving them water from their calabashes. The King emerged from his palace, surrounded by his elders and the noble ladies of the state, to survey the scene. Through the telescope, Ama saw Augusta amongst them.

Ama read nothing that day. She was preoccupied. She paced up and down the room. Real life had intruded upon the fantasy world in which she had been living. That night she turned away from Mijn Heer's advances.

"Is there something wrong?" he asked.

"It is nothing," she replied, turning over on her side, hugging herself and pressing her face into the soft pillow.

*****

De Bruyn and Ama were taking a light lunch.

De Bruyn had been to church that morning, leaving Ama behind as usual. She was curious to see how the whites worshipped their god, but Van Schalkwyk had not yet been able to convince the Governor that regular church attendance would be a good preparation for her conversion.

There was a knock on the door and Bezuidenhout, the new Commodore, entered. The Commodore was responsible for the management of the port at the mouth of the Benya and for coastal shipping. He bowed silently to Ama and apologised for interrupting the Governor's meal. A brig had anchored in the roadway and was signalling a request to send a party ashore. It flew the British flag and bore the name *Albany*.

"Albany? Albany? That must be that Irish blackguard Brew from Anomabu. What can the scoundrel want here? Signal back to ask if Brew himself is on board and what his mission is."

Two hours later Richard Brew, self appointed Governor of Castle Brew at Anomabu, was shown into the Governor's apartment.

"Ah, Brew," said De Bruyn, speaking English, "you must forgive me for not according you a more formal welcome, but your visit was quite unexpected. And on a Sunday, you know. This, by the way, is Pamela. Pamela shake hands with Mr. Brew."

"I am pleased to make your acquaintance, Mr. Brew," said Ama.

De Bruyn had been schooling her in European etiquette.

Brew did not release her hand. He looked her over frankly. She had put on one of late Elizabeth's less formal dresses. He looked her straight in the eye. She returned his stare for a moment.

"A pretty wench," he said, to no one in particular, "and you speak a tolerable English. What did you say your name was?"

Ama could scarcely make out his strong brogue. He paid no attention to De Bruyn who stood watching them.

"Mijn Heer calls me Pamela," she replied.

Still he held her hand. She stole a look at him. He was a large man, well dressed, too well dressed perhaps, in a laced coat and waistcoat, a shirt with a velvet collar, a silk cravat and patterned silk breeches. His eyes were bloodshot. He was not as old as Mijn Heer but his face had an unhealthy pallor.

"Where are you from?" asked Brew.

"Kumase," she replied.

"Kumase, eh? What is your language? Do you hear Fanti?" He gave her hand a final squeeze and returned it to her.

"Please, yes," she replied.

De Bruyn intervened to offer his visitor a seat.

When he was comfortably settled with a glass of port in his hand and the bottle on the table beside him, De Bruyn asked him, "To what do we owe the honour of this visit, if I may ask, Mr. Brew?"

"Just a social call, Governor, just a social call," replied Brew, "to strengthen the bonds which unite us African Europeans, marooned as we are here on this godforsaken continent."

"Come, come, Brew," replied De Bruyn, "I do not want to appear inhospitable, but your history and reputation hardly suggest that you would sail this distance just to pass the time of day with me."

"Good port, this," Brew nodded to him, sniffing the wine.

"Well, I will not deny that I have had my little differences with you Dutch in the past. But so have I had with the English Company.

"I am a man of principle, Governor. The principle I hold to most dearly is freedom, particularly the freedom to profit from my own God-given intelligence. I am not a company man, I admit it: I worked just long enough for the English Company to cure me of that affliction."

He paused to savour the port.

"Governor, I am by profession a trader. I do not have to tell you that if the trading paths to the interior are closed, there can be no trade; and if there is no trade, there can be no profit. And that is against my principles. So what I say is this: let the natives of the far interior make war; but on the coast there must be peace. It is to the achievement of that objective that I have devoted my energies. If sometimes that has meant stepping on your toes, Dutch toes and English toes, so be it. Do I make myself clear?"

"I recall, and no doubt you will too," said De Bruyn, "that soon after I took up my present office here, you detained a messenger of mine and placed him in double chains at your Castle at Anomabu. I had to suffer the indignity of requesting the intervention of the Governor at Cape Coast to secure his release from you."

"Oh that was a long time ago, Governor. Surely you do not bear me a grudge for that trivial misunderstanding after all these years? We are both old coasters, are we not? In these difficult times we need to pull together, not to drag dead horses from their graves. Your predecessor and I did good business together. The Governor at Cape Coast even had the cheek to reprimand me for selling slaves to you Dutch and importing goods from Amsterdam. I told him to go and fuck himself.

"My excuses, Madam," he said to Ama, "for the vulgarity."

"However, let me be frank with you," he continued. "I have not been well of late. A surgeon on a ship out of Liverpool gave me a thorough check-up last week and advised a sea trip. For the sake of my health. So I have left the shop in the capable hands of my assistant, Horatio Smith. You have met the young man? No? I shall send him to call on you. A capable merchant, if somewhat lacking in experience. My thirty years on this infernal coast have started to take their toll and I must begin to arrange my succession. A meeting might be useful for both of you."

Without waiting for a rejoinder from De Bruyn, Brew turned to Ama and, putting his hand over hers, said, in Fanti, "Tell me about Kumase. When did you come from there?"

"About a year ago, please," she replied, "or more."

"What were you doing there?" he asked.

Ama dropped her eyes.

"I understand. You were a slave. There is nothing wrong with that. Are you Asante yourself or a donko?" he asked.

"My people are called Bekpokpam. The Bedagbam kidnapped me and sent me to Kumase," Ama replied, wondering how she could bring this interview to an end without being rude to Mijn Heer's guest.

De Bruyn, meanwhile, was growing restive at his exclusion from this discussion in Fanti. The man's easy familiarity with Pamela upset him.

"I have some good connections in Kumase," said Brew. "The king's young cousin was my house guest for some years. Did you see the King while you were there?"

"I saw him often. I worked for the queen-mother, Nana Konadu Yaadom," replied Ama.

"Is that true now?" asked Brew, his mind working overtime.

He had dreams of acquiring a monopoly on trade with Asante. Young Smith would lead a mission to Kumase. This Pamela could be extremely useful to him.

"Mr. Brew, would you like to spend the night ashore? If not, it will soon be dark and you should return to your ship without delay," said De Bruyn, trusting that his curt welcome would induce Brew to refuse.

"Now that is most kind of you, Governor," replied Brew. "I should be most happy to accept your invitation. To tell you the truth, a sea journey may be good for the health, but the company on my brig is not the most stimulating. Human intercourse, you know, that is what life is about. One cannot spend all one's time reading books."

"I notice," he continued, nodding his head towards the glass fronted cabinet in which De Bruyn kept his library, "that you are something of a reader yourself. Dutch or English?"

"Mainly English," replied De Bruyn. "Are you fond of books?"

"In moderation," said Brew. "The golden rule. All things in moderation. Except for wine, women and good food. May I have a look?"

"I compliment you, Governor," said Brew as he examined the books. "A most excellent collection. Astley's Voyages. Dr. Johnson. Gulliver. Dean Swift was my countryman, you know: both of us from Dublin; Goldsmith too. Tom Jones. That's a romp, is it not? Poetry? No poetry? Pope? Addison?"

"No, poetry is not my strong point," replied De Bruyn. "Too much like hard work. My English is largely self-taught, as you will no doubt have noticed. I spent a year in London in my youth and what I know I picked up then."

"Ah, well, *de gustibus*, you know. I admit to a fondness for poetry myself. Who sends you your books?"

Even as he carried on this conversation Brew was scheming how to acquire the unusual slave girl.

"Captain David Williams, for one," De Bruyn replied. "*The Love of Liberty*, out of Liverpool. I am sure you have met."

"Williams? *The Love of Liberty*? Yes, of course," said Brew.

He had no recollection of the man.

"Some curious children's books too. You have a family here?"

"No, Pamela has been using those for her English lessons. The Reverend Philip Quaque kindly sold them to us."

"Quaque, eh? Impudent black boy that. I was a Christian before he was born, a proper Christian I mean, born and bred in the religion. Quaque is no more than a converted pagan, clothed in a thin veneer of civilisation. Yet he expects me to sit under his flat nose and listen to him pointing out my faults to me. He tried it once. I will not give him a second chance. Is he a friend of yours then, Quaque?"

CHAPTER 19

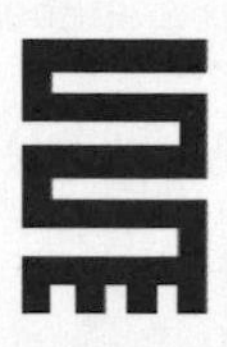

"Pamela," cried De Bruyn, rushing into the room in great haste one morning.

She was working at the table by the window.

"The *Love of Liberty* has just dropped anchor. You remember me telling you about Captain Williams?"

"My good Minister, you must excuse me," he told Van Schalkwyk. "You will have to curtail your lesson."

"Of course, of course, Director," said the chaplain, gathering up his books and throwing farewells to his pupil over his shoulder as he waddled out of the room.

The cannon began the salute. Ama covered her ears. The noise always disturbed her.

"Pamela, I hope you have my dress uniform ready," said De Bruyn.

"The slave quarters are full to capacity," he said, thinking aloud. "Williams has always been a good customer. If I play my cards right he might fill his holds at a single stroke."

Is that how he intends to keep his promise to improve conditions in the dungeons? Ama wondered as she laid his clothes out on the bed.

"Ama," he said when he had washed his face, "we must entertain Williams in style."

He was standing at the window staring out to sea. She stood behind him and put her arms around his chest.

"Calm down, Mijn Heer," she said. "Captain Williams is just another Englishmen, isn't he? What is so special about him? Why are you so excited?"

He turned and kissed her gently on the lips.

"Perhaps he has brought us some new books," he said. "Wouldn't you like that?"

He thought for a moment.

"I shall order a room prepared for him. After the rigors of the voyage, he will want the comfort of a female companion."

"No doubt," Ama replied, turning her face away.

He sees every female slave as just a vagina on two legs, she thought bitterly, not for the first time.

"Oh, let's not have that argument again," he said, reading her thoughts. "Here, won't you help me with these boots?"

"You are too sensitive. We didn't bring this custom from Amsterdam, you know: it was the Fanti kings who taught it to us. This is the renowned Gold Coast hospitality of which they are so proud. And I've told you before: the female slaves enjoy a night out, a warm bath, a good meal and a once-in-a-lifetime chance to sleep in a real bed with a soft mattress; and with a white man too. The other women envy the one who is chosen. Some of them haven't had a man in months. And when the lucky girl returns to the dungeon they are all agog to hear her story. Believe me: that's how it is."

Another cannonade. Ama's anger rose. *Did they envy me too, when I was stripped and humiliated like that in the courtyard*? she wondered. *Did they envy poor Esi when Jensen raped her*?

"I hope she cuts his prick off, that lucky girl," she mumbled to herself, taking a dislike to Williams even before she had met him.

De Bruyn was standing before the glass, pulling on his jacket.

"What did you say?" he asked.

Augusta's advice came to her. *I had better get a grip on myself. This is no time for an argument that will lead nowhere*, she thought.

"I beg your pardon, Mijn Heer, it was nothing," she replied.

"We will have him in for dinner tonight, just the three of us. I am sure you will like him. He is a most original man, always bubbling with interesting ideas. He brings a breath of fresh European air into this dismal corner of the world. He will charm you, just wait and see.

"I shall instruct chef to put on a real spread for him. That will make a change from maggoty ship's biscuits! And you will wear your best dress, I trust."

"How do I look?" he asked, but his voice was drowned by another blast from the cannon.

He kissed her again. Then he sought her eyes. She looked down.

"Is there something wrong?" he asked.

"No, no," she said, turning away. "Go and welcome your guest."

*****

Ama sat stretched out in her favourite armchair by the south window, reading.

Normally, wearing cloth, she would be curled up, but in this dress that was impossible. Mijn Heer had told her she would spoil her eyesight reading by candlelight, but she had just had to finish this chapter before the boring dinner party for the English captain. *They will talk, talk, talk,* she thought, *and most of it I won't understand.*

But, it occurred to her, *it might be interesting to practice my English on a real Englishman.*

She looked across at the tall clock. The pendulum swung back and forth. They were late. Mijn Heer had not been back the whole afternoon. He really was in love with this Williams. She felt a pang of jealousy. Then she laughed at herself. *Me jealous of a man, and an Englishman at that?* Mijn Heer was hers and hers alone. She had really conquered him. She thought of her namesake, Richardson's Pamela. *I've learnt a thing or two from her*, she thought. *How I would like to meet and talk with her. Or even just receive a letter from her. Mijn Heer says it is just a story book, that there is no real Pamela Andrews, that Samuel Richardson wrote all the letters himself, out of his head. I wonder if he is telling me the truth. Maybe I should ask Williams. He's an Englishman. He should know. Maybe he knows Richardson, or even Pamela herself.*

She put the book aside, rose, stretched her arms, yawned, took a deep breath and went to the mirror. Mijn Heer was right: white really did suit her. This was his favourite dress. Like the rest, it had originally been one of Elizabeth's, a ball gown he called it. There had been balls at the Cape. Mijn Heer had demonstrated to her how they danced the minuet. If that was a sample of the way the whites danced, she had told him, she didn't think much of it. But perhaps it was just that Mijn Heer was such a poor dancer. He was so stiff. She couldn't imagine him mastering the graceful movements of the *adowa*. In any case there were no white women for the men to dance their minuets with at Elmina.

Elizabeth's ball gown was made of a rich brocaded satin, sparkling white. The bodice was laced up tightly from behind, forcing her bust up against the low neckline. Mijn Heer loved her to wear it; he said the white cloth showed off the beauty of her black skin. But it was heavy and hot and uncomfortable.

Augusta had been teaching her to sew.

"Maame Augusta," she had asked her, "when you were married to Mijn Heer did you have dresses like this?"

Augusta had laughed.

"Of course not. There were no white women in the Castle in those days and no white women's dresses either. What would a Fanti woman like me do with such a dress? I would have been the laughing stock of Edina."

But she could see how Elizabeth's dresses suited Ama. As for the townsfolk, they used different criteria when it came to judging white men's wenches.

Ama had had an idea. She would take the dress apart, secretly, without Mijn Heer's knowledge, and sew it together again in a different style.

"That's a crazy idea," Augusta had reacted. "It might make Mijn Heer very angry."

Reluctantly, Ama had bowed to her veto.

Her hair had grown fast. When it was long enough, Augusta's youngest daughter, Kuku, had come to plait in the local style.

Now she took a piece of blue satin which Augusta had given her and wrapped it around her head in an elaborate turban. She wondered if Mijn Heer would like it.

Ama was still standing at the mirror when she heard the approaching voices.

"Pamela," called De Bruyn as he opened the door, "come and meet Captain Williams."

She could hear the liquor on his voice. She turned. His face was flushed. He continued his conversation with the visitor.

"Williams," he said, "shall we just summarise our afternoon's discussion before we settle down to eat?"

Then he saw her. His eyes opened wide, he rubbed them and looked again, up and down. He caught her eye, smiled and tilted his head in approval. Ama sighed with relief. He took her hand and gave it to Williams, who bowed slightly.

"I have been frank with you, Captain," continued De Bruyn. "I am overstocked. Ever since the Asante opened the road from the north, there has been a veritable flood of slaves. My dungeons are full. Yet if I were to refuse to buy, the dealers might take their business elsewhere, even to your countrymen at Cape Coast. So I am prepared to offer you a special deal: a bargain rate of six ounces of gold for a male, four for a female and three for a child. You make your own selection. What's more I'll take all your trade goods. There is only one condition and that is that you fill your holds here at Elmina. Accept my offer and you could be on your way to Barbados within a week."

"You tempt me," replied Williams, "but you must allow me to sleep on it. We can talk about price when my surgeon reports to me on his inspection of the stock. As to buying four hundred slaves at a go, most of them Cormantynes, I shall have to think about that very carefully. You know the problem. With so many of them all from one place and many probably speaking the same language, trouble is almost inevitable."

"But think of the advantages. You spend only a week in this insalubrious climate. The slaves are all fit and well when you set sail; not to speak of your crew. Should you be lucky with the winds, you might even arrive in Barbados without a single loss; and after a short voyage the slaves would be so healthy that they would command the highest prices."

"It's certainly an attractive proposition. Cormantynes do indeed fetch a high price in Barbados. However they are also well-known for their reluctance to be ruled," replied Williams.

"Let me make a further proposal. I have decided to repatriate five of my men, all experienced soldiers, to Holland. They are afflicted with some sort of skin ulcer which refuses to heal here. If you would agree to carry them to England, I would pay their passages. Five English pounds a head. They're all good men. and all quite well enough to use a musket or a sword."

Williams grunted.

"I must balance the pros and cons. Let us talk about it again in the morning."

"Agreed," said De Bruyn. "Now, Pamela, would you please ring for dinner, and I promise you that we will talk no more business."

Throughout this conversation Ama had kept her eyes down and her face immobile. She always felt humiliated when De Bruyn discussed the business of the slave trade in her presence. *He talks about us as if we were goats or chickens in a pen at the market*, she thought. But she had taught herself to swallow her anger. *Be charming to this Englishman,* she commanded herself, *however much you hate and despise him and his trade. After all, his business is no worse than that of Mijn Heer. And it is Mijn Heer who holds the key to your fate.*

CHAPTER 20

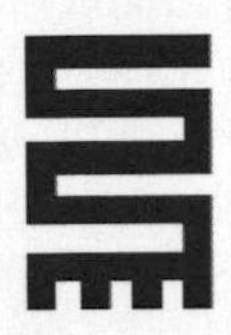

Ama awoke to find De Bruyn standing at a window, looking out to sea and breathing deeply as was his custom each morning.

"I drank too much," he told her.

Ama went silently about her ablutions.

"What did you make of Williams?" he asked her.

"If he is your friend, Mijn Heer, I must like him," she replied.

"That sounds to me as if you mean just the opposite. Yet he seemed highly impressed with you," De Bruyn called from the commode in the alcove.

Ama recalled an English proverb she had come across in Goody Two-Shoes. *When a man talks too much, believe but half of what he says.* But she made no reply.

"This morning," De Bruyn said, pulling up his trousers as he emerged, "I have promised to take our visitor on a grand tour of the castle and the town. Augusta has arranged for the King to receive us. Afterwards we shall lunch in the summer house in the gardens. Would you like to join us? I am sure Williams would be pleased."

Ama concealed her excitement at the prospect of a temporary escape from the confines of the apartment.

"Certainly, if that is what you want," she replied.

De Bruyn looked at her closely.

"Are you upset about something?" he asked.

"No," she replied, "What makes you think that?"

*****

"I have asked Pamela to join us I hope you don't mind," said De Bruyn

"Of course not," replied Williams. "She seems a sensible wench. However I must tell you that I disapprove in principle of teaching slaves and others of the labouring classes more than the bare minimum they need to perform their duties. It is in general prejudicial to their morals and happiness. It persuades them to despise their lot in life, rather than making good servants of them. Instead of wearing their yoke with patience, they become ill-mannered and intractable.

"But I must say that you seem to have trained her well. She appears to know where a woman's tongue is best kept."

"And where is that?" De Bruyn took the bait

"Chained and shackled within her mouth," Williams laughed; and then smiled at Ama.

Concealing her anger and acting stupid, Ama smiled back.

They began their tour on the flat roof of the West Bastion. De Bruyn gave Williams a lecture on the history of the castle, concentrating on the Dutch victory over the Portuguese. He explained the construction work in progress in the yard below; he boasted of the castle's fine brass twelve-pounders and other armaments; and with some pride described the orchards and vegetable gardens which lay behind Coenraedsburg.

They passed through the Council Chamber and then out onto an open gallery which ran round two sides of the Inner Courtyard. It was from this vantage point that De Bruyn had selected Ama from amongst the rank and file of her fellow slaves. Bringing up the rear, she paused and looked down. The deep arched recesses, filled with grilles of iron, looked familiar.

"Mijn Heer," she called.

He turned back.

"What is down there?" she asked.

"Those are the quarters of the female slaves," he replied. "Come, we are running late. Augusta will be waiting for us."

He was anxious not to get drawn into an embarrassing conversation before his guest.

Ama lingered. She knew the insides of one of those quarters, as he called the dungeons. Did she see black hands gripping the iron bars in the deep shadow? She could not be sure. Then, afraid that she would lose the two men, she hurried on.

She caught up with them on the North Bastion.

"Well, Williams, there you see the *Love of Liberty*, out in the roadstead. Here, take my spyglass. Everything in order? Now look down: you see the beach below? Pamela, come and look. We generally bring ships' cargo through the surf with our own boats but if they are not free or if the sea is too high, we get our bumboy to hire canoes. We use the gantry which you see here beside us to raise the goods up to the level of the doorway beneath us."

Intrigued by the wooden structure with its pulleys and ropes, Ama went to examine it.

"It is through that same doorway, of course," De Bruyn said to Williams in a low voice, as he watched her, "that we dispatch our outgoing cargo."

"How does it work?" called Ama.

"Quite simple, my dear," replied De Bruyn. "You use this handle to turn the windlass. The rope runs over that pulley, down to the lower pulley, up again around the upper pulley, down again, and so on, four times. Do you see the hook attached to the lower pulley? The goods are hung from that hook. Turn the handle clockwise and the hook goes up, and the goods with it. Turn it the other way and the hook goes down. Try it."

Cautiously, Ama turned the handle and saw the lower pulley and its hook move down. She opened her mouth in astonishment.

"Now turn the handle the other way."

The hook rose. She tried it again.

"Inquisitive wench," said Williams. "You wouldn't find an English girl asking such a question."

"Do you disapprove?" asked De Bruyn.

"In an English girl, I certainly would," said Williams. "Curiosity is unbecoming in the female sex. This girl's curiosity surely comes from your teaching her to read. An ability to read is prejudicial in any woman, in a slave doubly and triply so. It opens them to ideas unsuited to their station in life."

"Oh, I do not agree," retorted De Bruyn. "Teaching Pamela to read has certainly changed her; but it has also been a rewarding experience for me. Think of her as my Galatea and of me as her Pygmalion. You know the Greek legend, of course? She has become a better companion to me, better intellectual company, than any man in this castle. Your ideas on this issue are old fashioned, Williams. The times are changing, even in England; or especially in England. I get the sense of that from the novels you bring me. Think of Moll Flanders."

"Moll Flanders is a shameless harlot. De Foe set her up as a warning, not as a model for female behaviour."

"Richardson's women then. Anna Howe, Clarissa, the original Pamela Andrews herself."

"De Bruyn, you know I share your love of books. I suspect, though, that you take literature too seriously. I can understand that, considering the isolation of your existence here. But books are not life, you know. They are not even a poor reflection of life. Books are designed by their authors as fantasies, fictions, diversions; as distractions from the harsh realities of everyday existence. They are so designed for the simple purpose of earning a profit for their authors. It is a dangerous delusion to imagine that you can mine books for lessons on life."

"Do you include in that precept the Good Book itself?"

"Perhaps, perhaps not. I suspect, though, that a thorough search of the Bible, would provide you with justification for almost any course of action, perhaps even murder."

De Bruyn looked over his shoulder nervously.

"You English are outrageous," he said. "That is blasphemy."

They were descending the first of the three long open flights of stairs which led down to the main courtyard. Ama had been following the two men at a discreet distance, looking this way and that to disguise the fact that she was eavesdropping. She need not have bothered: they were so engrossed in their argument that they had forgotten the female person whose innocent inquiry had started it.

Ama's appearance, trailing behind the two white men, caused a stir in the busy courtyard. It was most unusual for a strange black woman to be seen emerging from the officers' quarters. The two men were paying no attention to her and her connection with them was not clear to the spectators. Her presence was an enigma.

Ama was concentrating on the steep stone steps and at the same time trying to catch the thread of the men's conversation. It was only when they reached the first landing that she lifted her eyes and saw the scene below. All activity had ceased. Every eye was trained on her. She stopped in her tracks. The two men, still arguing, were already on their way down the lower flight. Ama could not move. Her feet were glued to the flagstones. She wanted to scream, "Mijn Heer, Mijn Heer," but the words stuck in her throat. Her legs turned to jelly. She felt she must sink to the ground. If only the flagstones would open and swallow her. She recalled the palace of the Sleeping Beauty. All human movement in the courtyard had been frozen, all, that is, except that of the two men who continued inexorably on their way down the stairs. She did not know which way to look. She closed her eyes.

De Bruyn and Williams reached the next landing. De Bruyn suddenly became aware of the silence in the courtyard. He raised his eyes and then turned round to look for Ama. She stood there like a statue, a Galatea turned back into black ivory, and rooted to the spot on which she stood.

"Pamela," he called.

Ama looked at him appealingly. Still she could not move.

"Pamela," came a whispered chorus, an astonished echo, from the courtyard.

De Bruyn climbed back up the flight of stairs and took her by the hand. The spell on her was broken. She wanted to hang her arms around his neck but the presence of the onlookers would not allow it.

"What's the matter? Are you ill?" he asked and turned to cast a fierce gaze on the inquisitive throng below.

That lifted the spell on the watching traders and soldiers and they began to go about their business again, taking care only to twist their necks to keep the curious couple in view, Director-General De Bruyn and . . . who? There was a hubbub of excited speculation. Was this the slave-girl country-wife whom, rumour had it, De Bruyn kept imprisoned in his room?

Ama dug her nails into De Bruyn's palms.

"No," she said, "I'll be all right. Just stand by me a moment."

"Anything wrong?" asked Williams as they rejoined him on the lower landing.

"Oh just a momentary dizzy spell," replied De Bruyn. "My fault. I should have thought. The steepness of the steps perhaps. Ah, there is Augusta, now. Augusta, you have met Captain Williams before, not so?"

Augusta made the suspicion of a curtsey. Williams nodded to her.

"We will just take a quick look round the stores," said De Bruyn, "and then we will be with you. Pamela, will you join us or will you stay and talk to Augusta?"

"Augusta," she said in a hoarse whisper.

*****

"What!" exclaimed Williams as the store-man opened the door of the commercial magazine, "are all these for sale? A mixed lot, I'll warrant: muskets, carbines, blunderbusses, buccaneer guns, fowling pieces, pistols. What else, then? Do you sell cannon and mortars too?"

"What else? Elephant guns, dane guns, flints, fire steels, lead shot. Also swords. Gunpowder and cartouche boxes we keep elsewhere. Cannon, perhaps, on special order, but only to our closest friends," chuckled De Bruyn.

"Does it not put you at some risk, selling these guns to . . . them?"

"Not really," replied De Bruyn. "If you examine the weapons closely you will soon discern the reason. Warfare is endemic on this part of the coast. Most of the slaves who come to us are prisoners of war. If we did not sell arms and ammunition, there would certainly be less warfare and the supply of slaves might dry up. There is, however, a distinction between the quality of arms required for such local warfare as will ensure us a steady supply of slaves, and weaponry that might pose a threat to ourselves. Beyond that we do of course exercise some discrimination in the choice of our customers: we would not want even weapons of inferior quality turning up in the hands of potential enemies. I believe that the other European trading companies adopt a similar policy. We have no formal contract with them to that effect, but there does seem to be some sort of unwritten agreement of long standing.

"Let me illustrate. We have intelligence that the Asante, who are important customers for muskets, have recently made conquests in vast territories to the north of them; and that they are exacting large numbers of slaves in tribute. Pamela, though she is somewhat reticent about her origins, is evidently one of those. Some of those slaves they no doubt use for agriculture or mining, or as domestic servants; but many they send down to the coast in exchange for European manufactures, trade goods from the East and, you have guessed it, more arms and ammunition. So the wheel turns and turns."

*****

"Ah," said Williams as they crossed the second bridge, "a pleasant breeze off the sea. It is hot and humid in your courtyard. But what is that nasty smell?"

The two men walked ahead, with De Bruyn's personal body guards, Kobina and Vroom, smartly dressed in uniforms, in attendance. Kobina carried a musket and Vroom a cask of brandy on his head and a parcel of tobacco under one arm. The two women followed a short distance behind. Effibaa, carrying Augusta's stool, brought up the rear.

"Augusta," De Bruyn called back, "Captain Williams asks what that smell is."

"Stinking fish," she replied, thinking, *he knows very well what it is. Why does he ask me?*

"Well, I have to admit that there are parts of London which smell as bad," said Williams.

Augusta had dressed for the occasion. It was a singular honour for her to conduct the Director-General and his guest to the town. A small striped parasol protected her from the sun.

Ama was more simply dressed, in the same style but without the costly jewellery worn by the older woman. Though the slaves of the townspeople went bareheaded, Ama wore a headcloth. She walked a respectful step behind Augusta.

"Walk by my side, child, in the shade of the umbrella. You may be a slave but you are after all the Director's slave, and almost his wife. Behave like a free woman and perhaps you will soon be one."

"Maame Augusta, I am nervous," said Ama.

"Nervous? About what?"

"Maame, I have spent the past year in Mijn Heer's apartment. This morning is the first time I have been out. I am nervous about what your people will think of me."

"Don't be silly. You just keep close to me. Nobody will trouble you."

They had passed the open parade ground and were entering the wide street which led to the market square. De Bruyn, deep in conversation with Williams, looked round and waved. The women waved back.

"Maame," said Ama, "I saw the slaves arrive."

"Well?"

"I watched them with Mijn Heer's telescope. I looked at their faces, one by one, as they came up from the bridge."

Augusta turned her head to look at Ama.

"And so?" she asked coolly.

She had an uncomfortable foreboding of what was to come.

"They were dirty and exhausted, especially the men, from carrying those heavy chains around their ankles."

"We always give them food and water when they arrive. Then they have a bath and we give them palm oil for their skin. Did you see them the next day, before they were taken to the castle?"

"No," replied Ama, and continued, "when *we* arrived, we were taken straight into the castle."

"That was because you had already been sold," replied Augusta.

"Maame, they were very sad."

"Yes?" replied Augusta.

"Maame, where are they now?"

"In the castle dungeons, no doubt," replied Augusta.

"Maame, is it not wicked to treat human beings like that? I mean to chain them as if they were animals and then sell them to the Europeans? Are they not our own people, our own brothers and sisters?"

"Young woman, that is dangerous talk. I hope you do not talk such words to Mijn Heer."

"Maame, I am sorry if I have offended you, but when I looked at their faces, it was my own face I saw. It was as if I were looking into a mirror. Since then my sleep has been disturbed. I have had bad dreams."

"Ama, you must stop this talk at once. Let me tell you something. Three hundred slaves arrived. One hundred of those belonged to the King, whom you will see presently. Of the balance, sixty were mine and another twenty were for my husband. I made a special journey to the market at Simbew to buy them from the Asante. All three hundred have been delivered to the castle, but we, the suppliers, have yet to be paid. Mijn Heer says he must sell them before he settles his accounts with us. That is how we have always done business together. If you had ever been in trade, you would know the importance of giving credit to good customers. I do not distrust him. However, the sooner he sells them and settles his accounts, the better for all of us here.

"Mijn Heer is trying to persuade this English captain, Williams, to fill his ship with slaves from Elmina. If he is successful, we will be paid at once. That is why I have invited the two of them to visit our town and why, as you will see, we are showing Williams such special hospitality. The King himself will welcome Williams. He does not do that for every white captain who drops anchor at Elmina, believe me. But of course Nana has an even larger stake in this transaction than I have. It is important for us to make Williams feel good so that he will agree to buy many slaves.

"Have you understood what I have been telling you? Now, I do not want you to spoil everything by making speeches about your sympathy for the slaves. Do you think we are not also sorry for them? I don't need you to tell me that they are human beings, even if I would not go so far as to call them my brothers and sisters. But every one of them has done something to deserve his fate. Some have been defeated in war, others have fallen into debt, or been forfeited as pawns and so on. Some have even been sold into slavery by their own parents. That is life. In

Edina we depend on this trade for our livelihood. Where do you think I get the gold dust to buy these clothes, these ornaments? I will tell you. My profit from trade in cloth and other merchandise is nothing to me by comparison with what I make from trading in slaves.

"I hope I have made myself clear. I am sorry to have to speak to you so harshly, but I must warn you to speak no more of a matter concerning which you are ignorant and which, moreover, is none of your business."

She turned her angry face away. Ama's mind was in a turmoil. She felt humiliated, wrung out like a damp piece of cloth. She bowed her head. There was nothing she could do but apologise. She was near to tears. She bit her lip.

She said, "Maame, I beg you. I am sorry. I will not talk of this again."

Augusta looked at her and saw her distress.

"I did not mean that you should never talk to me about the slave trade. If it troubles you, you may talk. But only at a proper time and at a proper place. Now wipe the tears from your eyes and smile at me."

*****

Two male slaves, heads shaven, bare to the waist, each armed with a spear, stood guard at the gate of the palace. They greeted Augusta respectfully as the party approached.

"Now, Ama," said Augusta, "forget that you are a slave. As far as we are concerned, you are the Director's wife."

They passed through a covered porch into a single storied courtyard and then through a short passage into an enclosed quadrangle. Here the King held court with his elders each day except Tuesday, which was the day set aside for Tweneboa, the spirit of the Benya.

Opposite the entrance, on the far side of the courtyard, the elders, wing chiefs and family heads sat on stools under an awning. They were dressed in colourful calico prints, folded and wrapped calf-length around the waist. Each wore a necklace of beads and most a cap of deerskin or a European hat.

The King was at the centre, the only one seated on a chair, He alone wore his cloth over his shoulder. It was rich plain red velvet A heavy gold necklace, several gold bracelets on each arm and rings of the same material on every finger evidenced his status. His sandals, too, were encrusted with gold. An enormous red and green umbrella, embroidered with gold thread, gave him shade.

"*Àgòo!*" called Augusta, announcing their presence and asking permission to enter.

"*Amêê,*" came the acknowledgement from her husband, who was the *Omankyeame*, the official spokesman of the King.

Augusta led the visitors in single file to perform the customary greetings. Facing their hosts palm to palm from the right, the visitors shook hands with each of the elders in turn.

"Your Majesty," said De Bruyn in Dutch, "I hope you are well."

"Thank you," replied the King in the same language.

Chairs had been arranged under another awning on the opposite side of the courtyard. When the visitors were seated, slaves brought them palm wine.

Then the elders rose and threw their cloths over their left shoulders. The Omankyeame, his staff of office in his hand, led the King, followed by his umbrella bearer and the others to shake hands with the visitors. The slave attendants turned the elders' stools, and the King's chair, on their sides as they rose, setting them right only when their owners returned.

When they had again taken their seats and adjusted their cloths, the Omankyeame stood up and spoke in Fanti. He welcomed the visitors on behalf of the King and asked the purpose of their visit. Augusta translated this into Dutch for De Bruyn and De Bruyn translated into English for Williams. Then Augusta stood up and spoke, also in Fanti.

"Nana and respected nobles," she said, "we bring you no ill tidings."

There was a murmur of acknowledgement.

"His Excellency the Director-General of the Dutch company, Mijn Heer De Bruyn," she continued, "is well known to you. He asks me to greet the King on his behalf and wish him well."

She paused for her husband, the Omankyeame, to speak.

"Nana," he said, turning to the King, "the woman says that the visitors do not bring any bad news. She says that the Director greets you."

"This young woman is his wife," Augusta continued. "Her name is Ama Donko and her Dutch name is Pamela."

Another murmur.

"She speaks the Asante and Fanti languages. She can read and write in English as well as any white man."

The elders had heard about Ama, but this was the first time they had seen her.

"She can read and write in English as well as any white man," each repeated to his neighbour, nodding sagely.

Ama bowed her head in modesty. She had not expected this.

"Nana," the Omankyeame told the King, "she says the young woman is the wife of the Director. She says that this young woman can read and write in the language of the English."

"This gentleman is called David Williams," continued Augusta. "He is an Englishman and is the Captain of the ship which is lying offshore at present. We know that the Dutch and the English are rivals, but, in spite of this, the Captain is an old friend of the Director-General. He has come to our country to buy slaves. His holds are empty and he can accommodate as many as four hundred in his ship. Since he speaks only English, he has asked me to greet you, Nana, and to bring you the friendly greetings of the English King."

The Omankyeame told the King what his wife had said.

"Omankyeame," said Augusta, "the Director has brought Nana one anker of the best French brandy and a parcel of Brazilian tobacco and begs you to accept these gifts as a token of his esteem and that of Captain Williams."

"The King thanks the Director and the Captain and is pleased to accept his gift," said the Omankyeame.

Augusta signalled to Vroom and Kobina to deliver the gifts.

While she was telling De Bruyn what she had said to the King, more or less; and De Bruyn was translating for Williams, the Omankyeame again led the King and the elders to shake their hands to express his thanks.

When they had resumed their seats, the Omankyeame held out a pewter mug. A slave extracted the bung from the keg and filled the vessel with brandy. Adjusting his cloth with one hand, the Omankyeame poured a little of the drink onto the ground before him.

"Gods of the silent world," he intoned, "we are here. Tweneboa, spirit of Benya, greatest of the seventy seven gods of our nation, we greet you. Let gold flow. Let the sea and the lagoon be abundant with fish and the forest with game. We beseech you. Let the heavens give us rain and the soil give us food. Let there be peace and prosperity for all.

"Nana Kwa Amankwaa, founder of our nation, and all the great kings who have ruled us since and have gone before us: the King and elders of Edina greet you. We beg you to share this drink with us."

He poured some more of the liquor from the mug. The brandy soaked into the dry ground.

"We are gathered here today, the King and elders of the people of Edina, to welcome the white visitors, the chief of the castle and the captain of the ship who has come from over the sea to buy slaves. We have sold so many slaves to the Dutchman that his dungeons are full. Yet he says he cannot pay us until he, in turn, has sold the slaves to the white visitor. The captain has an empty ship. We beg you to use your powers to persuade the captain to fill his ship from the Dutchman's dungeons."

Another decantation.

"I have spoken what the King has commanded," he said and emptied the mug.

The vessel was refilled and passed from elder to elder. Each took a draft. Four glasses of the brandy were sent across for the visitors. Mijn Heer and Williams threw back their heads and poured down the drink. Ama took a sip. It burnt her throat and brought tears to her eyes.

The King was consulting the Omankyeame. Several elders gathered around them.

The Omankyeame stepped forward and spoke again.

"Woman," he said to Augusta, "Nana has instructed me to tell the white men that they are welcome and that their visit does him honour."

He paused for her to interpret.

"You have told us that the Captain has come to our country to buy slaves."

Again he paused.

"You should tell him that it is we who have supplied many of the slaves which the Director will sell to the Captain. The King assures him that these slaves are of the highest quality, healthy, strong and, above all, submissive to the will of their masters. The King says that he will be happy if the Captain will fill his holds with slaves from Elmina and so shorten his stay in these parts which are so unhealthy for white men."

Augusta was not sure that Williams would react favourably to this pressure.

"This is what the King's linguist says," she warned De Bruyn in Dutch, "but you might not want to translate all of it for the visitor."

"What does he say?" asked Williams, who was beginning to be bored by the tedious ceremonial, from which he was excluded.

"The King asks you to convey his highest regards to the King of England," De Bruyn replied, agreeing with Augusta's assessment, "and to assure him of the King's ability to supply to him as many slaves of the highest quality as His Majesty might require."

Williams laughed.

"Tell him that I undertake to pass on his message the very next time I meet King George."

"He has heard what you have said," said Augusta, "and he will think on it."

They sat for a few minutes. The brandy had begun to take effect on some of the elders and a heated discussion broke out. The King listened impassively.

Augusta rose again. "*Àgòo*," she called for attention. "My lords, the white men have asked me to thank you for your hospitality. They would like to stay longer. However they have pressing business to attend to. Therefore they request your permission for them to take their leave."

"The road is there: permission is granted," said the Omankyeame.

The visitors rose and after a final round of handshaking left the palace.

"Well, how did you find our King?" Augusta asked Ama as they emerged into the bustle of the market square.

Ama was about to make an unfavourable comparison with the pomp and pageantry of the Asantehene's court, but she thought better of it.

"He is a handsome man," she dissembled.

She no longer felt that she could be completely frank with Augusta. She was a slave, after all, and Augusta a slave trader; and the business of that morning's meeting had been the trade in slaves.

"Well, how did you find our King?" De Bruyn asked Williams.

They were again walking ahead of the women.

"He looks a great scoundrel to me," Williams replied, "but that is only an impression. You have a longer experience with the blacks than I have: how do you find him?"

"You are a good judge of character, Captain," said De Bruyn. "His Majesty thinks it no crime to cheat us, if he can get away with it. In this he is no different from his subjects: they will boast amongst themselves of their skill and ingenuity in deceiving any Dutchman. The only one of them that I can trust is Augusta and even she, who was once my wife, is not above taking advantage of me if she sees an opportunity."

CHAPTER 21

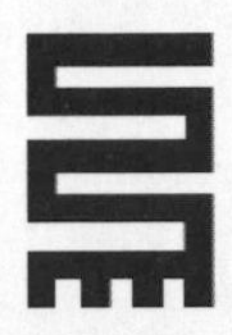

Sven Jensen, the Chief Merchant, ranked second after De Bruyn, above the Treasurer and the Commodore. Hendrik Van Schalkwyk stood fifth in precedence.

Jensen was an efficient administrator. As a trader he drove a hard bargain. De Bruyn was content to devolve upon him responsibility for most of the commercial activities of the Company. He had an ear for languages: of all the Europeans at Elmina, he was the only one who had picked up sufficient Fanti to trade without using a mulatto interpreter.

A handsome, at first sight charming man, the Dane was an inveterate, indiscriminate and shameless womaniser. He thought nothing of flouting the strict Company rules of conduct.

He was fond of telling the story of a visit he had paid to a house in the town where he was well-known. An old woman was sweeping the courtyard, her face lined with wrinkles, her flat, empty dugs hanging down before her bent body. Without waiting for an invitation, Jensen had taken a seat and started to employ his charm on the hag. She, however, was not to be taken in by his sweet words.

"First you fuck my daughter," she had said. "Then you fuck her very own pikin, my granddaughter, who never know a man before. Now, today, my daughter is not in the house and my granddaughter neither. You talk, talk like you also want to fuck an old grandmother woman like me, too."

"Get out, you shameless wretch, get out," she had screamed, driving him away with her broom.

Jensen was not above arranging a short term conjunction between a castle employee and a female slave. He rendered no service free of charge, but the nature of the payment was negotiable, in cash or kind, or merely in the form of an obligation set to mature at some future, unspecified date.

As poor Esi had discovered, he was not above paying a private visit to the female dungeons himself.

One of Van Schalkwyk's duties was to send to the Classis in Amsterdam a confidential annual appraisal of the spiritual progress of the Elmina community. There was seldom anything good to report. A reasonable attendance at church could only be ensured by fining absentees. There was a great deal of heavy drinking, and much bad language, both of which would have caused the elders of the Classis particular offence, had they known. Given the least lapse of security, the men would take a female slave, with or without her consent. Van Schalkwyk feared that if the Classis became aware of the extent of the moral depravity at Elmina, they would blame *him* for dereliction of duty, rather than the sinners for their sins. His report was largely constructed of wishful thinking. He was aware, however, that the gentlemen of the Classis were no strangers to human weakness; on the contrary, they thrived on it. So he found it expedient to lend his fiction credibility by spicing it with a few salacious titbits.

Van Schalkwyk had little to lose by disclosing at least part of the gossip about Jensen. He was aware of De Bruyn's dislike for the fellow and he was not averse to doing his friend a secret favour by cutting the Chief Merchant down to size. Jensen was, moreover, not a Dutchman and it was thus unlikely that he would have friends at court who might speak up on his behalf.

Van Schalkwyk sent off his report to the Classis; the Classis wrote to the Council in Amsterdam and in due course De Bruyn received a letter asking him to investigate the allegations made against Jensen. He called the Chief Merchant in and told him the contents of the letter.

Jensen immediately suspected Van Schalkwyk. He made no attempt to deny the charges. Instead he poured out a long stream of furious invective directed at the Chaplain.

De Bruyn let him boil, quietly enjoying his deputy's loss of composure.

"My advice to you," De Bruyn told him, when he had finished, "is to get married. Quickly. Without delay. I mean properly married, in church. I will issue the necessary instructions to the chaplain. I shall then be able to report the event to Amsterdam and to advise the authorities there of my expectation that the behaviour complained of will cease forthwith."

Jensen reluctantly accepted the Governor's advice and applied his mind to the selection of the wench who would be honoured with the title of Madam Jensen.

Some years before, a well-known Cape Coast harlot, by name of Taguba, had borne a mulatto child, a girl, whom she had named Rose. The child's paternity was unknown but, judging from her appearance was evidently European. When the girl was about eleven years old, she was seen by a factor at Cape Coast castle, who went by name of John Thompson. Taking a fancy to the girl, Thompson had paid a dowry to Taguba in return for a promise that the girl would be his when she reached a proper age for matrimony.

Jensen had visited Cape Coast on business and Thompson, meeting him for the first time and falling victim to his charm and flattery, had made the grievous error of boasting to his new friend of the beauty of his future wife. Shortly afterwards, Thompson had been promoted and sent to Sekondi as Chief Merchant there. Since he did not trust Taguba, he had persuaded her, in return for a further payment, to let him take the girl with him, solemnly promising that he would not consummate the marriage until after the girl's menarche. This, perhaps, was his undoing.

Thompson had invited Jensen to a farewell party at Cape Coast. Jensen had seen young Rose, Madam-Thompson-to-be, who already, in spite of her tender years, showed undoubted indications of the great beauty which she was to become, and who had, moreover, acquired from her mother precocious skills of coquetry.

At Sekondi, Thompson had looked after the girl with tender care, taught her to speak English and even taken the trouble to teach her to read a little and sign her name, *Rose Thompson*. He had had little else to occupy his idle time since there were no other Europeans in the vicinity to share his port and brandy. He had spoiled Rose by showering her with gifts of cloth and jewellery from his stock-in-trade, in the belief that this would encourage her to return his own undeniable, doting affection.

Jensen, having been instructed to marry, considered all the possible candidates. His light fell on Rose. After paying a professional call on his proposed mother-in-law and paying generously for her service, he discovered little difficulty in persuading Taguba to accept a further dowry in return for her daughter's hand. The two of them established an immediate understanding, each recognising in the other a kindred spirit.

Taguba then visited Mr. Thompson in Sekondi, allaying his suspicions by telling him how much she missed her daughter. In the course of the visit she contrived to have Rose kidnapped by accomplices and put aboard a canoe and sent to Elmina, there to be delivered into the now impatient clutches of Jensen.

Taguba, feigning mourning, returned to Cape Coast. Thompson, believing that his Rose had been panyarred and sold into slavery, immediately went mad and took to his bed. Soon after he was found there, murdered. Since Rose was now betrothed to Jensen, some suspicion fell on him. However, what little evidence there was, was entirely circumstantial, and in view of the separate and distinct territorial responsibilities of the judicial authorities at Cape Coast and Elmina, not to speak of the likely diplomatic complications should charges be laid, the suspicions remained just that. After some time the rumours subsided and Thompson was forgotten.

Rose, having acquired from Thompson sufficient rudimentary knowledge of the catechism to qualify for baptism, Van Schalkwyk joined her to the Church. The banns were put up and the date for the wedding was announced. It would be the first wedding to be held in the Dutch chapel since that of Jacobus Capitein and his white wife.

*****

Since it was he who had pressed Jensen into marriage, De Bruyn agreed to bear the cost of the wedding reception and offered to lend Rose the wedding dress of his late wife Elizabeth; moreover, he persuaded Augusta and Ama to make the necessary alterations, which they agreed to do in spite of their shared misgivings about Jensen.

Rose was brought to the Governor's rooms. The seams of the dress were ripped open and pinned to fit the slender form of the young girl.

Ama was fascinated by Rose's light complexion, her long brown hair, straight nose and blue eyes. But the girl was cheeky and Augusta had to reprimand her.

"Did they not teach you to respect your elders in Cape Coast, child? Or was it that white man, what was his name, in Sekondi, who taught you bad manners?"

Rose started to cry. She was still a child. Thompson had pandered to her every whim. He had treated her like a spoiled only daughter rather than his future wife. She had not loved him. Indeed, apart from her mother (and that with reservations), Rose loved no one but herself. But she had quickly come to realise that, unlike Thompson, Jensen would stand no nonsense from her. Now she began to miss her former mentor. When she heard of his murder, she wept bitterly. Then she finished crying and forgot about him. Her only regret was that she had had to leave behind all the presents he had given her; and that Jensen clearly had no intention of taking the risks contingent upon an attempt to recover them.

*****

The wedding was set for a Saturday afternoon.

Taguba's maternal uncle and family head, known as Kwesi Broni, agreed to give the bride away. Taguba and Kwesi Broni and a large party of friends and relations arrived at Elmina at dawn, just as the castle gate was opened. Jensen had set aside two rooms for them, one for the men and one for the more numerous women and children.

Old Kwesi Broni had persuaded the Chief Merchant at Cape Coast castle to let him have, on hire, a fashionable European suit, complete with buckled shoes, breeches, waistcoat, ornately embroidered jacket and powdered shoulder length wig, to which he proposed to add his favourite deerskin hat. He took his bath and his breakfast, attended by his granddaughter, the bride. Then he changed into this attire. After admiring his reflection in a looking glass he set out to inspect the castle courtyard and the town. He was followed by a chattering entourage of his extended family, who sang and danced from time to time, as the spirit moved them.

There was a long-standing rivalry between Edina and Cape Coast (or Oguaa, to give it its proper Fanti name) a rivalry which mirrored that of their respective Dutch and English patrons. In spite of this their townsfolk were united by many ties of marriage and clan. Uncle Kwesi Broni took the opportunity to pay his respects to his near and distant in-laws in Edina. Custom required that libation be poured at each port of call. Old Man, in consequence, became somewhat unsteady on his feet. As the time of the wedding ceremony approached, he had to be helped back to the castle and up the steep stairs to the church, where he sat down and promptly fell asleep.

In another room set aside for the purpose, Taguba and her sisters spent the morning dressing their daughter, doing her hair and adorning her with such paraphernalia and accoutrements as beads and bangles, necklaces and charms.

Jensen had invited all the officers above a certain rank to attend the wedding. He had no close friends, but all his drinking companions would be present. After the business with Thompson, he had decided not to send any invitations to Cape Coast castle.

However, Van Schalkwyk had thought this a good opportunity to reciprocate the hospitality which Philip Quaque had shown him. The Chaplain of Cape Coast castle had been borne over to Elmina in a hammock the previous day, accompanied by his personal slave. He would stay for a week.

Ama, never having attended a church service before, was excited at the prospect. It was not the religious aspect which intrigued her. She enjoyed the tales she read in the Bible, but she regarded them as no different from the rich fables she found in other books, nor indeed from the folklore of her childhood and the Asante Anansesem. Her intelligence rejected Van Schalkwyk's claim that the European god was the only one there was. She had grown up aware of the pervasive spiritual presence of her ancestors, mediated by the elders in the three shrines of the Owners of the Earth: the Earth Shrine, the River Shrine and the Fertility Shrine of the women. Unlike the ancestors, the gods were remote and impersonal.

In Yendi and Kafaba she had heard of a powerful god called Allah and of other gods who had their own shrines, priests and devotees. The Asante paid homage to their own ancestors, but also worshipped a supreme god, Kwame Onyankopon and an earth goddess, Asase Yaa, through a pantheon of minor regional deities who lived in rivers, rocks and mighty forest trees. And the people of Edina, as Augusta had told her, had seventy seven gods of whom the greatest was Tweneboa, spirit of the Benya river.

It seemed natural and proper to her that different peoples should each have their own gods. That applied, of course, to the Europeans as well. It would be strange if the whites were to worship Fanti gods. By the same token, she could not see why, far from home as she was, she should abandon the ancestors of the Bekpokpam for the god the whites called God or for the ancestor they called Jesus.

The chapel was a simple rectangular room, furnished with plain wooden benches. Two shuttered windows looked down into the inner courtyard of the female slaves and four more, two on each side, flanked the door which led out on to a landing with steps down to the roof of the North Bastion below and a view of the bay beyond.

The benches were already quite full when Ama arrived with De Bruyn. The Governor led her to the front of the room. They shook hands with Van Schalkwyk, who introduced them to his guest, the Rev. Philip Quaque, whom neither of them had met before. De Bruyn went off to look for the groom and Van Schalkwyk to attempt to explain to Kwesi Broni, now awake, but only somewhat sobered, what would be expected of him.

Ama was left with the Cape Coast Chaplain. They sat in awkward silence for a few moments.

Then Ama said, in Fanti, "You are welcome to Elmina, sir."

"Speak to me in English, child," the Reverend replied. "I neither speak nor understand that heathenish tongue."

"Reverend Van Schalkwyk," he continued. (She smiled at the peculiar accent with which he spoke the Dutch name.) "Reverend Van Schalkwyk tells me that you speak a passable English and that you have also acquired some skill in reading and writing. So speak to me in English, if you please."

"Please, sir," Ama replied in English, "I said that you are welcome to Elmina."

"I know what you said, child," he replied testily. "What is your name? Van Schalkwyk told me but I have forgotten."

"Please, sir, I am called Ama."

"Not your pagan name, girl," said Quaque. "Do you not have a Christian name?"

"The whites call me Pamela," she replied.

"Pamela?" he said. "That does not sound like a Christian name to me. I do not recall a saint of that name. Saint Pamela? No. My name is Philip, you see. I am named after Saint Philip who was one of the twelve Apostles of Our Lord. My late wife, my first wife, was called Catherine, after the holy Saint Catherine of Sienna. But Pamela has the virtue at least of being an English name. To have an English name is an honour and to have acquired a command of the language is a blessing, especially for a pagan. Now let me test you. Can you recite the Lord's Prayer?"

Ama looked nervously over her shoulder. The chapel was filling up. The ladies from Cape Coast sat chattering amongst themselves at the back. The Dutch officers, in their dress uniforms, had taken their seats nearer the front. Three of them sat immediately behind Ama.

She was shy. *Why does the man do this to me?* she wondered. But she had no choice. The world was ruled by men.

"Our Father," she began, in a low voice, almost a whisper.

"Louder," said Quaque. "You need not be ashamed of prayer."

She began again, a little louder.

"Excellent," he said, when she had finished. "I am most impressed. Reverend Van Schalkwyk is clearly a gifted teacher. He tells me that you read the Bible too. Which is your favourite book?"

De Bruyn had reminded her that it was Quaque who had sold him the children's books which had introduced her to English. Thinking to flatter the austere black minister, she flashed a smile.

"Goody Two-Shoes, sir."

"Goody Two-Shoes! What kind of book is that?"

He laughed an outraged, humourless, laugh.

"A story book, sir," she replied. "Mijn Heer, I mean the Director-General, told me that it was you who sent it, with many others, to help me to learn to read."

"Ah, yes, I remember now. It must be one of the chapbooks that Catherine brought out with her. Catherine was my first wife, you know. She was an English woman, a white. But she died within a year of coming to Cape Coast. This is not a good climate for whites."

For a few moments he was lost in thought.

"Goody Two-Shoes, did you say?" he asked, coming back to the present. "Well, I suppose if it was one of Catherine's there could be no great harm in it. But that is not what I meant by my question. For me there is only one book, the Good Book, the Holy Bible which contains the revealed Word of God. I see no purpose in delving into other books, except of course, the Book of Common Prayer. I advise you too to confine your reading to the Bible. I ask you again, which is your favourite book?"

Ama was saved from the necessity of a reply by the reappearance of Van Schalkwyk. Quaque, too, was not wholly displeased at the interruption of his conversation with Ama. He felt it his duty to raise with her the issue of her baptism and salvation from the sinful condition in which she was living with De Bruyn; but he was uncertain how to tackle the diplomatic problems which might arise. Now, with a clear conscience, he could set the issue aside for a more opportune time.

Soon the ceremony began. The congregation sang the opening hymn. Bombardier Trenks, who was the company map-maker, attempted an accompaniment on his old fiddle. His musical gifts, regrettably, did not match his cartographic skills. However the singing of the Dutch men made up in volume for what it lacked in grace, so Trenks' scraping was drowned out and little was lost. De Bruyn led Jensen in and, leaving him standing in front of the simple table which served as an altar, took his seat next to Ama. Jensen was resplendent in the white uniform with gold braiding and epaulettes in which Ama had first seen him. She remembered Esi and sighed. The *pig-god,* they had called Jensen. She squeezed De Bruyn's hand and looked at his profile. He did not react. She wondered where Esi was now.

Van Schalkwyk welcomed the visitors and announced the order of the service. Then, at a signal, Trenks led them into Handel's *Joy to the World* and Kwesi Broni entered, his suit a little the worse for the morning's wear, his deerskin hat perched jauntily on his wig and Rose clasping the extended crook of his arm. Rose looked beautiful in the late Elizabeth's reconstructed white satin wedding gown. Jensen, turning his head, saw the approach of the veiled apparition and for a moment swallowed his bile at having been forced into this ceremony. The Cape Coast women applauded and, forgetting where they were, broke into a rhythmic chant of praise, drowning out what remained of the hymn.

It was only when the bride and groom had been asked to sit and Kwesi Broni, too, had been shown to the seat reserved for him in the front row, that Van Schalkwyk managed, with some difficulty, to re-establish a semblance of order. Stung by the interruption, he chose to deviate from his prepared sermon, quoting, in both Dutch and English, John Knox's description of women as *weak, frail, impatient, feeble and foolish; unconstant, variable, cruel, and lacking the spirit of counsel.* However the censure was lost upon its target. The Dutch men, pleased that on this occasion at least, they were not the object of their predikant's invective, and without womenfolk of their own to intimidate them, murmured their agreement. Van Schalkwyk was flattered that they had heard him. All too often he suspected that he was preaching to deaf ears.

Ama wondered what Van Schalkwyk could be talking about. His sermon went on and on. She tried to recognise a Dutch word, any Dutch word, but soon gave up. It was muggy in the chapel and she began to feel drowsy. A fly buzzed at her ear and she lashed out at it. De Bruyn gave her a stern look. Her attention wandered and she dozed.

At last the preacher signalled the approaching end by summarising what he had said. De Bruyn screwed up his eyes in a conscious effort to focus his attention. If he remembered nothing else, the summary at least would allow him to make a respectable attempt at polite conversation on the sermon. He could not reveal to poor Hennie that he sometimes found it impossible to follow the thread of his tedious homilies.

When Reverend Quaque, in response to Van Schalkwyk's invitation, rose to read the lesson in English, there was another uproar. It was not that the Cape Coast women had much regard for the black minister; on the contrary they usually regarded him at best with suspicion and at worst with contempt; but he was, after all, a Cape Coast man; and he had not only mastered the white man's language and become ruler of the white man's church in his own home town, but he was now making his mark in the very den of their Edina rivals. They might understand nothing of what he said; after all he insisted on speaking only the *broni* language: yet they shared his triumph. And so they cheered and clapped, ignoring his withering glare.

The service proceeded slowly to its interminable conclusion and in due course gold rings were exchanged and Jensen lifted Rose's veil and kissed her, evoking ululations from the bored visitors.

Van Schalkwyk now brought the service to a close. As a challenge to the outrageous paganism of the visitors he led his countrymen in Luther's *A Mighty Fortress Is Our God!* which his compatriots, catching his crusading mood, sang with great gusto. The groom signed an improvised register and the bride followed with *Rose Thompson*, which was all she could write.

CHAPTER 22

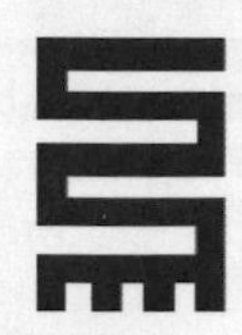

A passing ship brought news that the Dutch factor at Axim was seriously ill.

"I'd have to go even if it weren't for this crisis," De Bruyn told Ama. "It's two years since my last inspection."

"How will you go?"

"Bezuidenhout will take me in the brig."

"When?"

"As soon as possible. On the high tide tomorrow morning if the wind is right."

"Well I shall just have to manage without you."

"I'll come back just as quickly as I can. You will miss me, won't you?"

"Of course," Ama replied, kissing him on the cheek.

"I'll tell you what. We'll ask Hennie to brush up your catechism while I'm away. As soon as I get back we can have you baptised. Then we can start thinking about a date for our wedding."

*****

The brig Admiraal de Ruyter was moored in the Benya lagoon.

Ama went on board with De Bruyn. There was only one cabin in the little ship and since De Bruyn would be using it Commodore Bezuidenhout would have to sleep on deck with the Europeans and company slaves who made up the small crew.

Though Ama had never been on a ship before, she had often examined the tall masts and the rigging through Mijn Heer's spyglass. Now she ran her hands over a hemp rope and revived the shine on a brass bollard with the corner of her cloth.

"What a tiny room!" she said as they entered the cabin.

It's almost as small as the little store under Konadu Yaadom's stairs where Esi and I hid when Osei Kwadwo died, she thought. There was barely enough space for the two of them to stand beside the bunk.

"It's time to leave, Mijn Heer," said Bezuidenhout. "The tide has already turned and there is no guarantee that this off-shore breeze will hold."

Ama climbed down into the small boat and the bumboy rowed her ashore.

The brig weighed anchor, the draw bridge was raised and two canoes towed the vessel down the short canal to the sea. The seamen-slaves who were already up in the rigging unfurled the sails; the breeze caught them and as they filled, the ship became a living thing. The tow ropes were made loose and the paddlers swung their boats aside to make a way for the larger vessel.

Ama ran down along the rock quay, waving and shouting to De Bruyn. Then the brig had passed the end of the mole and was weathering the surf.

*****

Ama threw herself into her favourite armchair. She needed to think.

Tonight, for the first time since she had slept in De Bruyn's bed, she would sleep there alone. Before his return she had some hard decisions to make.

Christianity, from what she had seen and learned of it, meant little to her. But did it really matter? She would say *yes* and *amen* at the right places and then Van Schalkwyk would agree to marry them. That was not what concerned her. Nor was it that she did not really love Mijn Heer in the same way as she had once loved Itsho; he was kind to her and, in spite of their differences she was genuinely fond of him.

What troubled her was the thought of what would become of her once she had married him. He talked of retiring after Captain Williams' next visit and possibly joining Williams in a business venture of some sort in England. What was England like and how would she be able to live there, a black woman in a white man's country? Apart from what she had read in books, she had no means of judging, no experience which was relevant, no one she could look to for disinterested advice.

She rose and opened a drawer. From the bottom of a pile of neatly folded cloths, she took one that was old and torn. She shook it open and spread it over her shoulders. This was her only material memento of home. It was the cloth she had been wearing when she had been abducted, when Abdulai had raped her. The strip missing from one ragged edge was what Abdulai had torn off to bandage the finger she had bitten. She smiled. *That brute will carry the mark I put on him all his life,* she thought.

She took the cloth off her shoulders, crumpled it and buried her face in it. She imagined that she could smell the sweet fragrance of home, the smoke from the fire on Tabitsha's hearth, the aroma of the stew she was cooking, the dust of the harmattan, the sweat on Itsho's body when they lay together after making love in Tabitsha's dark room.

De Bruyn had said that he could never give her children. He was ageing and his eyesight was declining. In Holland or in England, he might go blind and she would have to look after him in an environment which was completely strange to her. Then he would die and she would survive him, alone, childless, without friends. Who would believe that he had given her her freedom then? She would be at the mercy of any white man who might decide to commit her again to slavery.

She thought of the Irishman Brew. Mijn Heer had said he had offered to send her to Kumase with his nephew. She had dismissed the idea and never given it another thought. Strange how it came back to her now. She stretched out on the bed.

Dressed in one of Elizabeth's dresses, she led the young white man whose linguist she was, into the Asantehene's court. As they made their entrance, she paused and laughed out loud, but no one seemed to notice. Koranten Péte looked closely at her. Her face was familiar. The white man spoke to her in English and she replied in the same language. Koranten Péte appeared to be astonished.

"Could this young woman who speaks the language of the whites possibly be the Ama whom I gave to Konadu Yaadom as a gift?" he was clearly wondering.

Then she noticed that Koranten Péte was not the one in charge. Sitting on the royal chair was Osei Kwame, Kwame Panin, her boy lover.

"Chief Executioner!" called Konadu Yaadom.

"No," said Osei Kwame, "I love her and I always will. Ama, please believe me: I had nothing to do with your banishment. Will you marry me? With your knowledge of the white man and his language, you will be able to keep Konadu Yaadom in check. I shall make you my principal adviser."

"I shall agree to be your wife only if you promise to give up your other wives, all three thousand three hundred and thirty three of them, set them free from the harems and find suitable husbands for them. And you must compensate them all for the years you have kept them locked up. You must free all the slaves in your Empire. The annual tributes from the subject states must no longer include slaves. You must agree that no one except convicted criminals will ever again be put to death by the executioners."

She was teaching school. All the royal children sat at tables busily writing. Osei Kwame himself sat in the front row and Konadu Yaadom and Koranten Péte were there too. Esi handed each a copy of Goody Two-Shoes.

Ama and Osei Kwame sat side by side, each in a hammock. Then they were riding on horse back at the head of a great caravan. Nowu, playing outside Tigen's compound, looked up and saw them. He rushed inside to warn Tabitsha. Ama ordered Damba to gallop forward to tell them not to be afraid. She dismounted and embraced her mother and then Nowu and then all the other children. Then she knelt before Tigen.

"My father, this is the Asantehene, Osei Kwame. He is my husband."

She was woken by repeated knocking at the door. It was the steward, bringing her lunch from the Governor's kitchen.

As she sat picking at her food, she tried to make sense of what she could remember of the dream. She had been thinking of Brew as she fell asleep: that is what must have set it off.

Her writing was making good progress. She was sure that she could write a letter to Brew.

"Richard Brew, Esquire,

"Governor,

"Castle Brew,

"Anomabu."

Anomabu. Bird's nest. She wondered what sort of a town it was that could have been given such a name.

"Honourable Sir,

"I hope you will recall having made my acquaintance during your recent visit to Elmina. Mijn Heer, the Director General, has told me that you might wish to employ my services as a guide and linguist for your nephew during his forthcoming proposed visit to the Asante King in Kumase. I should be pleased to accept your invitation. Please keep this matter secret from Mijn Heer and burn this letter as soon as you have read it.

"(signed) Pamela."

She wondered whether she should write *"Pamela De Bruyn, Wife to the Governor of Elmina,"* but decided that that would be untrue. *"Pamela, Consort to Pieter De Bruyn, Director General of the Dutch West India Company, Elmina Castle"* might do better.

She went to wash her face.

"Ama," she told herself, "you are still dreaming. Wake up."

*****

Every day Ama scanned the seas with Mijn Heer's telescope, searching for the Admiraal de Ruyter; but the day the brig returned she was engrossed in a book and it required Rose's repeated banging on her door to alert her to its arrival.

She rushed down to the quay. The brig's sails had already been furled. The breakers were sweeping the vessel towards the narrow canal entrance. As it passed the end of the breakwater, ropes were hurled out onto the quays. Slaves grabbed the ends and strained to slow the ship down.

There was no sign of De Bruyn. Bezuidenhout had the brig made fast alongside the quay.

"The Governor is ill," he told Ama in Dutch. "He has a high fever. We will put him on a stretcher and carry him up to his apartment."

Ama climbed the plank gangway. She knocked gently on the door of the cabin. There was no reply. She opened the door and went inside. De Bruyn lay on the bed which occupied most of the little room. His eyes were closed. He was bathed in sweat and his bed clothes were soaked. She wiped his forehead with the corner of her cloth. He opened his eyes and stared at her.

"Pamela," he whispered.

"Mevrou," Bezuidenhout addressed Ama politely, asking her to move out.

Bezuidenhout grasped De Bruyn under his armpits and a seaman took his legs. They manhandled him through the door and laid him on a rough improvised litter. Bezuidenhout bound him down with canvas straps. Four slaves lifted the litter with its passenger and passed it over the railing and down to six more who stood waiting on the quay. These raised the cross members to their shoulders and set off at a fast walk, up the hill and into the portal of the castle. Bezuidenhout followed.

All this time Ama had been hovering about, not knowing what to do, her mind confused by the sudden turn of events. Mijn Heer appeared to be seriously ill. She felt that she was, in fact if not in law, his wife and responsible for him. There was no surgeon in the castle garrison. She needed help and advice. To whom could she turn? Bezuidenhout was a stranger and, with only a few words of Dutch, she found it difficult to communicate with him. Jensen was not to be trusted: he would be happy to see De Bruyn dead. Rose was no more than a child. Van Schalkwyk was totally lacking in practical skills. Suddenly she was aware how isolated she was.

As they passed through the courtyard and up the stairs a silent crowd assembled to watch them. Death was no stranger to the castle but the usual victims were new arrivals from Europe. De Bruyn had been Director General for a long time. If he were to die there might be unwelcome changes in the administration. Few had any love for Jensen.

Ama caught hold of Vroom.

"Vroom," she said, "go and call Madam Augusta. Ask her to come at once. Tell her it is urgent."

She overtook the stretcher party on the last flight of stairs and, catching her breath, hurried down the wainscoted corridor to open the door. The doorway was not wide enough to allow the litter to pass. The slaves set it down outside. Ama pushed them aside and untied the straps which bound De Bruyn. He opened his eyes.

"They have tied you up like a rebellious slave," she told him.

He tried to smile but the effort was too much. His eyes closed and at once she regretted her weak joke.

The slaves lifted Director General, three on each side of him.

He has lost so much weight, Ama thought. *It is like lifting a child.*

She pulled aside the curtains of the four-poster and they laid him on the white sheets.

"Thank you," she told the six castle slaves in Asante, "you have been very good and gentle. When Mijn Heer recovers, I will ask him to reward you all."

"Yes, madam. Thank you madam," they chorused as they withdrew.

They had entered the most secret domain of the Dutch governor. There was a story to tell around the fire tonight.

De Bruyn's eyes were still closed. Ama looked at him. His face was flushed, his lips swollen. She felt his forehead. He had a high fever. She pulled the cord which would summon a servant. As she did so there was a knock on the door. It was the hot water she had intended to order. She poured some of it into the basin of cold water to take the chill off it. The water which they drew from the brick lined caverns was always cold, as cold, Mijn Heer would say, as ice. There was a foul smell about him. She stripped the shirt off him. It was covered with dried vomit. He opened his eyes. She saw now that the whites were bright yellow and streaked with blood. He retched. The spasm shook his body. He tried to raise himself but he was too weak. Ama put her arm under his far shoulder and helped him. A spurt of dark vomit, streaked with blood, soiled the sheet. He lay back exhausted and closed his eyes.

There was a knock on the door. It was Van Schalkwyk.

"How is he?" he asked.

Ama shook her head. She was near to tears.

"May I?" asked Van Schalkwyk .

"Of course," she whispered.

The Minister took a quick look at his friend. Then gripping the edge of the bed, he lowered himself to his knees and prayed silently.

"There is a ship in the roadstead," he told her when he had regained his feet, "a Dutch ship. The surgeon has come ashore to inspect . . . you understand? Jensen will bring him to examine Mijn Heer."

As he left, Augusta came waddling down the corridor, Effibaa in tow.

*****

"Wait outside," Jensen told them in Dutch.

"Wait outside yourself," Augusta told him.

Jensen glared at her but said nothing. Ama rejoiced at Augusta's confident rebuff.

Augusta had nothing to fear from Jensen. She was a free woman. Ama had never seen her so angry.

She spoke to Ama in Fanti, knowing that Jensen would understand.

"Will the man nurse the patient, wash him, change his clothes, feed him, sit with him day and night? This one would be only too happy if Mijn Heer were to die. 'Wait outside,' he tells us. Foolish man."

She blew a rude noise through her lips.

The ship's surgeon was looking at De Bruyn's tongue. It was bright red.

"Are you in pain," he asked.

De Bruyn nodded weakly.

"Where?" asked the surgeon.

De Bruyn lifted an arm and pointed to his forehead.

"And my back," he whispered.

When he had finished his examination, the surgeon took Jensen aside.

"It's the Yellow Jack," he said.

"That's what I thought," said Jensen. "I hope it is not contagious."

"Some say it is but my experience tells me they are wrong. I understand that he caught it in Axim. He must have visited some place there where there was a miasma, a poison in the air. Perhaps a marshy area."

"No doubt. We have cotton plantations there and I believe we grow some swamp rice too. Is there a cure?"

"None that I know of. Regular doses of lemon juice will do him no harm. If you have any grains of paradise or cardamom seeds, you might soak them in the juice. I will bring him an infusion of chinchona bark and orange peel in brandy when I come again in the afternoon. If there is no improvement in his condition by tomorrow, I might decide to bleed him. Otherwise there is only prayer."

When they had gone, Ama pulled up her armchair and went to sit by the patient. She took a book but when she came to the end of the page she found that she had no recollection of what she had read. De Bruyn twisted and turned and sometimes called out in his sleep.

"Pamela."

De Bruyn spoke with difficulty. She leaned over him.

"What did you do while I was away?" he asked her.

"Don't speak," she said, "I see how it exhausts you. You must rest."

"What did you do?"

"Well, the day after you left, I decided to give this room a thorough cleaning. I got some of the guards to help me and we moved all the furniture to the middle of the room. I swept and dusted and polished. Then I took everything from the cupboards and drawers and gave it all a good airing. I washed all your clothes and the bedding and the curtains. That took me a couple of days. Then we moved all the furniture back again. Are you listening?"

He opened his eyes and moved his head in the slightest of nods.

"Next I sorted out all your books. I wrote down their names and the names of the authors. And do you know what I found?"

His eyes were closed again. She squeezed his arm.

"Do you know what I found?" she asked again.

Again he opened his eyes.

"I feel so weak," he said.

*****

De Bruyn's fever fell and his face was less flushed. Ama began to hope for a recovery.

He was pale. His gums were swollen and bleeding and he was still vomiting black vomit streaked with blood; yet he felt a little stronger. He knew how ill he was. His inability to urinate in spite of drinking so much lime juice disturbed him. He got Ama to send for Van Schalkwyk.

"Hennie," he whispered, "I want you to help me make my will."

Van Schalkwyk nodded sagely.

"Pamela, do you have ink and paper?" he asked.

He helped Ama drag the escritoire to De Bruyn's bedside.

"This is the last will and testament of me, Pieter De Bruyn . . . Hennie you know what to write. I appoint you my sole executor."

When Van Schalkwyk had finished writing the preamble, he raised his head. De Bruyn was waiting for him.

"To the female slave, my dear Pamela, who has lived with me as my wife for the past two years, I give her freedom.

"To the said Pamela I give also all the clothing of my deceased wife Elizabeth, all my English books, all my furniture and china and silverware, my gold ring and five ounces of gold dust.

"To my first wife, Augusta, trader, of Edina town, I give five ounces of gold dust.

"To my good friend Hendrik Van Schalkwyk, chaplain et cetera, et cetera, I give my decanters and glassware, my chess set from Batavia, all my Dutch books, all my clothing, for distribution as he thinks appropriate to Company employees and others, and ten ounces of gold dust."

Van Schalkwyk looked up but De Bruyn cut his interruption short.

"To my only son Isaak De Bruyn, resident at Cape Town, I leave the residue of my estate . . . "

He was suddenly overcome by a paroxysm of retching and vomiting. At the same time his nose and gums began to bleed. Ama rushed to help him. Van Schalkwyk was glad to retire.

"I shall prepare the draft and read to it to you as soon as you are a little better," he told De Bruyn as he left the room.

In the evening Augusta brought Edina's leading priest. He had already slaughtered six cockerels and a sheep supplied by Augusta. Now he poured libation to invoke the help of the spirits of the ancestors and the seventy seven gods of the town in saving De Bruyn's life. That done he strapped a leather amulet on each of the patient's wrists and made him sip a herbal remedy.

"You should have called me earlier," he told Augusta as he took his leave.

The patient spent a fitful, restless night.

Since De Bruyn's return Ama had not had more than an hour's continuous sleep. When Van Schalkwyk came in the morning, she was exhausted.

Van Schalkwyk read the will to De Bruyn and helped him to scrawl his signature at the bottom. Then he signed as witness. Ama wrote "Pamela", as he instructed her, in the place provided for a second witness. Then Van Schalkwyk left, taking the will with him.

*****

Pieter De Bruyn fell into a coma four days after his return to Elmina from Axim.

Ama and Augusta kept a vigil by his bedside but both were so exhausted that they fell asleep. When they awoke at first light, the Governor was dead.

Augusta started wailing an improvised lament, "Mijn Heer, why have you left us. Mijn Heer, why did you die? You have left your wives widows . . ."

Ama put her hand on Augusta's shoulder and interrupted her, "Sister Augusta, Mijn Heer was a white man and a Christian. Let the Dutch bury him after their own fashion."

She felt a guilty sense of relief that it was all over. She had fought for his life but she had known from the first day that it would be a miracle if he survived. Whites had little resistance to Africa's diseases. She wondered how it was that Mijn Heer had lived so many years.

The visiting surgeon came and signed a death certificate. Van Schalkwyk came and prayed. They left Augusta and Ama to prepare the body for burial. When they had washed the corpse, they dressed it in De Bruyn's best uniform. That task finished, they bathed and dressed themselves in the new red and black funeral cloth which Augusta had sent for. Then they sat and waited. Early in the afternoon, castle slaves carried in the coffin the carpenters had made. They lifted the body into it and tacked the lid down.

In the courtyard the coffin was opened and for an hour the company staff filed by to pay their silent respects.

*****

As they wound their way back from the Dutch cemetery, the sound of musketry still ringing in their ears, Augusta asked Ama, "Sister Ama, what will you do now?"

"Maame, I am too tired to think of that. I told you that Mijn Heer made a will before he died. I heard Van Schalkwyk read it to him before he signed it, but it was in Dutch and I couldn't understand much. The Minister told me that in his will he granted me my freedom. I hope that that is true. But as to what I will do, I need to sleep before I can think of it."

At the front gate of the castle, Ama shook hands with Augusta and with the King of Edina and his delegation. She declined their invitation to join them in a funeral celebration, pleading exhaustion. While she was talking to them, she saw Jensen and his Rose, now visibly pregnant, enter the portal. She felt a slight sense of unease, but she was too tired to attempt to identify its cause.

Van Schalkwyk passed by and stopped to talk to her. Beyond Edina, the sun was a red ball, lighting up the western sky.

"I will go and see Jensen to fix a time to read the will," he said and patted his waist coat. "I have kept it here for safe custody."

When Ama reached the top floor she was surprised to see that the door of De Bruyn's room was open. Her apprehension increased as she went in. Jensen and Rose were surveying the candle-lit room and its contents with a proprietorial air.

"What do you want?" Jensen snapped at her.

"Please, sir, I am very tired. I had little sleep while I was nursing Mijn Heer. I thought . . ."

"Never mind what you thought. I am the 'Mijn Heer' here now. You will sleep tonight where you came from and where you belong."

There was a discreet knock on the open door. It was Van Schalkwyk.

"Ah, Jensen," he said, "I have been searching all over for you. They told me I would find you here."

"Mijn Heer Jensen, if you please. I act as Director-General until the Company Directors rule otherwise. What do you want?"

Van Schalkwyk blanched at the snub.

"Mijn Heer Jensen. Director-General De Bruyn made a will before he died. I have it here. He appointed me his sole executor."

He drew the document from his waist coat.

"I wondered if we might fix a time for it to be read to the officers."

"Let me see that," demanded Jensen.

Van Schalkwyk handed it over. Jensen took it to the escritoire, where there was a candle. He read the document.

"This is a forgery. I know De Bruyn's signature. He did not sign this. I recognise your handwriting Van Schalkwyk. I will have you arrested and charged with forgery."

As he spoke, he waved the will around and, by accident or design, the flame of the candle set the paper alight. He held it by one corner and let it burn.

"Oh, what a pity," he said. "An unfortunate accident. But fortunate for you. No evidence. Now it will not be possible to charge you. However, I can inform you right now that you will receive a formal letter giving you your notice tomorrow morning. Writing it will be my first official task.

"Do you think," he continued in triumph, "that I do not know the contents of the reports regarding me that you sent to the Classis? That was most unwise of you. It was your doing to land me with this whining baggage, this excuse for a wife. Now you will have your reward. You will take the first ship bound for Amsterdam."

"You can't do this," blustered Van Schalkwyk.

"I can do whatever I like. By virtue of the Company's rules I am automatically invested with all the powers of the Director-General; and in this establishment the Director-General is second only to God. Now get out."

As Van Schalkwyk beat a crest-fallen retreat, Jensen called for a guard.

"Take this slave to the female dungeon," he ordered, indicating Ama.

"Wait," Ama cried, as the guard came towards her. "Mijn Heer gave me my freedom before he died."

"Oh, he did, did he? Well then where is the evidence? Where is the completed form of manumission?"

"He ordered the Minister to write it in his will. I heard the Minister read it to him and saw Mijn Heer sign it, weak as he was."

"And where is this will, pray?"

"You have just burnt it," said Ama.

The enormity of her predicament suddenly dawned upon her. After two years of faithful service to Mijn Heer as his wife, she was to be hurled unceremoniously back into the dungeon.

Jensen was obviously enjoying her discomfort. She saw the cruel smile on his handsome face.

"You shit. You shit-arse. You rapist. You bastard. You pig. You filthy pig," she exploded.

A cloud passed over Jensen's face.

"Out!" he instructed the waiting guard.

"Lock the door," he ordered Rose.

"A pig, am I? A shit-arse? Is that what that stupid fool De Bruyn taught you English for? To abuse your betters? Now we'll shall see who is the pig, who is the shit-arse."

He grabbed her. She felt at once his overpowering physical strength. In a moment he had stripped her mourning cloth from her and then her beads. He threw her face down over the bed. She felt his trousers slip to the floor and heard him kick them aside.

"Itsho! Itsho! Help me," she cried, then, "Rose, Rose."

"Rose you come and watch this performance," commanded Jensen.

Then he entered her, not her vagina but her anus.

"Shit-arse, eh? Pig, eh?" he said again and again keeping time with his driving.

When he had finished he rested in her for a moment.

"Rose, my darling," he commanded his wife, "fetch me something to wipe my shit-arse prick with."

Rose opened a drawer and found there Ama's oldest cloth, her only painful memento of home.

Jensen withdrew and without waiting to clean his organ, threw Ama to the floor.

Ama had been raped before, twice, but never had she been so humiliated. She wanted to die.

"Who's a pig, now, shit-arse?" he demanded.

He pulled up his trousers. Then he kicked her in her naked ribs. She screamed in pain.

"Speak."

He threw the cloth at her and went to look at his dim candle-lit image in the mirror.

"Rose, shut your fucking mouth."

The girl was whimpering. Jensen washed his hands.

"Unlock the fucking door," he commanded.

She ran to do his bidding.

THE LOVE OF LIBERTY

African slaves were sold in Lisbon as early as 1441. The European discovery and colonisation of the Americas set the scene for the transatlantic slave trade, which lasted from early in the sixteenth century until the second half of the nineteenth. The slaves were all African. So too were many of those who sold them. The buyers and shippers were almost all Europeans. In the course of three hundred years, upwards of ten million black men, women and children arrived in the Americas as unwilling migrants. Millions more died on the journey to the Atlantic coast, and at sea.

They love liberty, go to war with their neighbours because they choose to become republicans, and insist upon the right of enslaving the negroes.
Robert Southey, 1807

CHAPTER 23

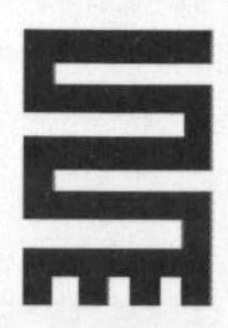

The Holy War in the mountains of the Futa Jalon lasted fifty years.

From time immemorial the Jalonke had been the owners of these upland areas: that is why their Susu brothers called them *Jalon-ke*. Descended from the rulers of the old Mali empire, they were aristocrats, soldiers, traders; and not too fond of physical labour.

When the wandering Fula cattle herders drifted in, the Jalonke gave them land to graze their livestock. In return they expected their tenants to pay a tax on every animal they slaughtered.

In the years before the war started, the Fula and the Jalonke lived together in amity. The Fula worked iron and wove cotton cloth and the Jalonke took these goods to the coast and exchanged them for salt. Sometimes the Jalonke made war on their Limba and Kisi neighbours and sold their captives to the merchants who lived near the mouths of the many rivers that discharge into the ocean along that coast.

The Fula worked hard and prospered. In the course of time they came to resent the taxes which their Jalonke landlords imposed on them.

Then the famous Fula scholar Karamoko Alfa returned from his pilgrimage to Mecca, inspired with religious zeal. Travelling across the great desert, suffering terrible thirst and in danger of losing his life to brigands, he promised Allah that if He permitted him to return to his home in safety, he would undertake to convert all the infidels in the Futa Jalon to Islam. The jihad was the fulfilment of his promise. The instrument he chose was his cousin, Ibrahima Suri, who had already proved himself a capable general. United by their faith, the Fula forces overcame their erstwhile patrons.

Many Jalonke fled to the coast. Others accepted the new religion but found it difficult to accept that those who had once been their tenants were now their landlords. They, too, fled. There were some, however, prosperous merchants and owners of cattle, who were more accommodating. The Fula were not ungenerous to converts who were prepared to co-operate. They appointed some of these men to rule the villages in which their brothers were kept in bondage. They even encouraged them to send their children to school, where they learned to read and write Arabic and to commit passages of the Koran to memory.

One day Karamoko came to open a new mosque. Testing the Koranic knowledge of the local Jalonke boys, he was so impressed with one youngster that he honoured his diligence by honouring him with a new name, that of the patriarch Ibrahima.

Allah bestowed many blessings on the young Ibrahima. It seemed that he could do no wrong. As he grew up, he prospered. He fought in many battles. By the time he was thirty he owned great herds of cattle, a veritable army of slaves, the maximum permitted quota of four wives (one of them a Fula woman), and an ever increasing number of children.

The Fula took to arms again and Ibrahima, now a general, joined their army, along with his slaves. But the slaves of the Futa Jalon were restive and as one great battle reached its climax, they began to desert, first in ones, then in tens and finally in droves. In the end their masters were left to fight on alone. Ibrahima was captured. Denied the customary opportunity to pay a ransom in exchange for his freedom he was marched off to the coast, fettered and manacled.

Chained he might be, but the first thing he did whenever the caravan stopped to rest, was to perform the *salat*. He prayed, too, all day long as they marched, carrying on a conversation with Allah, reciting passages from the Koran in an undertone, searching for a sign to explain his predicament.

"Allah knows best," he consoled himself. "Perhaps He is testing me. Perhaps He is punishing me for my pride and complacency. Now I perceive that all my wealth was as nothing in His eyes."

From Ibrahima's devout soul-searching there emerged in him a determination not to accept his bondage. He had learned the lesson of his humiliation. He believed that Allah now wished him to be free.

He knew the route well, having travelled it as a slave trader several times in his youth. He made his preparations and bided his time. While his fellow slaves and their guards slept, he worked quietly and patiently each night on his rusty shackles.

The camp from which he planned to escape lay in a clearing in the high forest, only a day's journey from the coast. He knew that if he should fail, he would not have another chance.

Waking, he raised himself on one elbow and looked around. The camp was quiet. He sat up cautiously. The moon had not yet risen and the fires had sunk low but there was enough light to make out the shadowy shapes of the guards. They all seemed to be asleep. He levered the shackles open and removed them from his feet, freeing him from the chain which bound him to his neighbour. An owl hooted and he froze. Then he prized the shackle from his left hand, leaving it hanging from his right. He worked out the course he would take. He would risk passing close to one guard whose cutlass lay beside him as he slept. The only other thing he would take would be a water bag. How he would survive in the forest he had no idea. All his thoughts were concentrated on one objective: to get away. He calculated that because they were so close to the coast his captors would not waste time attempting to pursue him.

Ibrahima closed his eyes and prayed. Then he rose slowly to his feet, gripping the shackle which was still attached to his right hand. He stood for a moment, his heart pumping, before taking the first step. Then, after what seemed an age he was on the path which led from the clearing to the latrines, cutlass in one hand and leather bag in the other. His feet were bare. He wore the same Mandinga coat and breeches of bleached Fula cloth in which he had been captured, though his suit was no longer the spotless white it had once been.

The path soon ran out. It was so dark in the forest that he had to swing the cutlass out in front of him, like a blind man's stick, to avoid walking into the trees. He had no idea where he was going, no landmarks to guide him. The forest smelt of rotting leaves, dank and sweet. He closed his ears to its strange night noises, concentrating on making his way between the trees. The canopy above him was so dense that even when the moon rose no light penetrated. He tried to keep going in the same direction, but he had no illusions: if he had misread Allah's will, he might end up back in the camp, having described a circle in the dark.

But it appeared that Allah was with him, for when dawn broke Ibrahima was free.

He drank deeply from a stream. Then he lay down and slept. When he awoke it was already afternoon. Every muscle in his body ached and he was famished. Yet before he did anything else, he washed his face and hands and, guessing which direction was east, said his formal prayers, adding thanks for his deliverance.

For the next few days he wandered in the forest, surviving off half-eaten fruit dropped by monkeys. Early one morning he lay on the bank of a stream and, exercising great patience, caught a fish in his left hand. He cleaned it with the cutlass and ate it raw. He disliked the taste, but lacking fire, he had no choice. The rusty shackle still hung from his right hand.

As he was washing after this meal, he was startled by the report of a distant gun-shot. Overcoming his immediate instinct, to flee, he waited apprehensively; but all was silence. He decided to investigate.

Some time later he came across the hunter, stretched out on his back under a tree, snoring. By his side lay a musket, a leather bag and the carcass of a small buck. Ibrahima gave thanks that there were no dogs. He took the gun first: if the hunter awoke, the man would be at his mercy. He was about to take the buck when it occurred to him that he would not be able to cook the meat. The hunter's pipe lay on his chest: somewhere he must have a firestone. Ibrahima decided to steal the man's bag, returning later for the carcass. All this time the hunter slept. *He must have been out hunting all night*, Ibrahima reflected. It was not until he was well out of earshot that he allowed himself the luxury of considering the fellow's reaction when he awoke from his sleep. Then, for the first time in many days he laughed out loud. The poor snorer would surely attribute the theft to malign and mischievous forest spirits.

The buck was heavy on his shoulders. He let it fall and sat down to rest. In the hunter's bag he found some stale corn-bread which he ate at once. But more important, there was a firestone in a little leather wallet, a sharp knife, some lead shot and a metal box half full of gunpowder.

He walked on until mid afternoon, setting a safe distance between him and the hunter and taking care to conceal his tracks. Then he put down his load, collected firewood and made a fire. He gutted and skinned the carcass, and hung the skin up to dry before setting a leg to roast on a rude spit.

There was a fallen tree nearby. The hole in the canopy had let in the sunlight and dense undergrowth had soon filled the clearing. Here Ibrahima collected branches and green leaves and built a crude smoking oven. He waited until dark to reduce the risk that someone would see the smoke rising above the canopy.

With food assured for at least a week he set about constructing a shelter. The fallen tree lay in the middle of the thicket. It was suspended in space, supported at one end by a profusion of tangled roots, torn from the ground, and at the other by its own splintered branches. He tested it by making a precarious ascent on the inclined trunk. Then he cut and trimmed a number of straight saplings. The lower end of each he placed in a trench; the upper end rested at an angle against the trunk. He wove more slender saplings in and out of the first to hold them together. Then he used his bare hands to squeeze mud into the interstices of this network. He smoothed the wall, inside and out, with the broad blade of his cutlass to. Finally he pressed broad leaves into the soft surface to protect it from the rain.

A week later he added a front wall of sun-dried bricks and a rough door of woven saplings. Now he had a snug one-roomed dwelling which was invisible from the perimeter of the clearing. It would keep him dry and protect him from predators.

During the months which followed, Ibrahima consolidated his tenure of his stretch of the forest. He devised and set traps for fish and animals and fashioned simple tools and furniture. He made cooking pots of clay and improvised a kiln to fire them in.

He no longer solicited Allah's help in his prayers, but rather gave thanks for his delivery from bondage into a garden of Eden. He seldom thought of home. His wives had been little more than servants and his relationship with his children had not been close. He had lived in a world of men, ruled only by Allah and by the Fula whom Allah had sent to bring His message to the pagan infidels.

Of necessity he soon abandoned any attempt to follow a *halal* diet; he even developed a taste for bush pig. And though he continued to share his thoughts with God, he no longer found it essential to pray in the formal manner five times a day.

What he missed most was the millet porridge which was the food of his childhood. He longed to cultivate a garden but he had no seed. Apart from meat and fish, and the fruit the monkeys dropped from the canopy, the only other food he found in the forest was wild yam and palm nut.

With his base assured, he took to wandering further and further each day. He was careful not to make paths which might lead another hunter to his hide-out but he learned to recognise landmarks to guide him back from his explorations. One day, by chance, he came upon the site of the camp from which he had escaped the slave caravan. He determined to lie in wait for a party of traders and to steal from them, while they slept, a basket of corn or perhaps some useful tool. He always carried his gun with him but he had tested it only once, and that, prudently, far away from what was now his home.

He took to camping out at night in the vicinity of the caravan halt. He would go there in the late afternoon and return to his home the next morning. He had long since put his white suit away and now wore a ragged garment which he had fashioned out of animal skins. In the gloom of the forest he was practically invisible.

For several days there was no sign of human life on the road. Then one day at dusk, just as he was beginning to believe that the route had been abandoned, Ibrahima heard drums. As they came closer he heard the familiar clank of the male slaves' chains. Unobserved, he watched the procession pass into the camp site. For the first time since his escape he saw women. Suddenly he became aware of the loneliness of his life and yearned for company and affection.

By chance, a young woman with a child strapped to her back soon left the clearing and passed along the path which led to an area which the travellers used as a latrine. She was alone. He could not be sure that she was a slave; she might be the wife of one of the guards. There was no way that he could know whether they shared a common language, for the light was too poor for him make out any identifying facial incisions. He had primed and loaded his gun in case of trouble. Now he was determined to take the opportunity which presented itself. The woman raised her cloth and began to shit.

"My sister, do not be afraid," Ibrahima said quietly in Susu, "I mean you no harm."

The woman started at the voice and looked around but Ibrahima was well hidden and since it was already quite dark she saw nothing.

"Do you hear me? Nod your head if you do."

She looked around again and then nodded her head.

"I was once a slave, but I escaped. Are you a slave? Nod your head if it is so."

She nodded her head again.

"I have built a house in the forest. I am a free man now but I live all by myself. I have food and shelter but I am lonely. If you will come with me, you will live as my wife. If you refuse, tomorrow you will reach the coast and there you will be sold to a white man and sent away over the great water, never to return. Will you come?"

She had finished shitting and was wiping herself with leaves. Her baby woke and began to whimper. At any time a guard might come down the path.

"Let me see your face, first," she said quietly.

Her eyes opened wide as Ibrahima stepped forward. Clad in his animal skins, with his ragged beard and long hair, his gun at the ready, he was indeed a strange sight.

"Decide," he said.

"I will come," she replied.

"I promise that you will not regret your decision. Now return to the camp. Wait until all the guards are sleeping. Then come back along this path. I shall be waiting for you."

*****

The woman was a Baga but she spoke fluent Susu. Her child was a boy, whose father had named him Tomba after his own grandfather, a revered Baga chief who had fought the slave trade until he himself had been captured and sold across the sea.

As Tomba learned to speak, Ibrahima taught him to call him 'Papa.' When he was four, Tomba's mother died in childbirth. Ibrahima was stricken with grief and blamed himself, but there was nothing to do but to dig a grave and bury the woman. Tomba cried for days, but Ibrahima soon became both mother and father to him.

So they lived together, Ibrahima and Tomba. Ibrahima taught his son all he had learned of forest lore. As Tomba grew up he quickly surpassed his step-father. He could imitate the sound of every animal and bird. He was an expert trapper and fisherman. There was no stretch of his territory which he had not explored.

One thing, strangely, Ibrahima did not teach Tomba, and that was the knowledge of Allah. He himself continued to pray from time to time, but living outside the community of men, a hermit, he found that he had no need for religious sanctions on his behaviour; the forms of Islamic observance became less and less important to him.

Years passed. As Tomba began to change from a boy into a man he became restless. He would go off and not return for days at a time. He would hide in the bush on the outskirts of some small coastal village, observing the inhabitants but too shy and fearful to present himself. At night he would walk along the sea-shore picking up shells in the moonlight and wondering at the never ending pounding of the waves. He had learned to swim in a creek near their home but he was scared to enter the sea alone and there was no one to encourage him. Sometimes he would creep into a dark village and steal what he could find: a discarded fishing net, a broody hen, mangoes, a hoe; or some other useful tool.

Then, when he was already a young man, he returned from one such expedition to find that Ibrahima had died in his absence. Dimly recalling that Ibrahima had buried his dead mother, he dug a shallow grave and laid his father in it. Now he was on his own.

*****

It was not until he woke the next day that Tomba realised the depth of his dependence upon Ibrahima.

Though they had never spoken much there had been a close bond between the man and the boy. It had never occurred to Tomba that Ibrahima was not his natural father. He felt guilty that the old man had died all alone while he, Tomba, had been gallivanting around the countryside.

He had no difficulty maintaining himself. The supply of fish and game in the forest was inexhaustible. He knew where to find wild yams and cocoyams; and when the rains came he would feast on snails.

He suffered from loneliness: there had always been Ibrahima to come home to; now there was no one. Lacking experience, he did not understand what it was that afflicted him. He took to spending longer and longer periods away from the little house in the forest which was all he had ever known as home. He would haunt the coastal villages and the slave caravans which continued, year in, year out, to make their dreary way down to the sea.

Ibrahima had tried to explain to him the nature of slavery. Reflecting on his past, the old man had developed a deep hatred for the institution. But Tomba had grown up in complete freedom and he could not imagine any other state; Ibrahima's explanations had meant little to him. There were many mysteries in life but it was not in his youthful nature to waste time on contemplating them. The slave caravans came and went. He would watch them pass. Sometimes he would steal from them while the guards slept. He looked at the chained slaves with curiosity; but he lacked the capacity to recognise their predicament. He was free but he was in no way devoted to freedom: he knew nothing else.

So a year passed, and then another year.

Then he fell in love.

The object on his attentions lived in a village set on higher ground near the mouth of a river. There was an abundance of fish in these waters. The villagers smoked the fish and harvested salt from a tidal pan in their territory. These commodities they exchanged for slaves whom the Mandingas brought down from the hinterland. From time to time a ship would anchor offshore – a sandbar blocked access to the river – and they would barter the slaves for cloth and guns, rum and a miscellany of cheap baubles. They were prosperous and content.

The only disadvantage of the village's location was that the river was saline for some distance upstream, even at low tide; and the ground water was brackish. The men could have fetched water by canoe; but the fetching of water was women's work and it suited the men to let the young girls of the village make several journeys a day to the nearest source.

It was one of these girls, returning from the distant stream, straight-backed, balancing a heavy calabash on her head, who had awoken such strange emotions in Tomba. He must have this girl. Yet, while he hungered for her company, he had no idea what he would say or do once she was his. His solitary life with Ibrahima had left him without social graces. It was not that he was selfish, just that he had never had a chance to absorb the subtle rules concerning acceptable behaviour that children learn while growing up within a community of adults.

Tomba's experience as a hunter had taught him patience and self-discipline: one unplanned move and the prey would be alerted and flee. So from his refuge in the bush he watched and waited.

One day the object of his desire was returning to her village in the company of her friends, gossiping and laughing merrily. Suddenly she realised that she had forgotten to retrieve a favourite bangle which she had removed from her wrist before wading into the stream to fill her gourd.

"Wait. Wait for me. Please don't move a step until I catch up with you. I shall only be a moment," she told them as a friend helped her to put down her calabash.

She had no warning. She heard nothing. She felt only a strong arm pinioning hers. An instant later a hand stifled her scream. Then she felt the fur of his jacket against her skin. For a moment she thought that she had been captured by some strange, unheard-of animal. Then she knew that she had been panyarred.

*****

Sami learned to love and value Tomba and the carefree, independent, self-reliant life they lived.

He was a real man. Stripped of his deerskin garments he had the body of a hero. His muscles bulged. His skin was dark, smooth and unmarked. He had no facial incisions and she could not make out what nation he belonged to but she guessed, from his complexion and his height that he must be a Baga. Yet he knew no word of the Baga tongue. He was a man of mystery and her life with him was a great adventure.

She had learned a little Susu from the Mandinga traders so from the start they could communicate. Tomba cherished her. He treated her better, she knew, than any husband from her own people would have done. Ashamed of his ignorance of the outside world, he questioned her endlessly about her village. Sami, in turn, was fascinated with his knowledge of the forest, which she had been taught to fear as the abode of wild animals and malevolent spirits, a place where only the bravest of hunters ventured alone.

After a year a girl-child was born to them. Tomba fell into a great panic when

Sami went into labour but he survived the shock and grew to love his baby daughter above all else.

The cloth which Sami was wearing when she was captured was now threadbare; and there was nothing for the baby to wear. Tomba made them both new clothes of deer-skin, but he realised that Sami hankered for finer stuff. One night he set off on an expedition. He had little concept of private property. The villages and caravans were a resource for him, just as the forest was a resource. He avoided Sami's village and chose the next one down the coast. The dogs were howling their praises to the full moon as he approached. Bribing them with bones, he entered the sleeping hamlet. Some careless woman had left a new cloth out to dry and forgotten to retrieve it. She had nothing to fear: theft within the village was virtually unknown and, in any event, impossible to conceal. Tomba took possession of the garment. But tonight he was unlucky: a young man returning from a secret assignation with his lover saw in the light of the full moon the apparition of a strange and frightening creature. Though it walked upright on two legs it had the hairy skin of a four-legged animal. It had wrapped a piece of cloth around its waist. The lover fell back into the shade of a wall, his heart pumping with fear. Perhaps this creature had murdered some innocent in her sleep to steal her cloth; but what was it, man or beast or evil spirit? He waited until it loped off into the forest. Then, as soon as it was out of sight, he gave the alarm. Soon torches lit up the village. The chief called the elders into an emergency session of the village council. No one in the village had been harmed and though it was true that there had been some mysterious disappearances of various items in the past, on this occasion all that was missing was the cloth of a careless woman.

Some doubted the lover's story and asked what he had been doing wandering the village at that hour. Perhaps he had stolen the cloth and invented this story to cover his tracks? He told them he had gone to empty his bladder.

Others recalled the mysterious disappearance of a young woman from the next village up the coast. The young men proposed pursuit, but wiser counsels prevailed and in the end they all went back to their sleeping mats.

But in this way the legend of the wild man of the forest was born.

Sami became more demanding and Tomba's raids became more frequent and more daring. He was cunning. He travelled considerable distances so as to spread his activities amongst several villages. Slave caravans were a favourite target, especially when they made camp in the forest.

News spread from village to village and the myth grew. Then Tomba was seen again by a vigilant caravan guard who slashed at him with a cutlass. He was lucky to escape unscathed.

The child was now beginning to talk, Mende to her mother, Susu to Tomba. She was a constant delight to him. He could spend hours playing with her.

Sami's family feared that their daughter had been panyarred and sold into slavery. They despaired of ever seeing her again. But when they heard the stories which spread along the coast, their hopes were revived. Her father set about organising an armed expedition to rescue her.

*****

Returning one day from a round of his traps, Tomba saw that the undergrowth had been slashed to make a path into his redoubt. His house had been demolished and his crops destroyed. Broken pots lay around. Nothing of any value remained, not a cutlass, not a knife, not a calabash of water. Even the puppy he had stolen for his baby was gone.

He paid scant attention to all this. Sami and the little girl were uppermost in his mind and they were nowhere to be found. He sat down on the bare ground and, in a state of utter despair, buried his head between his knees. He had no idea how long he sat, his mind a complete blank, unwilling, unable to face up to the reality of this new situation.

Then he heard a sound in the bush. He sprang to his feet and grabbed his gun. But it was only a hen which must have scurried off into the undergrowth to escape the assassin's knife. His dog whined. It was time for his meal and he was hungry. Tomba kicked it and it ran for cover, its tail between its legs. Then he was sorry. He took a knife from his bag, cut a leg off one of the hares he had trapped and threw it to the tyke. Then he sat down again and tried to think.

*****

The tracks led to Sami's village but in spite of keeping watch for long hours over many days, Tomba never caught a glimpse of her.

He was consumed by a deep, incurable anger. He resolved to avenge himself, to punish the perpetrators of the crime. His first task was to establish a new base. The place he chose was on a steep hill, well-wooded and riddled with caves. A leopard claimed the territory. Tomba shot him. After a year he was ready. He took two pistols and a musket and lay in wait for a caravan of slaves. When he judged that the guards were all asleep, he walked calmly into the tent where the master, too, was sleeping and put a hand on his mouth and a pistol to his temple. *This is too easy*, he thought.

"One false move and you are dead," he told the man. "I see you understand me well. Now get up."

Soon the party's arms lay piled on the ground and the guards and other free men stood cowering some distance away. The master lay on the ground before him.

"Order your men to unlock the shackles and release the slaves," Tomba instructed him.

When this was done, Tomba addressed the slaves. He had never spoken to more than one person before, but he spoke now without hesitation.

"I am the son of an escaped slave. I have come to free you from these criminals. I live in this forest. I am inviting you to join me. If you are prepared to work, you will not be short of food. I shall be your leader but not your owner. You will be free men and women. Those who refuse my offer will surely be sold to the white men and sent across the sea, never to return. Now who will join me?"

There was a moment of hesitation and Tomba had a fleeting sense that his enterprise had failed. Then one lad spoke up; and another. Soon they were all cheering and shouting Tomba's praise. He smiled.

"Undress the guards and take their clothes," he told them, "then shackle them and chain them. Run the chains around those trees. But do not harm them."

When this task had been completed he ordered them to take up their loads, together with whatever weapons and implements they could carry. By dawn they were at the foot of the hill he now thought of as his own.

*****

It took them time to recover from their ordeal. They were hungry and dirty. Some had been marching for a month. They had festering sores from the manacles. As they convalesced, he interviewed them, one by one, assessing character and identifying useful skills. There were many mouths to feed now, but there was seed and there were farmers. The rains would come soon and in a few months they would celebrate their first harvest. In the meantime, they depended on Tomba's skill as a hunter, trapper and gatherer of the edible vegetable bounty of the forest. The younger and fitter men soon began to help.

He could have taken his pick of the women, but he declined. The men and women soon paired up. Since there were fewer women than men, some women took more than one husband, contrary to all previous custom. They spoke many tongues but most understood Susu and since this was Tomba's only language, Susu became their lingua franca. Tomba allocated sites and on these there rose, at first rough shelters and later, more substantial dwellings with walls of stone and sun-baked bricks.

When they had recovered health and spirits and begun to fall into the routine of their new life, Tomba called the men together. He had not lost his pain and anger at Sami's abduction but he had taught himself to contain his feelings within broader ambitions.

"It is not enough that you have been freed. Every day more slaves are being brought down to the coast to be sold. The people who live by the sea have grown fat on the suffering of others. It is time for this to stop."

For the second raid Tomba changed his tactics. His men surrounded the camp. He fired the first shot into the air. Immediately afterwards each man with a gun followed suit. The slave traders believed that they were being attacked by a much superior force. Taken completely by surprise, they offered no resistance.

*****

Tomba's village grew.

There was limited space on the hill so he set up a satellite settlement on a similar hill nearby. The struggle against the slave traders became more intense. News of the raids spread. The caravan masters became more vigilant. In one battle, several of Tomba's men were killed.

The cost of tightening their security reduced the profits of the traders and they began to desert this stretch of the coast. The chiefs of the coastal villages became more and more desperate. They could survive on fishing and a little shifting agriculture on the fringe of the forest, but the luxury of the good old days seemed to have disappeared for good. As the white slavers got to hear of the consequences of Tomba's mischief, fewer and fewer ships dropped anchor offshore.

A meeting was called. Old feuds and territorial conflicts were set aside in the common interest. No single village had resources to match those of the brigands. A deserter who had taken unkindly to Tomba's iron discipline, disclosed the whereabouts of his hidden redoubt. The chiefs decided to dispatch an expeditionary force to destroy the interloper. It took them three days to agree who would lead the battalions. Once they had done so, they all got drunk to celebrate the forthcoming victory.

They underestimated the strength and determination of Tomba's forces. Their general was inexperienced and incompetent. Tomba's men ambushed the war party and killed every man.

At once he dispatched a small force to each village. As soon as the full disc of the rising moon became visible, the raiders slipped quietly into the target villages and fired the thatched roofs. Then they slipped away again, unseen.

The villages had suffered a devastating blow. The chiefs assembled again, this time in more sober mood. Their very survival was at stake. They decided to mobilise every active male.

When their meeting was in its third day a ship, which they recognised by its flag as English, dropped anchor some way offshore. It was the first such ship to stop on that reach of the coast for some considerable time. The chiefs at once dispatched an invitation to the Captain to join their deliberations.

*****

Tuesday, 10 a.m. Dropped anchor south of the mouth of the River Nunes. Gave orders for the long-boat to be prepared. Scanned the beach and observed what appeared to be a gathering of local notables. Amongst them the chieftain of the village at the mouth of this river, whom I recognised from my previous visits. A devious rascal if ever there was one. Almost at once a canoe was launched through the breakers. The principal passenger was a shifty-eyed mulatto who gave his name as John Smith. Strong scent of native liquor on his breath. Spoke passable English. Said he bore instructions to invite me to attend a meeting of the most important "Kings" of the region, which was that very day in session. The Negro potentates in question remained assembled on the beach awaiting my reply.

Tuesday 4 p.m. Went ashore in the longboat. Usual interminable exchange of courtesies and gifts. (I being the recipient of the courtesies and my hosts the recipients of the gifts). Using Smith as an interpreter, the "Kings" solicited my help in the conduct of a military adventure. The enemy, one Tambo or Tomba, I was told, had been raiding the slave caravans and setting the slaves free. A party sent to capture him had not returned. All slaughtered, most likely. On the same night the thatched roofs at several villages were set alight simultaneously. And mysteriously, since no one saw any of the arsonists.

Wednesday, 10 a.m. Sent ashore six men, fully armed, seven kegs of powder and a four-pounder with twenty balls. The condition of this military aid is that I shall have a selection of as many of the captives as I choose at a fixed price of no more than ten pounds apiece for a male, eight for a female and six for a child. Since I understand that Tambo or Tomba may have as many as a hundred men under his command, I may be fortunate to have an excellent bargain. The cost of the gunpowder will be recovered from the proceeds of the sale. The cannon will be returned.

Wednesday, 4 p. m. Ordered the carpenter to complete the preparation of the holds. He is the most competent man in an otherwise hopeless crew.

Thursday, 10 a.m. Watched the departure of the "army" through my glass. I counted three hundred men, about half of them equipped with muskets, the rest with spears, machetes and various other weapons.

Saturday, 10 a.m. The "army" returned after dark last night. Evidently successful. Will go ashore shortly.

Sunday 10 a.m. Conducted morning service at 8 a.m. Gave thanks to God for the successful prosecution of this little adventure. Some ninety males, females and children were captured in the battle. Ten bodies were found and an unknown number escaped into the forest. The leader, called Captain Tomba, was captured. He is reported to have put up a courageous and prolonged resistance, but that might well be an exaggeration designed to enhance the reputation of the victors. I have retrieved the four-pounder, resisting pressure to sell it to the local chief. Five of the attacking force succumbed and one of my men was slightly wounded.

The slaves are kept in open lodges, chained together in threes or fours under the care of a *grometto.* They are all in good condition, in spite of the war, but dejected in consequence of their defeat and capture.

Tomba is a young man, tall and strong and of a bold, stern aspect. He seemed to despise his fellows for allowing themselves to be examined by the surgeon. He refused to rise or stretch out his limbs when so commanded by the chief. This provided the latter with an excuse to subject him to an unmerciful whipping. The manatee strap left his back a raw mess of torn flesh and blood. The chief was consumed by rage and would certainly have killed the fellow, had he not considered the loss of revenue this would entail. Tomba bore the beating without flinching. I saw him shed an involuntary tear which he tried to hide, as if ashamed.

The surgeon having been instructed to complete his examination this day, we load tomorrow and expect to sail the next day.

CHAPTER 24

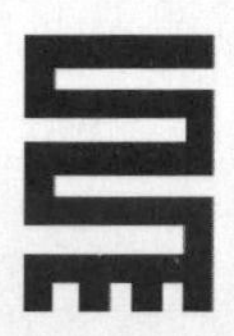

It was the breakers which brought Ama to her senses. The first big wave lifted the bow of the canoe and drenched them all with the cold salt spray. Then two rows of brawny arms thrust their wooden blades down into the water. They were singing, these Edina men. To them this was just another day's work.

The women lay huddled in the belly of the canoe. Coarse ropes bound them to each other and to the boards on which the paddlers sat. Not a week before, a desperate woman had jumped out of a canoe and drowned. The ropes were there to prevent a recurrence of that unfortunate, costly incident.

The young girl next to Ama threw up. Ama wiped the vomitus from her breast and strained against the cords to raise her head. The women's panic-stricken screams were lost in the roar of the surf. As the bow rose again, Ama caught a glimpse of the massive castle looming above the beach they had just left. The boat balanced for an instant on the crest. Then her head was thrown down against the boards and a wave of bilge water washed over her.

Fear rose in her throat as the bow rose yet again; for a moment they hung motionless in space; then the canoe rode down on the far side and the paddles drove them on to the next encounter. In spite of herself, Ama was exhilarated. She was alive again. It was if she had been reborn.

Then it was over: they had passed into the gentle swell beyond the breaking waves.

"It's rough today," said one paddler.

"But we came through it in style," said another.

"As we always do," added a third.

"By the grace of Onyankopon," said a fourth.

"I will insist that the white man gives us each a tot of brandy for our efforts," shouted the captain, who stood precariously at the stern, using a long paddle to steer.

The crew raised a cheer as they dug into the water. The canoe sped on its way.

The woman behind Ama said in Asante, "It is calmer now. Perhaps we are dead and have joined our ancestors."

"But where are they, then?" asked the young girl next to her. "I never thought death would be like this."

Ama thought, *I have fought and overcome; the danger has brought me back to life.*

*****

She had been as good as dead, for how long now, a week, a month? She could not tell. She had a vague recollection of being carried down the stairs, one man at her feet, another holding her under the armpits. She had lain motionless for hours, just where they had thrown her, in the female dungeon. Her whole body had been suffused with pain, her violated anus, her bruised ribs and her back and buttocks, where she had been bumped on the steps. But she had not groaned. She had just lain there, on the cold stone floor, her mind blank. Numbed, without fear, she had waited for death. She had felt no emotion of any sort, seen no vision of Itsho or of her mother Tabitsha. Nothing. No hunger, no thirst. Only a void; only the pain. She had not felt the damp rising from the bare stones. She was not aware of the other women in the dungeon and none of them had paid any attention to her. Each was drowning in a private quagmire all her own.

Vroom unlocked the padlock and opened the iron door.

"Out, out!" he commanded the women.

He was in charge of the gang of castle slaves whose job it was to swill and sweep the dungeons.

The women rose stiffly to their feet and filed out into the courtyard, blinking in the sunlight. Only Ama remained. Vroom rolled her over with his bare foot. Then he saw who it was.

"Sister Ama," he said.

"Sister Ama," he said again, "Sister Ama," but still she made no response.

She just lay there.

The castle slaves drew water from the great cistern which the Portuguese had constructed beneath the courtyard, filling tubs for the women to wash in.

"Here, you," Vroom ordered a young girl, "take this woman and help her to bath. Then rinse her cloth for her. Do you understand?"

The girl attached herself to Ama.

"It was my mother," she said, "my mother and my sister Amponimaa."

No one else would listen to her. She told Ama endless stories, stories about her mother and her sisters, stories about forest spirits, Ananse stories. At least Ama did not tell her to hush. But Ama heard nothing. The girl fed her with the gruel which was brought to them twice a day and helped her to the bucket. Ama did as she was told, but she saw nothing, said nothing. She was a living corpse. Even when the surgeon subjected her to the customary intimate examination, poking his fingers into her, flexing her arms and legs, using a whip to make her jump, forcing her lips open to examine her teeth, even when his assistant had pressed the red hot iron into her right breast, branding her for life with the ornately scribed letters "L-o-L ", she did not flinch.

Now, tied down in the belly of the canoe, all this came back to her in a rush.

*****

" Ere, Fred, eres a loikly un fer yer," said Joe Knox as he dragged Ama up over the lee gunwale. "Got a bit of flesh on er, this un as."

Ama thought that she heard English, but the accent was so strange that she could not make out the meaning of the words.

"Stan up straight now, an les get a look at yer," he ordered.

Bewildered, Ama did as she was told. She looked around her. Before her stood the tall main mast, stretching up into the sky. Stays and rigging ran out from it in all directions.

"Nice pair o tits," said Joe.

"Ere Fred, look at this uns boobs," he called, weighing each of Ama's breasts in a palm. "What dye think, eh?"

Ama stepped back and gave him an angry look; but she let the English profanity which rose to her throat die on her lips. Her mind was beginning to work again. It would be better if these white men did not realise that she understood their language. She took her wet cloth and rewrapped it under her armpits.

"Okwaseá. Foolish man," she spat out at him in Asante.

"Knox, stop foolin around," called the Bosun from the quarter-deck, cutting short Joe's reply.

*****

The women sat in the shade of the long boat. Ama ran a palm over the stubble on her shaven head and looked back towards the shore. There again, dominating its surroundings, was the massive edifice of Elmina Castle. It looked quite different from this angle. Suddenly, she was sure she recognised the windows of Mijn Heer's apartment. In her excitement, she grabbed the arm of the woman next to her and stretched out a finger to point; but then she drew back: who would believe her story, even if she saw fit to tell it? The woman stared at her. Ama smiled back weakly, embarrassed.

A ladder had been placed against the threshold of the open doorway halfway up the castle wall. On the beach below stood armed men, white men. One at a time, male slaves emerged from the dark interior and descended the ladder. When they reached the bottom, the whites shackled them together at the ankles, two by two.

A wave carried a canoe towards the shore, the crew working feverishly at their paddles. As it struck ground they jumped out and dragged the vessel a short way up the sand.

The guards forced the waiting slaves into the canoe and chained them to the seats.

Ama looked around. She had been aboard a ship only once before, when she had seen Mijn Heer off on his fateful journey to Axim. Now she was to be a passenger, of sorts, herself. She fanned her face with her hand. The air was still. The sky was clear and the sun stood directly overhead. Even in the shade of the long boat, it was hot. She dropped her damp cloth around her waist and then used a corner to wipe the sweat from her face. The cloth was faded and torn. It was the same cloth that she had been wearing when Abdulai had raped her.

What is it in the nature of men, she wondered, *that makes them treat women with such violence? Abdulai, Akwasi Anoma, Jensen. I am still young and yet already I have been raped three times. Jensen was the worst. These sailors seem bent on the same course. I shall have to watch out for myself. I hate all white men.*

She yawned and turned to look in the opposite direction, out to sea. For the first time she saw that there was a man trussed to the foremast, his arms stretched out and tied to a horizontal spar. *Like Van Schalkwyk's pictures of Jesus Christ*, she thought. *Even the loin cloth.* The sun fell on the man and his body shone with sweat. There were red welts on his black skin. Nearby there was a open-topped barrel, with a metal ladle hanging from the edge. Ama rose and walked the few steps to the barrel, a little uncertain on her feet as the ship rolled in the swell. She dipped the ladle into the water and sipped the contents to make sure it was potable. She drank the rest and filled the ladle again. Then, holding it carefully to stop the water spilling, she raised it to the man's lips. He drank greedily and thanked her silently.

The sweat was running into his eyes. She looked around for something to wipe his face with. There was nothing. She loosened her cloth and used it to mop his face, his neck, his arms and, gently, his whip-marked torso. Then she wound the cloth around her again.

"More water?" she asked him in Asante.

"Allo, allo, allo. Wots this now? Mary Madilin in person, is it now? Wipin the preshus feet o Cappin Jesus Tomba Chris isself, is it?"

This was Fred Knaggs. He whipped the ladle from her hand and put it back on the barrel.

Jabbing a finger at her, he said, "This ere water is fer crew, see? Not fer likes o yous. An if theres any feedin and drinkin o this ere Cappin Tomba to be done, twill be done by us, never by yous. Do you savvy?"

"Fuckin imprudence," he muttered to himself.

Ama looked at him blankly and returned to her seat. The women murmured to one another.

Knaggs looked towards the shore. It would be all of five minutes before the next canoe reached the ship. He turned to address the slaves sitting under the long boat.

"Honbil ladies and genkmunk," he said, pausing briefly to make sure that he had attracted the attention of his mates, "it is me great honner to interduce yous-all to the famous Cappin Tomba."

He drew blood from Tomba's chest with a precise flick of his whip. Tomba flinched. The women watched, uncertain of what was going on. Only Ama had some inkling of what he was saying.

"Until jus three weeks ago, this ere genkmunk wer known as Genral Tomba. But me an me mates, we made war on Genral Tomba. We whipped is tail an took im captive, we did an all."

There was applause and laughter from Fred Knaggs' mates.

"Ony the Genral were not content to be Private Tomba and when we invited im to be our gest on this ere noble ship, *The Love of Liberty,* e took a liking to it an decided e wud like ter becum er Cappin isself. Trouble is, *The Love of Liberty* already as a skipper as didna see fit ter ave isself put out of a job. So Cappin Tomba as ad to be taught a lesson, e as an all."

There was more applause and laughter.

"Fred Knaggs," called out the Bosun, "that'll be enough o that now. Now get back to work, or yerl be learning a lesson yerselves."

Ama leaned out to take a look at the speaker. He stood behind the rough wooden barricade which had been erected on the quarter-deck, blunderbuss at the ready. Beside him were two nine-pounders on swivels, trained on the main deck.

Why does the name The Love of Liberty strike a bell in my mind? she wondered. *Mijn Heer spoke the names of so many ships. What is so special about this one?*

*****

"Man overboard!" screamed Joe Knox suddenly, attempting to outdo his mate in waggery.

Indeed two of the slaves in the canoe had managed somehow to free themselves from the chain and, manacled together, had jumped into the sea. With only one free hand each, they could do little more than tread water.

"Swim, swim," shouted Ama, willing them to make for the shore; but the canoe swung round and they were soon dragged back on board.

The two culprits were the first to be pulled up onto the ship. At once, on the Bosun's orders, they were stripped of their remaining vestiges of clothing and securely bound to opposite sides of the main mast, bare buttocks facing outwards. Fred Knaggs was given the task of punishing them. His instrument was a cat o'nine tails, nine knotted log lines attached to a short handle. He swaggered around the mast, administering a lash to each man in turn, timing his strokes so that this was the first sight that greeted each new arrival as he gained the deck. And the first sound that each heard was the scream of the victim. The lesson was clear but it suited Knaggs to drive it home with a succinct homily after each stroke.

"That'll larn yer fer yer imprudence. Take that fer yer cheek. An' take that *on* yer cheek."

The victims' backs were soon a mess of blood and raw flesh.

The women set up a great moaning and groaning which rose in protest at each stroke of the lash and fell as they flinched in anticipation of the next. Ama stood up and moved out of the shade. The others followed. Ama took a hesitant step forward. The others did the same. She had no idea what she would do but she felt driven to stop this outrageous cruelty. The problem was solved for her by an imperious command.

"Knaggs, stop that at once!"

Ama recognised the voice. It belonged to Captain Williams, Mijn Heer's cherished friend. She recalled now that she had been struck before by the irony of the name he had chosen for his ship.

Williams spoke angrily, but in a low voice, to the Bosun. By now the canoe had discharged the last of its load.

"Cap-tain, cap-tain," came a voice calling from the canoe.

Williams strode across the quarter-deck.

"Cap-tain," called out the other captain with a broad smile when he caught sight of his counterpart.

"We finish. Soon dark. Tomorrow."

Williams raised his hand to his forelock in an informal salute.

"Cap-tain," the man called out again.

"What is it?" Williams called back.

The captain of the canoe patted the cupped palm of his left hand with the back of his right hand several times, meaning "I beg you." Then he lifted his loosely clenched right fist to his mouth and made as to drink.

"Bosun," said Williams, "give the man an anker of rum."

*****

The seamen unshackled the men, one pair at a time. Then they stripped them of their clothing. The garments were added to a heap which would in due course be washed and stored for distribution on the eve of their arrival in Barbados. Under the watchful eye of an armed guard, Butcher, the surgeon, carefully re-examined each naked man. At his command, two of the crew grabbed a slave and tossed him into the air. He made no effort to land on his feet. They did it once, twice, again, giving him a last chance to qualify for a free passage to the New World. Each time the slave crashed to the deck. Butcher ordered that the faulty goods be sent back to the vendor. While this was going on, the shackles were thoroughly checked and re-riveted where necessary. A piece of tin embossed with a unique number was fixed to each leg-iron. African names were difficult for the Europeans: it was much easier to do the book-keeping if the slaves were numbered.

At last Knox handed each man a short length of coarse blue cloth and a cheap wooden spoon. This was the slaves' equipment for the journey: a loin cloth and a spoon each and a shared set of shackles. The women and young children were allowed more freedom: all they got was a loin cloth and a spoon.

Once Butcher had completed his inspection, the new arrivals were herded to the centre of the main deck. Captain Williams stood on the quarter-deck, four steps up.

"Do any of you understand English?"

There was no answer to his question.

Arbuthnot, the chief mate, who was standing alongside him muttered, "We should have called at Cape Coast first, to take on a linguist."

He knew from long experience how difficult it was to manage the slaves without the help of honest and competent interpreters.

"When I want your opinion, Smith, I'll ask for it," Williams told him.

Arbuthnot looked down at his boots.

When Williams had first taken him on as second mate, on a previous voyage, he had told him, "Arbuthnot, eh? I reckon that's too long a name for a second mate. 'Mis-ter Ar-buth-not.' That's all of five syllables. Much too long in an emergency. If you want the job, you'll have to answer to the name of Smith. Understood?"

Williams turned to the slaves.

"Well, I don't expect you would answer in the affirmative if you did, but I will say what I have to say to you anyway, because I am sure that if any of you do understand, you will pass my message on to your fellows. And, in due course, when we get to Cape Coast, we shall take on a linguist to tell you all this in your own languages.

"I am the Captain of this ship. On this vessel my word is law and subject to no appeal. But I am a just man. I pride myself on my fairness. My crew will tell you that I am a hard and demanding master. That is true. But I do not believe that any of them will accuse me of being unjust. If you follow the rules, you will have no trouble from me.

"If you break the rules, if you try to escape, if you refuse to eat, if you raise a hand against any white man, you will feel the full impact of my anger. Tomba, over there, has been punished because he is a stiff-necked fellow and refuses to do what he is told. He has chosen the wrong adversary, I can tell you. I will tame the beast. By the end of this voyage he will either be as gentle as a lamb or he will be dead.

"These two new arrivals have been given a good beating because they tried to escape. That I will not tolerate. If any of you should jump overboard and survive the teeth of the sharks, you will feel the teeth of my cat, I can assure you. You are now in my charge and I will deliver you to your destination, safely and in one piece, come hell or high water.

"If, on the other hand, you co-operate, I will protect you. If anyone on this ship should abuse you in any way, send your complaint to me through your overseer. I promise that the matter will be fully investigated and that justice will be done."

The slaves were restless. Ama looked around. Judging from her companions' expressions she guessed that none of them understood what this white man was talking about. Most of them, indeed, did not seem to realise that his harangue was addressed to them. They began to talk amongst themselves.

One man said loudly in Asante, "This man has eaten too much okro. The words are pouring from his mouth like loose shit."

There was laughter. Williams paused. Knaggs and Knox moved in, flicking their whips. Cowed, the men looked down at the irons on their feet and fell silent. Williams continued.

"Life on this ship will not be pleasant. We will be very overcrowded. That is true not only for you, but also for these white men, my crew. They have to sleep on deck, whatever the weather. I am the only person on this ship to have a cabin to myself. I know that you will not be comfortable in your quarters. However, it is up to you to make the best of it. Remember always that cleanliness is next to godliness. Keep your quarters clean and you will not be afflicted with disease, with smallpox or the flux.

"I know that many of you fear for your future and that some of you believe that you are being taken across the sea to be eaten. Nothing could be further from the truth. On the other side of the ocean you will be given work, often work that you already know well, such as tilling the soil; you will be given regular meals, clothing and a house to live in. Your conditions will be immeasurably better than anything you have experienced in Africa.

"I hope that we will all have a peaceful and trouble-free voyage and that you will reach Barbados, for that is where we are bound, in good health. Are there any questions?"

"No questions, it seems. Bosun, see that they are given their victuals. Give the men also a small draft of rum. Then show them to their quarters and bring those down below up for their dinner. And you may release the malefactors."

*****

The two seamen removed the hatch cover and put the ladder in position. One of them went down into the first hold. A third, armed with a pistol, stood by in case of trouble. The new men were helped down the stairs in their manacled and shackled pairs. To Ama it appeared that they were making the descent into some dark and terrible underworld. She recalled Van Schalkwyk's graphic descriptions of the torments which awaited sinners and unbelievers.

Then it was the turn of the women. One of the whites unlocked the padlock and swung the heavy door open. Another made the women form a line. They were exhausted and dejected, many of them in a state of deep shock. Resistance did not occur to them and they complied docilely with the young man's gestured instructions. Ama fell in near the back of the line. She was curious to see where they were going and peered past the shaven heads and bare backs; but beyond the open door there was only darkness. She fingered the brand mark on her breast. The scab was itchy. She examined her fellows. All had been relieved of their own cloths. Like the men, each now had a short length of coarse blue linen. It was barely long enough to wrap once about the waist and tuck in. Some had made a loin cloth, tucking the ends into their beads. One older woman, careless of all modesty, or perhaps more modest about her shaven head than the regions below, had fashioned hers into a head cloth. *She must be mad, poor thing,* thought Ama.

She had tried to stop them taking her own old cloth. It was the only link she had left with home. The one called Knocks had torn it from her with some lewd remark which she could not understand. *Knocks,* she thought, *what an unlikely name.*

The line moved slowly forward. Ama looked back towards the shore. Near the beach, small boys were riding the waves on broken pieces of a wrecked canoe, totally oblivious of the disaster which had struck Ama and her companions on *The Love of Liberty*. Over the roar of the surf Ama thought she heard fragments of their innocent shouts and screams. Today was just another ordinary day. To them the slave trade was part of the scenery, part of their little world. So it had been before they were born and so it would always be.

Five more ships were anchored in the roadstead. She had observed the activity on just such ships through Mijn Heer's spyglass. At the stern of the nearest one the sun glinted on a gilded representation of itself and she could make out the word *Amsterdam.* All the sails on the three masts were furled; a large flag hung limply from the top of the mizzen. On deck she could see some white seamen going about their business, but no blacks.

She noticed for the first time the crosses on the castle's roof. *So much for Jesus Christ*, she thought.

They were approaching the door.

"What more punishments have these white monsters prepared for us?" asked the woman in front of her of no one in particular. She spoke Fanti.

Ama replied, "I think they are just sending us into a dungeon. It surely cannot be worse than the one we have left."

"I wish I could believe you, my sister," replied the woman, "but since I was panyarred I have learned that things never get better, they always get worse. I fear that it will continue like that until we reach the white man's country and they slaughter us to serve in their palm soup."

"Palm soup? White men?"

Ama laughed.

"Sister," she said, "white men do not eat palm soup. And I can assure you also that they do not eat human flesh."

"How can you be so sure? If they aren't taking us across the sea to make palm soup of us, what are they taking us for? Answer me that."

Ama had no chance to reply for it was now the woman's turn to go inside.

"What is your name?" she called back.

"They call me Ama," Ama replied as she prepared to follow.

"Wait, please," said the white man at the door.

Ama looked at him. He was young, younger perhaps than she was. His hair was a strange red colour such as she had never seen before. The sun had burned his pale skin a deep crimson, almost the colour of a tomato, so that he seemed to be on fire. She wondered why he had said, "Please." It was unusual: the language of these people seemed so full of violence. And there was no way that this boy could know that she understood English. Seeing that she was looking at him, he lowered his eyes. She toyed with the idea of addressing him in his own tongue. What should she say?

"Send in the next one, George," she heard from the darkness within.

CHAPTER 25

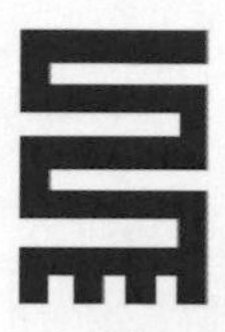

The air inside the hold was still, hot, humid and foul. Light penetrated only from four tiny vents set above each platform and from the open door. The floor was full of women, women squatting, women lying down, one or two standing with their heads just grazing the boarding above. It seemed to Ama that a hundred pairs of eyes were gazing at her.

"Here," said the white man, steering her in the right direction, "make yer way across to yonder platform. Orders is: new arrivals on the upper deck."

He followed her across, but she had already put a knee up and was levering herself on to the platform. She was on her hands and knees.

"Down ye go then," said the man, giving her a gentle push on the buttocks and pointing the way.

As she crawled, Ama wondered why he had spoken at all. He could hardly know that she understood English. Was she the only one, or were there others who also knew the white man's language?

She crawled towards the women on the far end of the shelf. *Like some four legged animal in the bush,* she thought. She stopped to peep through a vent hole.

"Ama, this way," said the woman who had been before her in the line.

"Ei, my knees," said Ama.

"*Kòse,*" said her friend, "Sorry. Human beings were not created to walk on their knees like that."

"All right, you lot. Out," called the white man, gesturing to those whose presence they had come to meet.

There was a rush towards the narrow doorway. Each woman, Ama saw, was clad in a narrow strip of the same blue cloth which had been given to her.

"They are going for their food," said Ama's new friend.

"How do you know?" Ama asked .

"One of them was complaining that we had delayed them and she was hungry."

"I don't know how anyone could develop an appetite in this stench. It is enough to make one vomit," said Ama.

Now the floor of the hold was empty. Ama jumped down and started to explore. At least here she could stand upright. The floor sloped away from her and then back again as the ship rolled in the light swell. She pressed her palms against the boards of the ceiling just above her head. Then she danced a few steps of adowa. It was strange the way the ground was constantly rising and falling beneath her feet as she danced. Her stomach seemed to be rising and falling inside her too. For a moment she felt she must throw up. But the nausea passed. She took off her cloth and holding one end in each hand she traced the graceful movements of the dance, celebrating the departure of the terrible darkness which had afflicted her.

"Take care, my sister," warned her friend.

Ama wrapped the cloth around her waist.

"Take care of what?"

"The white man showed us our place. He will punish you if he finds you walking around."

"Oh, don't mind him," Ama replied.

The room was bare. The principal feature was a round wooden pillar. Nearby stood several wooden buckets, narrower at the top than at the base. She went to examine one and withdrew quickly, holding her nose. It was full of shit.

Near the back of the hold there was a heavy door. She gripped the bars of the grating and tried to shake it. There was a steep stair leading down on the other side.

"*Àgòo,*" she cried. "Is there anybody there?"

A reply came in a language she could not make out. Then the head of a child appeared. There were others behind him.

"Small boy, I greet you," she said, smiling. "How many of you are down there?"

The boy spoke shyly, but she could make nothing of what he said.

"Stay well," she told him and took her leave.

"There is a room there, with young boys inside," she told her friend who was sitting with her legs dangling over the edge of the shelf. "Poor things."

The woman's head was wedged against the boards above.

"This place stinks," said Ama. "I pity those who have to sleep next to the latrines. I wonder how we shall ever get used to this smell."

The woman grunted, "It will get worse, mind my words."

"I'm sorry, I forgot to ask your name,"

"I am called Nana Esi."

Ama was silent. Following her example, several other younger women had jumped down.

Ama had a thought.

"My sisters," she called out, "if you want to go somewhere, you had better go now. You may not get a chance when the others return."

"I had a friend called Esi," she said to Nana Esi.

Nana Esi waited to hear more, but Ama was in a brown study.

"What happened to her?" she asked at last.

"I don't know. I wish I did. She was my best friend. Excuse me, I am going to take my own advice before the others come back."

She hadn't given Esi a thought since Mijn Heer's death and what came after. The poor girl must have gone through this same experience. She too had been raped by that monster Jensen. Now Ama felt a pang of guilt. Perhaps she would meet Esi again in the white man's country. She held her nose and tried not to breathe as she sat on the bucket.

The older woman who had used her only garment for a head cloth was standing nearby. Suddenly she began to shake violently. Almost at once she fell to the floor, twisting and turning. Other women came to look at her but did nothing.

"Hold her," cried Ama from her seat. "She will hurt herself."

She looked around for something to wipe with but there was nothing.

Lucky it was a firm shit, she thought.

The convulsions stopped and the distressed woman rose to her feet. Now she started to laugh, a wild, animal, incoherent laughter. From time to time she paused to take a breath or was overcome by another shaking fit. Then the laughter resumed. It went on and on and on. At last she began to cry out.

"Fools, fools," she cried again and again, gripping the grating on the outer door.

The noise drew the surgeon, Butcher.

"What's going on here?" Ama heard him ask.

The door opened. The woman was dragged out and the door closed again with a bang. Ama went to it and looked through the grating. The woman lay on her back on the deck. Two seamen sat on her, fixing manacles and handcuffs.

"Send her back with the first canoe," said Butcher. "There's no way we're going to give this one a free trip to Barbados."

*****

The other women returned from the deck.

They were followed by the surgeon and six white seamen, who hung lamps on the bulkhead.

Butcher addressed them in a loud voice, "Soon this hold will be full. It is time that you learned how we want you to arrange yourselves. The men will show you how you are to lie."

They began to line the women up according to Williams' plan. Their first customers were confused. The men spoke to them, then used sign language and finally man-handled them into position, each lying on her right side, facing into the back of her neighbour. Once they realised what they were required to do, the other women complied without resisting, as if this were some kind of game they were playing.

"As for the mind of the white man, it is a mystery," said one.

"*Me broni*," said another to a young seaman, "*wo ho ye fe se anoma*," meaning, "My precious white man, you are as beautiful as a bird."

There was an approving roar of laughter from those who understood.

Ama watched, wondering again why the white men bothered to speak to them at all. She vowed to keep her mouth shut: there was no way that she would become their *okyeame*.

Then the white men left and the women rearranged themselves before they settled down for the night. There was still plenty of space to stretch.

*****

The next day was a Sunday. Williams would have liked to continue loading his ship, but the Dutch company's rules about the observance of the Sabbath were inflexible.

The women were allowed out onto the quarter-deck soon after dawn. An awning had been rigged for them and they were not uncomfortable in the shade. Tomba's people sat to one side. Ama greeted them with the formal morning salutation. They replied with smiles in a language which was totally strange to her.

"Do none of you hear Asante?" she asked.

One older woman raised her open palm to her ear; another spread her palms and cocked her head. There was laughter and some animated conversation.

Ama tried her mother tongue, Lekpokpam, without much hope and with a similar result. She looked over her shoulder. None of the Elmina party appeared to be watching her and none of the crew were nearby.

"What about English?" she asked in a whisper.

"English," came a loud reply.

Ama's heart gave a leap. If one of these women understood English the two parties would be able to communicate. But who had answered? She raised herself to her knees. The English speaker was waving to her. She was a slim young woman with a mischievous smile. Her companions paid no attention to her. She moved aside to make room for Ama.

"You hear English?" Ama asked.

"English," she replied with a grin.

Then she pointed to the crew on the main deck.

"Man," she said.

Then she pointed to herself and said, "Wo-man."

Inspired by a sudden thought, she pointed to Ama and said, "Wo-man, A-frica wo-man," and laughed.

"You must know more?" Ama asked.

"Man, *Ing-lish* man," she said, pointing as before.

"Wo-man," she said again, pointing to herself; and then after a pause, added with a sly laugh, "Fokkie-fokkie. Man, wo-man, fokkie-fokkie. Ing-lish man, A-frica wo-man, fokkie-fokkie."

And she laughed yet again. The woman sitting next to her looked at her with disdain. Ama rose, disappointed. This was not her hoped-for linguist.

Then, as one person, the women around her suddenly rose to their feet.

"Tomba, Tomba," they cried.

Tomba, who had been led out, shuffling the irons which held his ankles, turned and raised his manacled hands up high, acknowledging their greetings. He spoke a few words and at once his guard flicked his cat at him. They saw the lacerations from the beating he had received and there were cries of sympathy. Then the guard forced him on his way to the forecastle, where he and the boys took their food. The boys came out of the door below and followed.

"Kwaku, Kwaku," called Kwaku's mother, struggling forward to the edge of the quarter-deck.

The boy is barely ten years old, thought Ama. She saw him respond to his mother's call and begin to sob. The guard flicked his whip and the boy withdrew. He was the only Akan. His mother had not seen him since they had been brought on board. The others were all Tomba's boys. They turned to wave to the women as they passed and there were calls to them too.

The food was in large round trays. As they settled down in a circle around the two trays, Ama heard the voice of the surgeon, Butcher.

"For what you are about to receive," he intoned, "may the Lord make you truly thankful. Amen."

The boys knew what was expected of them.

"Amen," they chorused.

*****

The men were brought up from the bowels of the ship and chained to iron rings.

They looked around, bewildered, as they ate.

Once, back home, long ago, Itsho had hacked off the top of a termite mound. Ama was reminded of the confused panic of the subterranean insects, suddenly exposed to the light and to the appetites of the compound chickens.

Of each pair of men, one had a right hand free and the other a left hand.

"These white men may know how to make ships, but their customs are uncivilised. It is bad enough that they keep us in chains, but to force us to eat with our left hands, that is the ultimate humiliation. It is against all custom," Ama heard one of them complain.

When they had herded the male slaves back into their dark abode, the crew assembled on the main deck.

Captain Williams emerged from his Cabin and Arbuthnot called for silence.

"Our Father," Williams intoned.

"Which art in heaven," responded the crew in their various accents.

Silently Ama mouthed the familiar words; but when she came to "as we forgive those that trespass against us . . ." she stopped. *Why should I forgive them when they persecute us so*? she wondered. She loved the music of the words, but the sense offended her. *They say their god is all powerful. If that is so he must have ordained what they are doing to us.*

Then the service was over. Half the crew jumped down into a waiting canoe. Amongst them Ama recognised the ones called Knox and Knaggs.

*****

Ama woke early the next morning. It was dark in the hold but she could see a glimmer of dawn through the barred door.

She slipped off the platform and picked her way through the bodies. She wanted to piss but the thought of the smell of the buckets put her off. It pervaded the hold; but when you were sitting on the bucket it was overpowering. She would wait. On Sunday afternoon she had watched the man they called Chippy busying himself with the construction of a platform cantilevered from the side of the ship. There were steps up to it and then a wooden seat with holes in it. Ama guessed that this was to be a latrine: you would sit over the hole and your shit would drop straight down into the sea.

Butcher passed by the door, rubbing the sleep from his eyes.

Catching sight of Ama, he asked in dialect, "What, missus, so eager t'be let out of yer prison?" and unlocked the door.

"*Owura, medaase*," she thanked him in Asante, wondering what his reaction might be if she said, "Thank you, sir," instead. Then she improvised sign language to ask him if she could use the Chippy's new facility.

"Sure, sure. Go ahead," he said, "but take care you don't fall through the hole!" and laughed at his feeble joke.

Ama climbed the steps up over the gunwale cautiously, nervous of the height. *What would Butcher do*, she speculated, *if I should suddenly fall into the sea and start swimming for the shore*? Williams had spoken of sharks. She looked down to the waters below. She had never seen a shark but Mijn Heer had told her what damage they could inflict.

Amongst the canoes which had hoisted their sails to catch the morning's offshore breeze, she picked out one with white passengers. It was the crew returning from their night's carousing ashore. They were evidently somewhat the worse for wear. Two were bare to the waist.

"Where's yer shirt?" asked Arbuthnot of one as he clambered over the gunwales.

"Sold it," came the mumbled reply.

The Mate shook his head wearily.

Then he grabbed the last man aboard by his wrist.

"Where's Knaggs?" he asked.

The seaman looked around for support.

When none was forthcoming, he said sheepishly, "Arrested."

"Arrested?" asked the mate. "For what?"

"Murder," said the other grimly.

"Murder, is it?" asked Arbuthnot. "Then hadn't ye better be reporting to the skipper?"

Ama tried to conceal her interest, but her dissimulation was unnecessary. The white men spoke as if the blacks did not exist.

The women began to come out of the hold in ones and twos, making their way up to their customary places on the quarter-deck.

Captain Williams emerged from his cabin with Butcher.

"Bloody Jensen," he said. "In De Bruyn's time this couldn't have happened. His men were never allowed out into the town after dark. Jensen is unpopular and he is canvassing for support amongst his garrison by relaxing the rules. We'd better go ashore and find out how bad things are with the Dutch sergeant. Bring your instruments: you may need of them. And that demented woman: bring her along too. But truss her well: I don't want her causing any trouble. Jensen will have to give us a marketable replacement."

*****

When Williams and Butcher returned in the late afternoon, they had Knaggs in tow.

"Get to work, you rapscallion," Williams told him as they came aboard, "or I'll be docking you a week's pay rather than a day's. And hear me well. I am tired of your villainies. Test me once more and I'll clap you in irons for the rest of this voyage. You're a bad influence."

As soon as the Captain and the Surgeon were out of sight, Knaggs was surrounded by his minions.

"What happened, Knaggsy, ole feller?" asked one.

They were standing just below the quarter-deck. Ama moved closer so that she could hear.

Knaggs was swollen with pride.

"There was this ere Dutchy," he told them. "Said e were a serjeant. We was drinkin punch together, nice an friendly like. Well, then e teks it into is ed to say sommat nasty bout our King George."

"Whatid e say, then, Fred ole chap?"

Fred scratched his head.

"Don' rightly know," he replied. "Twere in is lingo. But twere insulting, take me word fer it."

"Whatid yer do then?"

"I tol' im where ter get off, course."

"An then?"

"Silly fool challenges me to a jool, wit swords, min' you. I grees an we goes roun the back."

"Someone gives me this sword and says 'one-two-three.' But Fred Knaggs din wait fer 'three.' No, not Fred Knaggs. At 'two' I drives me sword strait inter the fool's belly. Then e falls on is back, grievous wounded, blood an intestins flowing from a ole in is ernatermy. An Fred Knaggs standin oer im wit me sword. 'Teach yer ter insult King George,'' says I.

"Then e begs me not ter finish im off.

" 'Release yer sword, then,' says I, an e lets it go.

" An I does the same. Thas me, Fred Knaggs, magaminous. I coulda killed im right there, but I lowed im is life, misrable Dutchy bastard."

There was applause from the sycophants.

"Three cheers fer Fred Knaggs," said one, but Fred put his finger to his lips, said, "Shh," and pointed in the direction of the captain's cabin.

"What happened then, Fred?"

"Silly Dutch buggers assaults me. Like ten of em, all together. But Fred Knaggs gives em as good as e gets, e does. Only I were overcum by strength o numbers. By rights, King George should give me a medal, fer defendin Is Majesty's honner."

" Ear, ear. A medal fer Fred. But what'd they do wi you, Freddy boy?"

"Stuffd me in a filthy, smelly dungeon. Fit ony fer niggers, it were. An it *were* full o darkies too. Not a honnest Hinglishman hamongst them. I thought they'd slit me throat, bot they din do me no arm. An there I stays till Doc Butcher cums ter fetch me."

"What'd e say?"

"'E says Ise lucky ter get orf. Dutchies woulda put a nalter round me neck, e says. Them were is very words. E says Ise lucky cos Dutchy serjeant's wounds is suprafishul an e were able ter sew is belly up, like."

"Knaggs!" came a roar from the first mate.

Fred Knaggs was in trouble again.

Ama had got the gist of all this. She was bursting with the news but in order to tell the story to her friends, she would have to admit to understanding English. And if the slaves knew that, it would only be a matter of time before the English, too, knew. So she bit her tongue and kept her counsel.

*****

Ama kneeled against the gunwale and rested her elbows on the rail. Overhead the gulls screamed and wheeled. Beyond the breakers and the rocks lay the mass of Cape Coast Castle. The latest arrivals had told of the terror in the dungeons there, underground, damp, dark, unventilated and infested with rats. Like Elmina, only worse, she guessed; if that were possible.

It was Sunday. She had been aboard *The Love of Liberty* for over a week. On the second day she had persuaded one of the canoe-men to take a message from her to Augusta.

"Tell her, I beg you, that Ama has been sold to the English and is on this ship. Tell her that I beg her to buy me back."

"Ama? Every seventh woman is called Ama, my sister. How will she know you from every other Ama who has been unlucky enough to fall into servitude? What makes you think that she will remember you at all?"

"Oh, she will remember me. Just tell her that I am here, I beg you. Tell her, Mijn Heer's Ama."

"Mijn Heer's Ama, you say?"

Once he had caught a glimpse of the late governor's almost mythical consort. She had been dressed in one of Elizabeth's gowns. A fabulous beauty, he had thought then.

"How I'd like to get my prick between that one's legs," he had told his mate; and they had laughed at his bawdy fantasy. Now here was this slave woman with her shaven head, wearing only a narrow piece of coarse blue cloth.

"You must be joking, my sister."

"I was never more serious. Please, please, tell her."

She had watched out for him the next day. Now he looked at her with more respect.

"I told her. She said she wondered what had happened to you. She thought you might be dead. She is pleased to hear that you are still alive. She says to tell you that she has heard that it is the new Director himself who ordered that you should be sold. She says that you know that she and the new Director are not on good terms. It will be very difficult, but she will see what she can do."

Every day he had come with another message. She was doing her best. It was extremely difficult. There were problems. Jensen had granted her an interview only to shower her with such insults that she had walked out on him.

"Tell Auntie Augusta that the Captain of this ship is an old friend of Mijn Heer's; that the last time the Captain was here she took him to see the King. Perhaps if she could get a message to him, he would do her a personal favour."

Then Williams had decided that he had had enough of Jensen's arrogance. Perhaps he would get a better deal from his own countrymen at Cape Coast.

The women had been sent into their hold to give the sailors room to work on the deck. Ama had felt the ship heave and creak as the wind filled its sails. That was in the morning. The same afternoon Williams dropped anchor off Cape Coast. When they were allowed out on the deck again the sails had all been furled as before. They were anchored opposite another, different, castle.

Conditions on board had steadily worsened. There was little ventilation in the female hold. More and more women were crowded into the small space. By midnight the air became so foul that it was difficult to breathe. By the early hours of the morning the smell from the buckets was overpowering.

The women, at least, were allowed to spend the day in the light and fresh air. For the men it was much worse. They were kept constantly in irons and allowed up only for a short time twice each day. Loaded guns pointed at them as they ate. Tomba's men who had already been on board for several weeks, looked really bad. Ama could see how they were suffering. And they were clearly unhappy at having strange men from Elmina and Cape Coast appointed as their overseers. The women were strictly forbidden to speak to the men; but only the threat of the cat could dissuade Tomba's women from communicating with their country-folk. Ama guessed that they were giving them news of their leader. She wondered how it was that these people seemed to have such a sense of solidarity. She resolved to learn their language and hear their history.

She interrupted her own reverie. It was time to consider her options.

She might make herself known to Captain Williams. That was unlikely to do her any good. Indeed it might do her harm. She remembered his prejudice against the education of slaves and women. He would surely be suspicious of her.

She looked out at the edifice of Cape Coast Castle. With its cannons facing out to sea it seemed to threaten even at that distance. She knew no one in Cape Coast, except perhaps the drunken relatives of Jensen's Rose. Then she recalled the Rev. Philip Quaque. They had talked at Rose's wedding. He would surely remember her. With him, the fact that she knew English might be a point in her favour. Perhaps he would buy her. He might even employ her as a teacher in his school. She had heard that he was second in status only to the English Governor.

She felt a thrill of excitement. This was a real chance, if only a slim one. But how could she get a message to him? She might ask one of the canoe-men, but any message that might recall her to Quaque's memory would be so complicated that it would almost certainly arrive garbled. If only she could get her hands on ink and paper!

Ink and paper! That would mean stealing into the Captain's cabin. She wondered whether he left his door unlocked when he went ashore.

In the midst of these speculations she heard a muffled conversation. Turning, she saw that Knaggs and Knox and three of their cronies had gathered at the foot of the quarter-deck stairs. They were keeping their voices low. She could make out nothing of what they were saying but it looked as if they were up to no good. One of them climbed the steps and surveyed the territory. Then he beckoned and the one called Knox joined him. Knox looked carefully around. Then he let his eye wander over the ranks of the slave women, some sleeping, some sitting quietly. Ama sensed danger. Slowly she moved out of their field of view. Knox appeared to come to a decision. He pointed to one of the women. Then he and his companion strode across and grabbed her, each taking an arm. Knox stuffed a rag into her mouth to stifle her screams. Some women stood up, alarmed. The sleepers awoke, still not aware of what was happening.

The two white men dragged the black woman down the steps and over to the main mast. They forced her to stand against it. Knox's accomplice pulled her arms round to the back of the mast. Ama could see that the woman was wide-eyed with terror. The gag prevented her from crying out loud, but Ama sensed her muffled scream as her arms were brutally twisted. Knox fumbled with his trouser cord for a moment and then he was inside her. But she twisted to one side and in that movement expelled his organ. He took a step back and slapped her face so violently that her head struck the mast. She stopped resisting. Joe re-entered her. His mates cheered.

"Fuck," they cried in unison at every thrust, "fuck, fuck, fuck . . ."

But even in their excitement they modulated their voices, looking back at the quarter deck from time to time. Then Joe made his final triumphant thrust. He withdrew and his accomplice released his hold on the woman. She slumped to the deck and the man dragged her to one side.

"You next, Fred," said Joe Knox, licking his lips as he pulled up his trousers.

All this time Ama had stood gripping the shrouds of the mizzen mast, unable to act. Now, as Knaggs bounded up the steps, she moved forward, determined to mobilise the other women. If they did nothing to defend themselves now, they would surely be raped one by one, whenever these men chose. Knaggs was in a hurry. Williams or Arbuthnot or Butcher might appear on the scene at any moment and he was already carrying a suspended sentence for the previous Sunday's exploit. But he was aroused. Old Joe had had his Sunday afternoon screw and nothing would stop Fred Knaggs from having his. He grabbed the first female at hand. Ama saw that it was a young girl, one of Tomba's people, so young that her breasts were barely formed. Ama struggled to make her way through the crowd of women. They were protesting vociferously but doing nothing else to prevent the outrage. Ama saw that she would not reach Knaggs in time to try to drag the girl from his clutch.

Without thinking, she called out, "Fred Knaggs!"

He paused, astonished at hearing his name called out in a female English voice.

"Who called me name?" he demanded.

"I did," said Ama. "Unhand that girl at once, you villain. You ought to be ashamed of yourself. She is young enough to be your daughter."

For a moment Knaggs was immobilised by his astonishment. He recovered quickly and threw the girl aside.

"Young enough ter be me daughter, are she? But yous aint then, is yer?" he said.

Ama was now standing defiantly before him. He grabbed her wrist and dragged her off behind him. He was immensely strong. Ama felt quite helpless. He propped her up against the mast.

"Lay off," he said to one of the men who volunteered assistance, "Fred Knaggs 'll andle this un isself."

The women were shouting abuse at him, but he paid no attention.

Ama felt disembodied, as if she were a spirit, floating above, watching these events from on high. Her mind was sharp. The man was strong but he was foolish and he could not be aware that this was not the first time a man had tried to rape her. This time she was determined that things would turn out differently. He lent his chest against her, pinning her to the mast, as he released his trousers. He was panting. Then he took half a step back and thrust his lower left arm against her neck, again pinning her to the mast, while he sought to guide his organ into her with his right hand.

It is now or never, Ama thought and, mustering all her strength, she drove her knee upwards into his crotch, crushing his balls. Knaggs staggered back, bellowing with agony. He was doubled up, his trousers around his ankles. Now

Ama was white with anger. She felt her heart pumping. If she had had a knife she would have driven it into him and ripped his belly open. Seeing that he was defenceless, at least for a moment, she took the only chance she had to drive her advantage home. She grabbed his penis and wrenched it as if to pull it off his body. The man screamed.

"Knaggs," came a man's stentorian voice.

It was Williams.

Knaggs was in no condition to answer. He was down on his knees, holding himself and sobbing. His friends drifted away.

Ama picked up her cloth and wrapped it round her. She stepped round Knaggs and started up the steps to the quarter-deck. Williams was standing at the railing. Then she felt her knees buckle beneath her.

CHAPTER 26

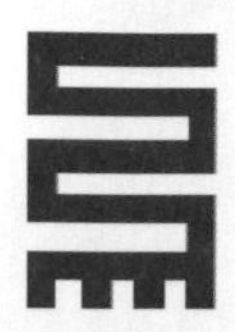

When Ama came to she was lying on the floor in the Captain's cabin. Butcher was kneeling over her, wiping her face with a damp cloth. The room was small. Above her she saw the boards of the ceiling; beside her, the legs of a chair and a desk.

"She is coming round," she heard the surgeon say.

Then Williams' red face loomed over her.

"Give her a piece of cloth," he said. "I can't have the wench naked in my cabin."

"Can you sit up?" Butcher asked.

He helped her to her feet.

"Here," he said, handing her a folded length of cloth from a pile which stood against the wall, "wrap this around you."

She did as she was told. Every muscle in her body ached. She lifted the cloth to examine her knees. The skin had been grazed off both.

"Let me clean those wounds," said Butcher, getting down on his knees. She winced as he sponged the raw flesh.

Now Williams spoke.

"The men tell me that they heard you speak to Knaggs in English? Is that so?"

She nodded, but said nothing.

"I am sorry about what happened this afternoon. Do you understand me?"

Ama looked him in the eye and nodded again. He dropped his gaze and fiddled with documents on his desk. She saw paper and quills and ink; a side table covered in charts and instruments; on the wall a brass chronometer and a barometer; and behind glass doors a shelf full of books.

"Knaggs will be severely punished. The scoundrel has given me trouble since his first day on board. He will have plenty of time to reflect on his sins. And I will see to it that there is no repetition."

He paused and looked up at her.

"You were loaded at Elmina. Why did you not reply when I asked whether any slave understood English?"

Ama said nothing.

"Do you not understand what I am asking you? Answer my question."

She looked him straight in the eye again. Again he found an excuse to look elsewhere. She saw that he was angry. She took her time.

"Captain Williams," she addressed him at last, "do you not know me?"

She saw him start. He pursed his brow. He looked at her face, but he did not recognise her.

"You are . . .?"

She waited for him to finish, but he just continued to look at her.

"Mijn Heer called me Pamela. You may remember that you were our guest one evening."

"Butcher," said Williams, "pull up a chair. Then wait outside."

"Sit down," he said as the surgeon closed the door behind him.

Ama noticed that he didn't say "please." *Is it his general lack of manners*, she wondered, *or is it because I am black, a woman and a slave?* She sat down. The pain in her knees was worse. She squeezed her leg above the wound.

"I am sorry that I didn't recognise you, but . . ."

He waved his hand in a gesture intended to indicate that she would surely understand the reason.

"I was shocked when I heard that De Bruyn was dead. He must have told you that we were planning to do some business together? Tell me what happened."

"He died," Ama replied.

She saw him thinking, *I know that, stupid,* but all he said was, "Of what?"

"I do not know the English name. I think I heard him say he had the yellow jack. He went to Axim and brought the sickness back with him. I nursed him as best I could. Augusta helped. You remember Augusta? But we could not save him."

"He was a good friend," mused Williams.

"But tell me: how do you come to be here?"

"Mijn Heer made a will, giving me my freedom. Jensen," (she spat the name out,) "tore it up. He . . . he sent me back to the dungeon from which Mijn Heer had taken me. What happened afterwards, Captain Williams, sir, I think you know better than I do."

She bared her breast and pointed to the brand mark. He dropped his eyes. She wrapped the cloth around her and tucked the end in. Williams pursed his lips and drummed his desktop with his fingers. Ama eyed the ink and paper, thinking, *sister Ama, you dislike this man so much that you may do or say something against your own best interests*. She closed her eyes: the afternoon's events had exhausted her. Suddenly she saw Itsho. She would have liked to speak to him but if she did so Williams would think her mad.

"Would you like a drink?" Williams asked her suddenly. "A little rum or brandy, perhaps?"

He had risen to his feet and was pouring for himself. Ama's instincts advised her to refuse. She disliked the taste of liquor and it was only to please Mijn Heer that she had taken a little something from time to time. She started to say "no, thank you," but choked the words back as she changed her mind. *Maybe*, she thought, *it will give me some strength. And what do I have to lose, after all?*

He poured her a stiff rum. She took the glass and poured a draught down her throat, trying not to taste the vile stuff. The fire inside her brought tears to her eyes. She saw that Williams was watching her.

"Pamela," he said, "I may call you Pamela, I suppose? I see your situation and I have been turning over in my mind the question of how I might possibly help you. But first, I must make it quite clear to you that, much as I may regret it, I accept no responsibility whatsoever for your predicament. Indeed I recall telling De Bruyn that he was wrong to teach you English. It has turned out badly, just as I expected and predicted. He civilises you, sets you apart from the backward, superstitious trash, like your fellows in the holds and, indeed, my own crew, scum like Knaggs; and then, by his own carelessness, he dies and leaves you unprotected and unprovided for."

"You must understand that I have little room for manoeuvre. I do not own this ship; neither do I own its cargo. The owners live in England, in a great city called Liverpool. They seldom venture beyond the city limits, and none of them, to my knowledge, has ever been to sea. But it is to them, the promoters of this venture, it is to them and them alone, that I am answerable. They are bankers. Their business is money and the making of it. Consequently, as my employers, they expect me to make a tidy profit for them. So it does not lie within my power to set you free. And even if I did have that power and sent you ashore, what chance would you have? You would only end up being sold again."

He lies, thought Ama.

"Captain," asked Ama when he paused, "what if someone in Cape Coast would agree to buy me?"

He sipped his rum.

"That is most unlikely. The authorities in Cape Coast are in the business of exporting slaves, not importing them."

"Would you let me write a letter to the person I have in mind?"

"And who is that, if I may ask?"

"The chaplain, Reverend Philip Quaque."

"Quaque, eh? Yes, I know the gentleman. And what makes you think that he would want to purchase you?"

Ama put on a show of humility.

"I thought he might put me to teaching the children in his school, sir," she said.

Williams laughed. Ama thought: *I have never heard a laugh so totally devoid of humour*.

"No, that would not do. The Governor would not permit it. I know that he shares my views on education for Africans. He disapproves of it. And neither he nor I would want to be establishing any precedents. Precedents: do you know the word? It means 'examples to be repeated in the future.' Do you understand? No, that would not do at all."

"But I have another idea which might suit you as well, if not better. I know a clergyman in Barbados, by the name of Jones. A Welshman like myself, but a Dissenter. He too runs a school, a school for the children of slaves. I think he might be persuaded to do me a favour. Teaching the children in his school would be better than ending up on a plantation. How does that sound to you?"

Ama nodded her silent assent. She thought, *what choice do I have? I am this man's slave, his chattel. He can do as he likes with me.*

Williams continued, "I would expect some service from you in return for this favour."

Ama dropped her eyes.

"Do you not want to ask what it is that I would want from you?"

I can guess, she thought, but she said, "I am your slave."

As the words left her lips, she heard in them a note of insolence. She sensed that Williams had heard it too; but he chose to take the remark at its face value.

"The Cape Coast linguists are all employed," he said. "There are too many other ships here at present. I would want you to act as interpreter for Butcher and the first mate. I would see to it that you got special treatment as far as food and so on is concerned. Do you agree?"

"I am your slave, sir, " she said again.

"Wait outside," he said. "If Mister Butcher is there, please call him in."

She stopped before the door and removed the cloth he had given her. She held up the ends and folded it in two; then she doubled it again.

"What are you doing?" he asked. "You may keep it."

"Thank you," she replied, and put the cloth back on the pile it had come from.

*****

"Butcher," said Williams to the surgeon, "there are so many ships trading here right now that it might take some time to arrange for a linguist. The wench outside understands and speaks good English; better, I have to admit, than any of our illiterate crew. Give her a try. Get her to speak to the slaves in their own lingo. Tell them that if they behave themselves, we shall treat them kindly and feed them as well as we can. Warn them that if they try anything on, it will only be the worse for them. You know the general drift. Do you understand?"

Butcher nodded.

"Then call her in."

"Pamela," said the Captain when she entered the cabin, "I think you know Mister Butcher. He is the ship's surgeon and as such he is responsible for keeping the ship clean and everyone on board in a good state of health. I have told him that as you understand and speak a good English he should employ you as his interpreter, his linguist. He will tell you what to say and you will translate his words to the slaves. Do you savvy, miss?"

"Yes, Master, I savvy," replied Ama.

"Then wait outside," he told her.

What a shit that man is, she thought. Then it struck her that she might, must, turn this assignment to her own advantage and perhaps that of her fellow slaves too.

The short tropical twilight had come and gone. There was a full moon. The air was quite still. The white pile of the castle was reflected in the water, the image shifting in the swell. The women had been sent back to their prison. Ama had missed her afternoon meal but she felt no hunger, only a sense of exhilaration. *Perhaps it is the liquor*, she thought. She closed her eyes and tried to conjure up Itsho's image, but he would not come. She had shunned him: perhaps he had deserted her.

Butcher came out of the Captain's cabin.

"Come on," he said.

As he let her into the female hold, he told her, "We'll start tomorrow."

Then, holding up his lantern, "Do you need a light? Will you find your way in the dark?"

She ignored him and felt her way, step by step, across to her place on the platform.

*****

Next morning it seemed that every woman wanted to greet Ama.

As soon as they had settled in their places on the quarter-deck a formal delegation of Tomba's party came to thank her. Ama stood up. Each woman made a little speech before shaking hands with her. The more eloquent of the brief orations earned shouts of approval. She could only guess at the meaning of their words. At last they brought the young girl whom Ama had saved from being raped by Knaggs. She alone was too shy to speak. Ama saw now how young she really was and felt a glow of satisfaction at what she had done.

"Where is your mother?" was all she could think to say.

The girl misunderstood and answered in her own language, "Yes."

Ama tried again.

"Do you see how the bad man is being punished?" she asked, pointing to the front end of the ship, the part they called the forecastle.

Knaggs sat there, shackled hand and foot and chained to an iron ring set in the deck, as if he, too, had become a slave. *In that respect, at least*, Ama thought, *Williams has been true to his word.* The girl smiled at her now and nodded. Then she allowed herself to be led away.

At last Ama was left alone to think.

If only I could get access to the Captain's cabin, she mused, *or if he would leave me there alone for long enough to write a short letter to Quaque. Quaque, it is true, is little more than a black Englishman. The chances that he will do anything for me are slim. But I must try.*

A canoe came alongside with a consignment of new slaves. The captain was standing just below her watching idly while his cargo was discharged. She greeted him respectfully in Fanti.

"This your work is very difficult," she flattered him.

"You speak the truth," he replied, unmindful of the irony of discussing his trade with a slave woman. "The white man does not recognise it. It can be dangerous and it requires great strength and courage; yet the money they give us is a mere pittance."

"I can see the strength the work requires from the size of your muscles."

How easy it is to manipulate a man, she thought, as he held up his arm to display his biceps. *He probably has grandchildren already. Yet he is as vain as a young man in his first heat.*

"My master," she said to him, "do you by any chance know a man called Philip Quaque? I believe that he is something in the castle."

"What! Osofo Broni? Of course I know him. When we were small boys we used to swim together in this same sea here."

The last of his cargo was being hoisted up on to the deck. She would have to hurry.

"Master, I beg you. Could you send him a message that I am here on this ship? Tell him the girl he met in Elmina Castle who speaks his language."

"You mean Fanti?" he asked as he cast off.

"No," she replied, "I mean English. The white man's language."

He almost overbalanced as he turned to look back at her. It was if he was seeing her for the first time. The canoe was already several lengths away. He raised a hand and waved to her.

"Good bye," he shouted in English, demonstrating to his own great satisfaction that he had brains as well as brawn.

*****

"Wot was you talkin bout?"

The question was spoken in a stuttering voice that could only be that of an Englishman. She turned and recognised the young man with red hair and a red face. She had heard him called George. He was the one who said, "Please," when he gave a slave an order. Ama dropped her eyes and said nothing. He didn't seem to mind.

"I seen how you dealt with Fred Knaggs," he said. "E ad it comin to im, the bastard. I ony wish it ad bin me wot give im is cumuppance. You was very brave. Ain't many a man on this ship wot'd tackle Fred Knaggs; an you on'y a girl an all."

He dropped the armload of tangled ropes he was carrying and sat down with his back against the gunwale, near Ama so that he could talk to her but not so near that his crew mates might notice and rag him.

"It's a hard life, ain it?"

He took a knife and an iron marlin spike from his belt and laid them out beside him. Then he looked up and caught her eye. Ama averted her gaze.

"Well you don't ave to answer if you don't want. I cin hunnerstan you might not want to old a friendly covversashun with one of your hopressors, like. I'd be the same if I was in your position. Not that mine is much different, mind you."

He looked up again; and again Ama dropped her eyes. He spoke with a broad twang and stuttered and she had to struggle to grasp his meaning.

"I knows you hunnerstans me though, cos I 'eard you call out to Fred Knaggs, I did. 'Fred Knaggs!' you said, 'Un'and that there girl at once, you villin.' Jus like in a book . . . I cin read, d'you know?"

He spoke the words with pride. Then he was struck by conscience. What he had said was not quite true.

"Well," he said, "a few words, at least. Me paw ad ter take me outer school fore I ad a chance to lern proper, see. But I cin figger good, that I can.

"Why'd e take me outer school? You may well arsk. Twas poverty. Me paw explained it all to me, 'e did.

"'George, me lad, 'e says, 'I'se goin to ave ter take ee outer school, me boy, an put ee to work. Otherwise 'tis workhouse fer us all. See, me wages is jus nine shillins an tuppence. Yer mother brings ome another two shillins an yer sisters two shillins tween em. Makes thirteen shillins an tuppence. I reckons we be needin all of sixteen shillins if we're not to go ungry. There's rent an firewood an clothes an all. An a shillin a week fer yer school fees. An then there's yer mother with child agin.'

"So e taked me outer school, me dad, e did. Saved a shillin. An I earns two shillins feedin the pigs an cleanin out the sties."

"What's your name," Ama asked him.

"George, miss, George Atcher," he replied.

He looked at her wide-eyed.

"Cor, miss. You speaks like a real lady, you does."

He had untangled the bits of rope. Now he concentrated on arranging them before him on the deck.

"A lady speaked to me once," he said, turning the memory of it over in his mind.

The only ladies Ama could place were Elizabeth, whose clothes Mijn Heer had given her to wear; and the mistress of her namesake Pamela, who was an old woman and died at beginning of the book. Surely this George could not be equating her with the likes of them? It was a puzzle.

"How did you come to be working on this ship?" Ama asked.

His sunburned face turned an even darker shade of red. He busied himself with his ropes.

"I ave a sweet'eart, I ave," he said at last. "Mary Rose er name an right pretty she are. Ony er ole man won low us ter marry. Cos o me family's poverty, see. So I ups an eds fer Liverpool ter make me fortune, so's I cin marry Mary Rose. I'd ten shillins saved, so I decides ter take the coach. Never took a coach before. That were me undoin. Coach were waylaid by seven 'ighwaymen in a wood. Guard kills three of em before me wery eyes, before e were killd isself. So when I arrives at Liverpool, I ad not a single penny ter me name.

"There were this Irish landlady wot offered me bed an board whiles I looks fer employment. Er usband runs a pub. Fuller pretty girls wiv painted faces. They calls 'em ores. Give em a shillin an they'll . . ."

He blushed and giggled.

"You know," he said, assuming she would understand.

"Well I didna ave no shillin, but the landlady she lent me one. Just ter ave a try, she said."

He giggled again. The memory had given him an erection and he brought his knees up to his chest in case Ama should see the bulge under his thin cotton trousers.

"Cum end of' the month an I still adna found no employment. Twas then that me landlady turns nasty, she does. Sez tis jail fer me less I pays up. I didna know which way ter turn. Then they brings this ere agent, they calls im, an e offers me this job. See the world, e says. Good pay, e tells me. Well, truth is, I didna ad no choice. They makes me sign me name on a paper. I couldna read it proper but they tells me if I die everyfing goes to the landlady, all me wages an all. So ere I am in Guinea. An me ole fokes an me sweet'eart never knows wot's become o poor ole George.

"It's a hard life, it is an all."

*****

Butcher led the way to the hatch.

"Bruce, Alsop," he called.

Bruce and Alsop knew the drill: it was their duty to ensure the surgeon's safety during his daily inspection. They opened the scuttle and hooked the steps in position. Each had a cutlass securely attached to one wrist with a cord and a loaded pistol in the other hand.

"Here, take the lanterns," Butcher called down to them as he put a foot on the top step.

"Come. Follow me," he told Ama.

He offered her a hand but she declined his help.

"What did you say your name was?" he asked.

"They call me Pamela," she replied.

"Well, Pamela," said Butcher, "I will tell you what to say and you must explain it to them in their language."

"They speak many different languages," said Ama.

"Oh," said Butcher.

He paused.

Then he asked, "How many?"

"I don't know, but many."

"And how many languages do you speak?"

"Six well and I can try in three or four more," Ama lied, "but it will take me time to translate your words into all of them."

"Oh, no problem about that," said Butcher, astonished at her linguistic claims.

He hoped that this "Pamela" would help to bridge the gulf which lay between him and the male slaves. With the women he could sometimes achieve eye contact; with the men, never. He was disturbed by the suspicion that they didn't regard him as a fellow human being.

The men's hold was worse than the females'. Ama was again reminded of Van Schalkwyk's Christian hell. The room was full of men, black men, half naked, sitting, lying, reclining on their elbows, every pair of eyes staring at the whites, staring at her. Sweating. *Like sinners suffering eternal torment. All that is missing is the lake of fire and brimstone and the unquenchable furnace. What sins could deserve such punishment?*

She saw Butcher put a hand over his nose. *Yes,* she thought, *and we have only been in here a few minutes. Yet these poor souls spend all their days and nights immersed in this fetid witches brew of sweat and shit and foul breath.* She swallowed hard and overcame a strong urge to vomit.

There was silence, broken only by the gentle creaking of the ship's timbers and the incontinent groans of an afflicted soul.

"*Agyei, agyei, agyei,*" the man called over and over again. "Father, my pain."

Bruce and Alsop cleared a space for them to stand. The men rattled their shackles and chains in a united gesture of defiance.

"What is it you want me to say?" Ama asked.

"Tell them I am the ship's doctor. They know me, they see me every day. It is my job to see that they keep well, that they receive enough food and water and that they keep clean and healthy. Start with that."

She cleared her throat. Then she spoke in her own language.

"My fathers, my brothers," she said, "my name is Ama. I hear the white man's language and because of that he is using me as his tongue."

"Speak louder, we cannot hear you well," came a voice from the dark depths of the hold.

She repeated what she had said, raising her voice.

"I am glad that someone has heard me," she continued. "I must speak quickly or the man will be suspicious. Soon this ship in which we are imprisoned will leave our shores and sail out into the great ocean. I do not know where they will take us or what they will do with us. Some believe that when we reach their country they will kill us and feed our flesh to their wives and children."

There was a murmur. Clearly there were several Bekpokpam men. She hoped that they were of better metal than those whom Abdulai had captured.

"We have all lost our families. We have to be family to one another. The women and children in the female hold are depending on you men. You must rise up against the white men and send the ship back to the shore so that we can escape. Now I see the white man is becoming anxious. I will speak to you again. Pray to our ancestors for help."

She paused.

"That took you a long time," said Butcher.

"That is how our languages are," replied Ama. "I have told them in one language but only a few understood, I think. Shall I try another?"

"Yes, yes, go ahead. Take all day if you like. Tell them they must use the buckets to shit in at night. Anything to try to reduce the stench in here."

He pushed past Alsop and stood on the second step, hoping that there would be some fresh air near the hatch.

Ama tried again, in Asante. This time she drew a greater response.

From the darkness a deep voice chanted the Asante war cry, "*Asante Kotoko; kum apem, apem beba!* Asante porcupine; let them kill a thousand Asante warriors; a thousand more will replace them."

That raised a cheer. She thought: *it was Asante that sent you here and yet you are still proud to call yourself Asante.*

Butcher sat down on a step in the square of light beneath the open hatch. He kept his hand over his nose. He looked pale.

Ama called out the customary greetings in Dagomba and added a few stuttering words of apology that she could say no more. In Gonja she could manage even less. But in each case there were shouts of acknowledgement and encouragement.

"Mister Butcher," said Alsop.

The surgeon opened his eyes.

"Get me out of here," he gasped. "This stench will kill me."

"Come, miss," said the one called Bruce, taking Ama's arm.

*****

Bruce and Alsop brought the men up on deck for air and exercise.

All the blacks looked the same to them, but they could pick out the overseers by their whips and the scraps of clothing they had been given. The first overseer led out his group of ten, in their manacled and leg-ironed pairs. On the quarter-deck, the barricade was manned by seamen with their guns primed and trained on the slaves. Butcher unlocked the irons of the first overseer and his fellow prisoner. He gave each man's body a cursory examination. The overseer wore a battered cloth cap as his mark of office. He was a small muscular man with bulging eyes.

"Ask him," Butcher instructed Ama, "if he has any complaints."

Ama passed on the question in Asante. It was as if she had opened a flood gate. A torrent of anger and abuse poured forth.

"Complaints? The white devil brands us with his iron, strips us of our cloth, imprisons us in that wooden coffin, without air, without water. He feeds us on food which I wouldn't give to a pig. He makes us live like swine. Would you treat a dog the way he treats us? What have we done to him to deserve this? And he asks if we have any complaints."

"Father, I beg you, please be calm. We will not escape our fate through anger.

We must watch and wait and take whatever opportunities present themselves. Our time will come."

"It would have been better," the man told her sadly, "if I had been killed to water the grave of Osei Tutu. At least my spirit would have had some rest."

"What does he say?" asked Butcher.

"He is very angry about the conditions in the hold," said Ama.

"Tell him that it is not in my power to do anything about that but that I will pass his message on to the captain. Tell him my job is only to keep him and his people well. Ask him if he or any of his group are suffering from any sickness."

"The white man asks if you are sick."

"Of course I am sick. What does he think? I am sick in my head, in my stomach and most of all I am sick in my heart."

Butcher saw him point to the parts of his anatomy as he named them. He smiled and went on to complete his examination of the last of the ten men.

"Now tell them to dance," he ordered.

"Dance?" she asked him, uncertain whether she had heard him correctly.

"That is what I said. Dance. They need exercise to keep them healthy."

"My father," she addressed the overseer diffidently, "the white man says you must dance."

"Dance?" he asked her incredulously. "Dance? Is he the Asantehene and I his clown that he tells me to dance? Shall I dance *adowa*? Or would he prefer *kète*?"

He turned his head and spat on the deck.

"Tell him I will dance at his funeral."

Bruce, a tall, bony Scot, whose head was shaved just like the slaves', produced a fiddle and struck up a vigorous Highland fling. He danced a few steps by way of illustration. The slaves stood silently and watched. The overseer shook his head in disbelief.

"Is this what the white man calls dancing?" he asked Ama. "It must be the Dance of the Goats."

Those who understood Asante laughed. One youth sent out a great guffaw. He slapped his naked thighs. Then he stepped out a grotesque, obscene parody of Bruce's performance. Tomba's men joined in the merriment. They had few enough opportunities. Ama could not suppress a smile. Bruce stopped his fiddling and looked at the surgeon.

Butcher was becoming impatient. He still had another ninety slaves to examine before he went ashore to inspect potential purchases. He called for reinforcements. They surrounded the slaves and began to flick their whips at their bare feet. The men danced.

"Play, you Scottish bastard, play. And let them dance until they drop! No chop for them until they've had their exercise."

*****

Ama was assigned to help Butcher to identify the sick. The cases which he adjudged to be most serious he transferred to the sick bay in the boys' hold.

She learned the drill quickly.

"Ask them," Butcher ordered her.

"The white man wants to know if anyone is sick," she told the men, "or if you have any other complaints."

"My young sister," the small Asante overseer with bulging eyes called out, "do not waste our time. You must get us tools to break these irons and you must show us where the white men keep their weapons. Then we shall overpower them and kill them all."

There was a desperate cheer and a rattling of irons from the men who understood. The others, Tomba's people, joined in.

"Nana," she replied, "Nananom, my grandfathers, my fathers. I am only one. I am a just one young woman. I cannot make a miracle. All the time I am watching and plotting. But the white men's eyes are not closed. As soon as an opportunity presents itself, I shall take it. Please believe me. And pray to our ancestors to give me strength."

She felt they were accusing her.

"What are they saying?" asked Butcher.

"They are complaining about the crowding, the smell, the heat. They want water to bath. They are dissatisfied with the food," she replied.

"And what did you tell them?"

"I advised them to be patient. I told them that you do not have the power to deal with general complaints like that."

"My sister," came the voice of a young man, "we hear that you are sleeping with the white man, the captain. Is it true? Are you not ashamed?"

Ama felt the blood rush to her head. She was angry.

"*Abrante*," she replied, addressing the questioner as a young man, an equal, even an inferior, "I am sure that you are a brave warrior! But you speak with the wisdom of a foolish youth. What you have heard is untrue. But if it were true, if I were to decide to submit my body to the Captain, do you imagine it would be for pleasure? You would like me to steal the keys to their armoury. How do propose that I get access to those keys. Eh? I am asking you."

"If you have no answer, I advise you to hold your tongue and let the men of mature years speak for you."

"Well spoken," came another voice. The men clanked their irons. Ama felt vindicated.

"What was all that about?" asked the surgeon, shaking his head in bewilderment.

"They are angry. The one who spoke holds me responsible for his predicament. He says I am the tool of the white man. I told him that I am also a slave, that you are only using me as your voice. I told them that it is only the King who holds the knife."

Butcher was puzzled. What was she talking about?

"Only the King holds the knife?" he echoed.

"It is a proverb. They will understand. It means that on this ship all power rests with the captain."

"My sister," came a voice from the dark recesses of the hold, "I hope that you are not reporting what my brothers have said to the white man."

"My brother," Ama replied, "to you I speak only the truth; to him only lies."

There were cheers and laughter. Ama was glad of the support but she was still aware of an undercurrent of mistrust.

"Pamela, I hope you are translating everything they say for me."

"Of course," she replied.

"You are doing well. I don't know how I would manage without you," Butcher sighed.

Two of the guards unlocked the irons of the sick men and helped them up the ladder and onto the deck. There Butcher examined them one by one. Ama interpreted. Even Tomba's people seemed to understand her better than they did the white man, though she could only communicate with them in an improvised language of mime and signs.

"Where is the pain? Does it hurt when he presses you there? How many times have you shat since morning?" she asked.

Many of them were afflicted with an inflammation of the eyes.

"You see," Butcher told her, "they are all suffering from the same complaint. The infection is spread by the miasma; it travels from one to the next through the air. There is little we can do to prevent it."

The surgeons on slave ships were often incompetent charlatans. Many of them were driven to drink by the nastiness of the work. Butcher, however, had something of a vocation for medicine. He believed firmly in the new scientific methods. He had attended some of Dr. Hunter's lectures in London and acquired the elements of comparative morphology and pathologic anatomy. He had even observed some post-mortem dissections. He carried with him on board a copy of Dr. Lind's essay "On the Most Efficient Means of Preserving the Health of Seamen."

The seamen themselves swore by the old remedies they had learned from their mothers, dung tea, crab eyes, the flesh of a viper and an owl; and for toothache, the eyes of a pike. Butcher humoured these archaic superstitions though he secretly despised them.

He hated this work. If it had not been for a financial disaster which had driven him deep into debt, he might have been conducting a successful medical practice in London, rather than confronting the impossible task of preserving the health of four hundred slaves until they could be sold in Barbados.

In spite of his knowledge of diseases and their treatment, he had at his disposal only a small stock of basic remedies. He used brandy and lime juice for most complaints of an internal origin. To the sores which afflicted the slaves' skin he applied palm oil, which was cheap. In the most serious cases, he made poultices containing the herb camomile.

He believed strongly in the prophylactic action of a liberal dose of malaguetta pepper added to the slaves' diet as a means of suppressing the incidence of the dreaded white flux.

The disease he feared most was small pox. He would have liked to have inoculated every slave but the procedure was new and dangerous and the ship's owners had not only decided against it but had strictly forbidden their surgeon to practice it. He would have to handle smallpox, if it chose to descend upon *The Love of Liberty*, with no more than quarantine, palm oil, a doubling of the patients' meagre water ration and a healthy dose of prayer.

Butcher's principal concern was the detection of infectious diseases. He pretended to no special expertise in health problems peculiar to women; so when it came to dealing with the female slaves, he was happy to allow Ama to handle most complaints. Calling for volunteers, she assembled two teams of experienced older women, one for the Akan speakers and one for Tomba's people. But since these had to work without access to either the herbal remedies with which they were familiar or the support of spiritual healers, which was an essential component of their repertoire of medical arts and skills, they could do little more than comfort the sick and pray to their ancestors.

Fortunately for them, the women seemed more healthy than the men. Denied the females' regular access to light and fresh air, the males were afflicted with illness in disproportionate numbers.

Twice a day Butcher summoned Ama to join him on his visit to the sick bay. If there were new patients to be admitted, he led them in a dreary procession through the empty female hold. Those who could still walk were required to help their fellows. The others were dragged or carried by slaves in a better state of health, or, reluctantly, by white seamen. George Hatcher was the only one who regularly volunteered. His mates regarded this task as suicidal and the chief mate had to force them to it. Everyday conduct on board was governed by many rules and Arbuthnot had the power to exercise his discretion as to punishments for minor infringements. The threat of a week's attachment to the sick bay party was a considerable deterrent.

Ama observed Butcher carefully. He was a creature of habit. He carried a bunch of large keys on a chain fastened to a ring in his leather belt. With one key he opened the door from the main deck to the female hold; another unlocked the door to the steps which led down to the boys' room and the sick bay; others were for the hatch covers.

The surgeon tried to examine Tomba. But Tomba hated every one of the agents of his humiliation with a deep and abiding hatred. The man would just not co-operate.

Ama recognised him at once. She knelt by his side. She did not wait for his greeting but gave the customary respectful answer.

"*Yaa agya*," she said in Asante.

He looked at her with a cold stare. She was not one of his people. He did not recognise her. Nor did he understand the words she spoke to him.

"Tomba. Do you not remember me?" she asked him. "My name is Ama. It was I who wiped your forehead after they had whipped you up there."

She mimed the whipping and the wiping of his forehead. Then he knew her. The merest hint of a smile broke his features.

"So now you know me?" she smiled at him.

He raised his manacled hands and grasped her hand. Then he smiled broadly and nodded his head repeatedly. She saw again what a fine, handsome man he was.

Butcher had been watching them. Now put his hand lightly on her shoulder.

"Pamela," he said, "you are a magician. For weeks now I have been trying to get through to this poor fellow, but he just ignores me. And in a minute you succeed in breaking down his resistance. Ask him, please, ask him if . . . ask him if, given his condition, I mean, you know . . . ask him if he is well or if any illness afflicts him."

Tomba turned a blistering look on his oppressor and Butcher winced, almost as if he had been struck.

Ama said, "I do not speak his language."

"Just do your best," Butcher said and retired to occupy himself with the boys.

"He is not such a bad man," Ama said to Tomba. "Sometimes I think that the good ones amongst them are as much prisoners as we are. Here let me see what damage these irons have done to you."

The skin on his ankles and his wrists had been rubbed away by the rusty manacles. *Strange that beneath our black skins*, she thought, *we are pink, almost the colour of the white man.*

"Mr. Butcher," she called, "may I have some of your ointment and bandages, please?"

She chatted away to Tomba as she worked on him. Not since Sami's abduction had he felt the gentle touch of a woman's hand. He warned himself not to permit this woman's kindness to undermine his stern resolve to have no part in his own oppression; but then he weakened. What choice did he have, after all?

Aware of the feelings she had aroused, Ama stood up. She fetched him water to drink and then turned to join Butcher, who was having more success with the boys, whom he was keeping amused by making a coin disappear and then pulling it from the ear of the youngest of them.

"Which of you is Kwaku?" she asked them.

Every day, when the boys were taken on deck for exercise, Kwaku's mother called out to him, plaintively.

A hand shot up into the air.

"Please, miss, it is I."

"These other boys," she asked him, "have you learned to speak to each other at all?"

"Small," Kwaku replied, flattered at having been singled out for attention. "They are teaching us and we are teaching them, too."

"You have done well," she said. "Learn as much as you can from them. I need to talk to Tomba and I count on one of you to be my tongue and my ears. Do you understand? Now what message shall I give your mother?"

CHAPTER 27

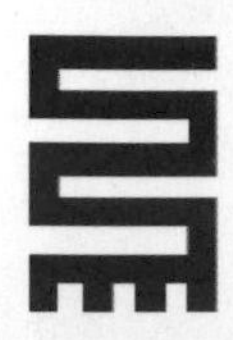

By the time she had finished her work with Butcher, Ama was exhausted.

She found some shade on the quarter-deck, lay down and fell at once into a deep sleep. She dreamed of Itsho. He stood in the patchy shadow of a thorn tree. She could see that it was him, but when she called out to him he did not answer; and when she tried to approach him she found she could not move.

When she awoke, it was dark and she was alone. She had missed the afternoon meal and she was hungry. She leaned over the gunwale and looked out at the castle, its sordid secrets hidden deep in moon-shadows. The small beach to the east was lit up with the torches of the night fishermen. Not for the first time she considered escape. She could so easily let herself down a rope and slide quietly into the sea. If they had not missed her by now, they would not do so before dawn. She shivered. She could swim a little, flapping her arms around, but she had never before swum in the sea and the shore was far away. She thought of the sharks and shivered again.

There was laughter on the main deck: the seamen were relaxing now that the slaves had been locked up for the night. Then there was a cough just behind her.

"Don't move!"

She recognised Williams' voice. His speech was slurred, as if he had been drinking. She kept quite still. Then she felt cold metal sticking into her bare back.

"Captain Williams," said Ama.

He stepped back.

"Oh, it's you, Pamela."

He uncocked his pistol. He was dressed in slippers and a red silk gown. He had a towel over one shoulder.

"What are you doing here? Why aren't you in the hold? I trust you were not planning to visit the sharks?"

He laughed his humourless laugh. She could smell the liquor on his breath.

"I fell asleep," she said. "When I woke it was already dark."

"When did you last have a bath?" he asked abruptly. "You stink."

Ama swallowed a tart reply.

"You had better come along with me. Tonight you are in luck. I came up on deck just now to take my bath, but my olfactory organ tells me that your need is greater than mine. The only person on this ship who is permitted to bath with fresh water is Captain Williams. Sea water does not agree with my delicate white skin, you see. There is the water, warm water I'll have you know, and here is soap and a towel. When you have finished, I shall be waiting for you in my cabin."

A piece of sailcloth had been hung over a rope in a corner of the deck to give the captain some privacy while he bathed. Ama slipped behind it.

What luxury, she thought as she soaped herself. Then: *you have sold your soul to the white devil, Miss Pamela*. And then again: *to hell with you all. I will survive. I shall survive.*

She went down the steep stair and knocked gently on the door. There was no answer. She tried again, a little louder. Still no answer. She tried the door. It opened. Williams was busy stowing bottles and glasses into an open cabinet.

"You told me to come. I knocked but there was no answer."

"Sit down," he said.

"You had better wrap yourself in the cloth I gave you the other day," he continued. "You see I have taken a little brandy this evening and I am at least two and a half sheets to the wind. If you sit there naked like that, I might be tempted to emulate your friend Knaggs. This is a lonely job, you know."

He was standing with his fingers spread out on his desk.

"You have seen the punishment I inflicted on Knaggs, I believe?"

Ama said, "I only used one jug of the water. There is plenty left in the basin if you want to take your bath. And thank you. I haven't had a real bath since Mijn Heer died. You had better go now if you are going, or the water will be cold."

"You have a confounded cheek, speaking to me like that. Have you forgotten that you are my slave, my chattel?" he grunted as he took a fresh towel and his gun.

Ama waited for him to reach the top of the stairs. Then she quietly closed the door.

The ink and quill and a bowl of sand were lying conveniently at hand. Nervously, she opened a drawer in Williams' desk and found a sheet of paper.

She looked at the quill. It needed sharpening, but she could see no knife. She had no time to waste and would just have to manage. Her hand shook as she dipped the quill in the ink. She had written exercises for Van Schalkwyk before but this was the first time she had had to write a real letter.

"The Reverend Philip Quaque," she wrote at the top of the sheet.

"Sir,

"I am called Pamela. I hope and trust that you will remember that we met at Elmina during the wedding of Jensen and Rose.

"After Mijn Heer De Bruyn died, Jensen sold me to Mijn Heer's friend, Captain Williams. I am writing this to you from . . ."

She heard a sound and stopped to listen. *Williams surely can't have finished his bath already?* But it was nothing, just a ship's noise. *I must hurry.*

"I am writing this to you from Captain Williams' ship *The Love of Liberty*, now anchored off Cape Coast Castle.

"I beg you to save to me. If you would buy me, I would serve you faithfully for the rest of my life. I could teach the children in your school to read and write. I must close now. I beg you sincerely.

"Pamela."

She sprinkled sand on the paper to dry the ink. The stairs creaked. This time it was not a false alarm. She whipped off the cloth he had given her and concealed the letter in it. As the door opened, she was holding the bundled cloth in her hands.

"Oho," said Williams as he saw her.

He had wrapped his towel around his waist and was carrying his gown. He put the gown down and Ama did the same with her bundle.

*****

"This is a hard job," he told her when he had finished his business with her.

They were squeezed alongside each other on the narrow bunk, both naked and sweating.

"A hard job and a lonely one."

Ama said nothing. She had allowed him to have her. Overcoming the dislike she had felt for the man since their first meeting, she had simulated lust and excitement. *The loneliness you complain of means nothing to me,* she told herself. *I have degraded myself in your bed for one reason only: to serve my own best interest.*

He squeezed her breast. Then he kissed her. She could feel his penis rising against her thigh.

"What, again?" she asked him, trying to make some space between them. "Already?"

He laughed.

"I haven't slept with a woman since I left England. And that was no more than a brief sordid interlude with a prostitute. You are an expert lover. You have awakened my desire. I want to fuck you again and again."

"It is time for me to go back to my place," said Ama and tried to climb over him.

"Eh, eh. What is your hurry? We have the whole night."

He forced her back alongside him.

"It is hot here," she said, "and your bed is not wide enough for two."

Her mind was on her letter to Quaque and how she might take it away without being detected.

"But more comfortable than the boards in the hold, surely?"

Ama said nothing.

"What would you say if I asked you to move in here with me?"

"So that you could use me during the voyage and then, when you get to your country, sell me at a good profit?"

"I have already promised you that I will sell you only to a good master. Probably my friend Jones, in Barbados."

"Sir, I don't want to go to Barbados. I want to stay in my country."

"I have told you before. That is completely out of the question."

Ama was silent.

"I ask you again. Will you move in here with me and keep me company during the voyage? I will treat you well. You will be better off than my seamen, even than Mr. Butcher, who, like them, sleeps on deck. You will eat from my table. And have regular baths. What do you say?"

"Is it up to me to say yes or no?"

"Of course. Why do you think I asked you?"

"Then my answer is no."

"Why not, for goodness' sake? Are you crazy? "

"I would prefer to be with the women, that's all."

"Will you at least come to me when I send for you? Please don't refuse me, Pamela. I need you."

"Sir, as you told me, I am your slave. I must do as you command."

"In that case, I command you."

*****

When Ama came out of the female hold the next morning, she had her letter concealed in her blue cloth.

There was an unusual bustle of activity on board that morning. Ama rubbed her eyes as she came into the light. She heard shouts and looked up. There were several sailors high up in the rigging, working on the ropes and the sails.

The cook summoned them to take their morning meal. This was irregular: as a rule they were fed in mid-morning, not at dawn. As soon as she had eaten, Ama went to her place at the gunwale nearest the shore, to keep watch for the canoe captain to whom she would entrust the delivery of her letter.

A ship which must have been lying a safe distance offshore during the night approached, carrying just enough sail to bring it to a convenient anchorage.

Williams hailed the captain.

"What news?" he shouted into his speaking trumpet when they had exchanged names and greetings. "Where are you from?"

Captain Eagles, the master of the brig *Bluebird*, property of the old trading firm Vernons of Newport, Rhode Island, cried back, "From Anomabu. The Governor there, Miles, is visiting in Cape Coast. I have come to call him back."

"That sounds like trouble."

"Richard Brew is seriously ill. You don't have a doctor on board by any chance, do you?"

The *Bluebird*'s crew were dropping their bow anchor and preparing to swing out their longboat.

"I certainly do. Doctor Butcher, a surgeon as good as his name!"

Williams laughed at his own stale joke.

"If you are heading that way, you might like to stop and see if Doctor Butcher can be of any service."

"I certainly shall. As you can see, we are about to sail. I have a young nephew working for Brew. Also called Williams. I brought him out on my last voyage. Did you come across him?"

"Of course. Excellent lad. A pillar of strength in Brew's establishment."

Eagles was now in the boat and his crew had their oars raised and ready.

"Are there stocks at Anomabu?" Williams asked.

"Not many slaves but plenty of promises. There were eight ships in the road when I left late yesterday. But I must go now. We shall meet again soon no doubt. Perhaps even later today."

As Ama listened to this conversation her hopes fell. It was clear that, unless Williams decided to backtrack along the coast after calling at Anomabu, she would not be able to send her letter to Philip Quaque. But Anomabu presented a new opportunity.

Williams was standing alongside Arbuthnot, quietly issuing instructions, which the mate transmitted to the Bosun, who in turn called them out to the men in the sheets.

"Knox, Hatcher. Get the females back into their hold," the Bosun barked out.

Ama stepped out of the line and stopped behind Williams.

"Captain Williams," she said quietly.

"Not now," he snapped. "Can't you see that I am busy?"

"Sir," she said quietly, ignoring his reprimand, "I couldn't help hearing your conversation. I know Mr. Brew. Would you let Mr. Butcher take me ashore with him to help?"

Williams said nothing. He just pointed to the line of women proceeding down the stairs and cocked his head in that direction.

*****

In the early afternoon the funeral procession wound out of Castle Brew, which lay hard up against the high white walls of its official neighbour. Then the Castle cannon blasted out a salute and each ship added its noisy respects. Ama was already half deaf by the time it was Arbuthnot's turn to give the order to fire. She closed her eyes and squeezed her hands over her ears, trying to block out the sound, but it was no good. Then, at last, it was all over. For a moment only the gulls and the lapping of the swell on the boards of the ship disturbed the silence. And the ringing in her ears. She hated the noise of the guns so much. *Why do they do it?* she wondered. *Perhaps they have to give notice to their god, sitting up there in his heaven, that another dead white man is on his way?*

It was now late afternoon. The conversation of even the most talkative of the women had run dry. Soon it would be time for them to be sent back into the hold for the night. Ama was bored. Not for the first time, she thought of asking Williams to let her have a book to read. But she was afraid of the reaction of the other women. They would think she was a witch. She stood up and stretched. Above her, in the shrouds, she saw George Hatcher, climbing. He paused to rest on the main top platform. Then she heard him call.

"Mis-ter Ar-buth-not."

The Mate appeared. Hatcher pointed along the coast but his shout was lost in the onshore breeze. Ama walked around to the opposite side of the deck to see what had attracted his attention. A great blackness had risen out of the sea. To the west the sun was dropping to the horizon in a cloudless sky. But there, approaching rapidly from the east was this monstrous tower of darkness. It announced its advent with an extraordinary flash of forked lightning and a clap of thunder louder than a cannon shot.

Arbuthnot's voice rang out. With the old man and half the crew out of reach ashore, his first real test of command had come at last.

"Get the women back into their kennel. Run up the try-sails on the fore and main masts. Secure the guns. Batten down the hatches," he ordered. "Look lively there now!"

The women tripped over one another as they were herded through the narrow doorway. Inside the hold their apprehension was almost palpable.

"Curse the white man that he should bring us onto this miserable ship to drown," called one.

Another began to scream wildly.

Then the door slammed shut behind them. Moments later a piece of black sailcloth was nailed over the barred grating on the door. The narrow beams of red light from the four small vents seemed only to accentuate the darkness.

The first squall swept up on them swiftly and fiercely. One instant the ship was rocking gently in the swell. The next it was if they had been seized by a giant hand, viciously twisted, lifted and then tossed down again into the depths. Ama's head struck the boards above her. A moment later she felt herself thrown off the platform, airborne. Alongside her other bodies were hurtling through the darkness. Her cloth went its own way. Instinctively she threw out her arms to cushion the inevitable impact. The floor leaned away. Women who only seconds before had been lying at the end of her trajectory, had rolled away into a heap under the far platform. She landed on the bare boards. The impact took her breath away. Her momentum and the slope of the floor took her onwards, sliding and rolling until her progress was halted by the tangle of screaming limbs and naked torsos. Now the ship righted itself and began to keel back to port. Ama clawed the darkness, desperately searching for some anchor in this maelstrom of terror. But all she found was the limbs of her companions in hell, and these were as free in space as her own. Last to arrive on the heap, now she was the first to be propelled back against the port wall. Trying to scramble to her knees she struck her head on the unseen edge of the platform. Then she was lying against the hull, buried beneath a pile of bodies. She struggled to free her arms. Her face was pressed down into another's belly. There was no air. She panicked and felt herself losing consciousness, her life slipping away. Then the ship began to roll back to starboard and she was free. So it went on, a terrible shaking of human bodies on and on, back and forth, port to starboard, starboard to port, forward and aft, aft and forward again, on and on, without end.

Up on deck the seamen hung on to the shrouds, drenched by the waves which threatened to sweep them overboard and scourged by the fierce cold wind. Night had fallen. From time to time lightning exposed a brief picture of their world to them; then they were lost in darkness again until the next flash. Hatcher called out to Bruce who was nearest to him but his words were carried away by the angry screaming and roaring of sea and wind. Arbuthnot had lashed himself to the wheel. He strove to keep the fragile ship's head into the sea as she laboured through the violence of the freak storm. There was little else he could do: such men as he had were beyond his command. He was not a religious man but now he prayed, shouting the Lord's Prayer into the teeth of the wind, again and again.

Inside the battened holds, insulated from the sounds outside, screams of pain and terror rent the air as the slaves were thrown back and forth. Bowels and bladders were involuntarily evacuated. Limbs broke, skulls cracked.

The Love of Liberty had been driven by the north-east gale. Now at last the anchor dug into the sea-bed and the ship was brought to a sudden halt, propelling the women back towards the door.

And then, almost as suddenly as it had arrived, the squall had passed. The sea still heaved but there was no longer any wind. Now the black cloud deposited its burden. The rain came down in a sheet, washing the seamen's matted hair into their eyes and setting up a deafening drumming on the decks.

Inside the holds, the flicker of a flash of lightning penetrated the vent holes, briefly illuminating in its narrow beams a scene of utter devastation. The women were, without exception, in a state of shock. But now, at least, as the storm abated, the survivors could hold their places against the pitch and roll of the ship. Slowly, amid anguished groans, the living began to disentangle their limbs.

In the ornate reception room of Castle Brew, with its glass chandelier, its twenty three Windsor chairs, two settees, four mahogany tables and two bureaux; its bookcases with volumes by Pope and Swift, Addison and Cervantes; with its four looking glasses and sixty six pictures of various sizes; in this ornate reception room the ten visiting captains, dressed in their best, their laced waistcoats and shirts with velvet collars, their patterned silk breeches and silk stockings, sat and drank through the night, drank the late Richard Brew's liquor, drank toasts to the late Brew's memory, drank until there was nothing left to drink. To a man they were deeply concerned at the fate of their vessels but in view of the weather, there was nothing to be done until the dawn; and so they drank.

And in Anomabu town, the fishermen and traders huddled together under their thatched roofs, flinching at each lightning flash and moving the brass basins to catch the leaks.

Ama crept along the floor, over prone bodies, scared to stand, stretching out an arm to locate the platform. When she found it, she dragged herself up. There at least there was some space. She propped herself against the hull and set about examining her naked body. There was a huge swelling on her forehead where it had struck the edge of the platform. Every muscle ached and her skin felt as if had been scraped all over with a sharp cutlass. But at least no bones seemed broken. She stretched out on the hard board and tried to sleep. Gradually the groans subsided and the exhausted women drifted off.

CHAPTER 28

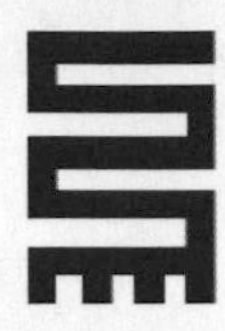

Ama was awoken by the noise of a splash. Struggling to her knees and looking over the gunwale, she was just in time to see the last body hit the water. Five female corpses floated naked on the surface of the sea, sightless eyes staring at the sun. The gentle swell washed over them, jostling them against each other and bumping them against the ship. One of them was Nana Esi. Ama closed her eyes and retched.

The fin of a great white shark sliced the water. She caught a glimpse of a mouthful of teeth fastening onto a leg. Then the first body was dragged down into the depths, leaving just a little crimson whirlpool in its wake. Ama screamed. All at once the water was alive with sharks, tearing the remaining corpses apart in a frenzied orgy of competition. The sea was threshed red; severed heads, limbs and human guts were everywhere as they tore the flesh apart. Ama sank back onto the deck and beat her head against the boards, unable to contain the violence of her sobbing.

*****

The first pair of naked men was carried up on to the deck. One was already dead and his companion was too weak to walk. Jack Tar uncoupled their irons and dragged the corpse away.

Silently, Williams cursed himself for having left the ship in charge of his inexperienced Mate. Then he cursed Brew for timing his death to coincide with such a damaging freak storm.

"Look sharp, now," he called, seeing his favourable balance sheet reversed by the cruel blow inflicted on him by perfidious nature.

Many of the seamen had, like Williams, spent the night of the storm drinking Richard Brew on his way. Those who had been left on board had also had a sleepless night. They were all weak, hungry and exhausted. Williams, refreshed by his few hours' sleep in the morning, urged them on regardless.

Ama dragged herself to the barricade to watch. Butcher stood back now and shouted orders. All hands except the cook and his assistants were applied to the task of extracting the men from the hold, unlocking and removing their irons, sluicing the blood and shit off their bodies, sorting the living from the dead and the living from the living.

Butcher conferred with the captain. What they were doing was contrary to all conventional wisdom. The situation was fraught with danger. The whites were heavily outnumbered. But Williams was anxious to ascertain the extent of the loss he had sustained. He decided to gamble. The slaves were in poor condition, weak and exhausted from the trauma of the previous night. He took the precaution of strengthening the guard. A bombardier stood by the quarter-deck guns with a lighted brand held high to let the slaves see his readiness to inflict an awful vengeance upon them should they venture to riot.

Ama became aware of someone beside her. It was the young girl whom she had saved from the clutches of Knaggs.

"So, Mara, you also survived the storm?" Ama said to her.

The girl replied with such a sweet smile, that Ama could not help but laugh at her innocence. She put an arm around her and held her close.

A sudden cacophony of voices drew her attention back to the scene on deck. The fit and curious women joined her at the barricade. As they watched, one male slave and then another sprang onto the port gunwale and dived overboard. The guards lashed out with their whips and swung their pikes and cutlasses, forcing a way through; but the other slaves did their utmost to obstruct their passage, all the time shouting encouragement to those who had escaped. Before the crew could take up their stations and enforce order, six men had leapt into the sea.

The women rushed to the gunwales, urging the swimmers on.

Williams' face was crimson.

"Lower the boat," he screamed.

The slaves, free of their shackles, their spirits roused by the intrepid behaviour of their comrades, barred the way and jostled the crew.

Williams drew a pistol and used the butt to force his way through. Reaching the gunwales he fired into the water ahead of the first of the swimmers, intending to impede his progress until the long boat could be launched. The women jeered and hooted at him. Williams turned. Arm outstretched and eyes narrowed, he took aim at them. They drew back, screaming in alarm. He turned again to the swimmers. The women resumed their imprecations. Williams re-loaded and fired. The swimmers dived. Then, as Williams was re-charging his gun, one of them, surfacing, seemed the spring out of the water. He threw up his arms and screamed abuse at the captain.

The crew of the long boat recaptured two of the escapees. Two more they pulled in, dead. Ama saw one sucked beneath the swell, after which there appeared a red track in the sea, which widened, faded and then was seen no more. The last one might have reached the shore. Ama fancied that she saw a naked man standing on the distant sandy beach, shaking a fist at Williams.

Williams now had the Chief Mate arm all the crew. He would normally have considered this foolhardy, an invitation to mutiny, but he sensed that the incipient revolt of the slaves had evoked strong sentiments of solidarity amongst the whites.

The two recaptured escapees were brought back on board, and the corpses.

On Williams' orders the crew shackled the watching slaves in pairs and chained them.

"Where is the girl Pamela?" he asked.

Bruce took her by the arm and dragged her forward.

"Come along now, Madam Desdimony," he told her.

"Ask them," Williams told Ama, indicating the two bound escapees, "how they came to mutiny."

"Ask them yourself," she replied sullenly.

He turned to her, his eyes dark. Then, slowly and deliberately, he raised his right hand and slapped her viciously, first, with his palm, on her left cheek and then, with the back of the same hand, on the other.

"Ask them," he told her again, using the same words as before, "how they came to mutiny."

Ama stared at him with hatred and contempt. She would have liked to have raised a hand to wipe her face but Bruce held both arms. Calmer now, she reflected that this was a battle she could not win. She looked at the two men. Both were clothed only in the ropes which bound them. One stood with his head bowed. The other, a man perhaps her own age, stared at her insolently.

She spoke in Fanti, assuming that because they could swim well, the men must be from the coast.

"The white man tells me to ask you why you tried to escape."

"Tell your husband," replied the proud one, "that he is a great rogue, firstly to buy us and secondly to carry us away from our own country. Tell him that we are resolved to regain our freedom by any means possible. Tell him that we would rather die than succumb to his wickedness."

"He says to tell my husband . . ."

Ama spat the words at Williams and paused for them to sink in; but Williams merely narrowed his eyes. She translated the man's words.

"Tell him," replied Williams, "and tell all his fellows who are assembled here, that it was not I who deprived them of their freedom. Tell them that each one of them either committed some heinous crime; or he was captured in a war that was not of my making; or was sold into slavery by his very own family."

He paused for her to translate.

"Tell this scoundrel that even if he had succeeded in reaching the shore, his countrymen would have been waiting there for him. They would have captured him at once and sold him again either to me or to some other. Or he would have been killed to make fetish for his heathen gods.

"Tell them all what they have been told before, that if they behave themselves and give no further trouble, I will treat them well. Tell them that in the country where they are going, no one will kill them for fetish. Of course, they will have to work, but in return they will be given better houses than they have seen in Africa, they will be given fine clothes, they will be well fed.

"Ask him if he has anything to say."

"My brother," Ama told the man, "the white man asks whether you have anything to say. Consider carefully. If your answer is proud, he will surely have you killed. If you beg him, there is at least a chance that he will spare your life."

"Wife of the white man, tell him what you like."

Ama said, "He says he has heard what you have said. He begs your mercy. He speaks for both of them."

Williams merely nodded.

"Bring the first corpse," he said.

Knox tied a rope under the armpits of the dead man. Then he threw the other end out over a spar on a gallows tree the Chippy had constructed and brought it back with a grappling hook. He held it firmly, taking the strain as the corpse was thrown overboard, to hang suspended from the rope. Then, as he paid it out, the naked body descended slowly to the surface of the sea.

"Tell him," Williams told Ama, "that I have heard his plea. Tell him that this once I will be merciful. Tell him and tell the others, that if I have any further trouble from them I will feed them alive to the sharks, just as I feed the corpses of their dead fellows."

"Bring them to watch," he told the guards, "and when they have seen, send them back to the hold."

They brought the slaves to watch in batches. Knox held the end of the rope. For the education of each batch and in order to make his bait last as long as possible, he teased the sharks by allowing them to take a bite and then raising what remained of the dead man's body just beyond their reach.

"May I go now?" Ama asked.

*****

The Love of Liberty set off on its steady, dreary eastward way, calling at every fort and trading post along the coast.

Williams lived in constant fear, particularly at night. His nephew, whom he had taken on board at Anomabu, declined his offer to sling a hammock in his cabin; so he locked himself in and slept alone with a loaded pistol close at hand. But neither the gun nor rum nor laudanum helped him to sleep.

Butcher, often busy ashore examining potential purchases, left much of his work on board to Ama, with Bruce and Hatcher usually in attendance.

As Williams bought more slaves, so conditions in the holds deteriorated. The floor and platforms of the male holds were completely covered in bodies. Sometimes Ama could not find a place to put her bare foot as she moved about amongst the men. Each day they were packed more and more tightly together.

Bruce had a good ear and was picking up a few words of the language.

"*Pini do! Pini do!*" he would cry, meaning, "Shift up! Shift up now!"

So that was the name the slaves gave him, Pini-do.

"*Pìni do! Pìni do!*" some wag would greet him in a falsetto voice, mimicking Bruce's broad Scots mispronunciation. And the wag's fellows would laugh and repeat the refrain.

"How can you laugh?" Ama heard one of the men ask his shackle-mate.

"How can I laugh? My brother, how can I not laugh? If I cannot command my spirit to laugh, I might as well send it back to whence it came. I must laugh in order to survive. And I shall survive. At least I shall survive long enough to kill a white man on this ship. When I have done that, then, and only then, they can do what they like with me. Until that time I am not ready to die; and until I die I shall continue to laugh."

Only Hatcher they treated with a certain reserve, sensing the healer in him. Bruce stood guard, ready to shoot at any sign of trouble, but Hatcher stayed with Ama, quietly going from man to man each day to identify the sick, examining their sores, feeling their foreheads for fever. And it was Hatcher who would unlock the shackles and the handcuffs of a man who had died in the night, throw the corpse over his shoulder and, bent almost double beneath the low soffit, carry it away. The men would make a path for him. Someone would sing the first words of a dirge and the others would join in. But when the young Englishman had manoeuvred his burden up the steps and out of sight, they would hammer their shackles on the boards and break out into a harsh tumult of angry curses. Then Ama would stand silently amongst them, afraid of the violence and hatred which was in their hearts and in her own.

*****

Williams sent for Ama.

"Sit down," he said when the door had been closed behind her.

She remained standing.

He looked up from his desk. He had been writing in his logbook.

"Now, Pamela. Don't be silly. Please sit down."

He took up his pipe and began to scrape out the ash.

"Look. I am sorry. I know I slapped you. I shouldn't have done it. It was in the heat of the moment. Can you not understand the pressure I was under? Now I need to talk to you. Won't you please sit down. And wrap yourself. It disturbs me to see you naked."

Ama took the cloth he indicated and threw it over her. As she took it, she noticed a bunch of keys hanging on a hook near the door of the cabin. She recognised it as that which usually hung from Butcher's belt. *So that's where they are kept when he goes ashore,* she thought. She sat down on the edge of the chair.

"What happened?" he asked.

"What happened?"

It was the first time she had opened her mouth. She could see him fighting his anger at her insolence.

"Yes, what happened? In the hold last night."

"One of the women died."

"How did she die?"

"What difference does it make? Slaves die every day on this ship. Her body has already been fed to the sharks."

"Her neck was broken."

Ama said nothing. She was struggling to take control of herself.

"She hanged herself," she said at last.

"Why on earth would she want to do that?"

Ama lost her temper.

"Captain Williams, do you really want to know the answer to that question?"

"Of course. Why else would I have I asked it?"

"Then tonight please take off all your clothes. Borrow a strip of blue cloth. Here, try this one for size."

Ama tore off her own and threw it onto the desk.

"Join your slaves in the hold. Just for one night. Then you will know the answer."

"You must be joking," was all he could reply.

*****

One seat of misery was followed by another. After Senya Bereku it was the English lodge at Shidoe and after Shidoe, the Dutch one at Nyinyanu.

They came at last to Accra. When Williams dropped anchor he found that a war between the proxies of the Dutch of Fort Crèvecoeur and those of the Danes of Christianborg, had produced a glut of slaves.

Within the space of a week he was ready to set sail.

The slaves were fed and sent back to their holds. Their quarters were diligently searched and the hatches firmly secured. The long boat ferried the seamen ashore for their last carouse before the rigors of the Middle Passage. Williams alone, amongst the officers, remained on board. He issued a tot of rum and a pistol, powder and shot to each of the six crew who had been selected for guard duty. A chest full of loaded and primed pistols was placed on the quarter deck and two of the nine-pounders were made ready. After a final inspection Williams retired to his cabin.

The sun set. Darkness descended on the sea. The guards dozed. Time passed. The moon rose, a great yellow orb in a sky full of stars.

"Pamela!" Williams shouted.

Ama woke suddenly, as from a bad dream.

"Where is the wench?" she heard him mutter.

He stood in the doorway, his bulky frame silhouetted against the moonlight.

"Pamela!" he shouted again.

The women were stirring. Ama felt embarrassed, humiliated. *Uncouth bastard,* she thought.

"I'm coming," she called back in something between a whisper and a shout.

"Ah, there you are," he said as she stumbled through the door.

His speech was slurred. Ama could smell the rum. She rubbed her eyes. Then she saw the moon, low and enormous, its elongated reflection moving on the water. She went to the rail to get a better view. Williams was swearing at the keys as he tried to insert first one and then the other. Ama turned to watch him. *This is my chance,* she thought. She looked around. There was a guard at each hatch cover. Asleep, all three of them. She heard snoring from the quarter-deck and craned her neck. Three more, also asleep.

"Here, let me help you," she told Williams.

"Oh no you don't."

He paused to belch and then continued with his fumbling.

"I know what you're up to. Keys ish for the captain. Only for the captain. Unnershtand?"

For a moment she thought he had read her mind. Then she dismissed the thought. As he turned she saw how drunk he was. She flinched as he groped for her breasts. Then his foul tongue was in her mouth. She freed herself and pushed him away.

"Not here," she whispered. "The guards will see us."

He suffered himself to be led down to his cabin. Ama's mind was racing.

"Lie down and let me undress you," she told him.

"I want to fuck you," he said and belched again as he climbed on to his bunk.

"Do you think you'll be able to get it up, in your condition?" she taunted him as she pulled his trousers down.

"Fuck you . . . Shtick my prick up your cunt," he said.

"Stick," she told him, "not shtick."

Now she knew what she would do. He was lying on the bunk, naked.

She spat on her hands.

"Yesh, yesh," he groaned. "Now, now, now. Now!"

"Aah," he sighed, his eyes already closed.

Ama covered him with a sheet. Then she sat down to wait. When he began to snore, she rose quietly and picked up the bunch of keys from the floor, where he had dropped them. She moved to the chair behind his desk, his chair. Slowly, watching him all the time, she pulled the top drawer open. Her heart pumping, she felt for the pistol she knew he kept there. She had never touched a gun before. Carefully she took the awful thing out. She forced herself to think. *Calm down*, she told herself, *there is no room for a single careless mistake.* When she was calmer, she got up, unlocked the cabin door and transferred the key to the outside. The candles flickered and she hesitated for a moment. Then she took up the gun and the bunch of keys and put them down on the first step. Taking a last look around, she blew out the candle, left the cabin, closed the door and locked it.

*****

She paused in the shadow of the awning, watching the sleeping guards, alone and afraid.

Nervously, she searched for the key to the door of the female hold. Inside, she closed the door quietly behind her and paused to recover her calm.

Then she made her way over the tightly packed naked bodies, searching at every step for a place to put her foot, breathing "Sorry," to the mumbled curses and moving on again.

A narrow beam of moonlight from a vent fell on the door to the boys' hold. She unlocked it and left it ajar. Below, it was dark, pitch dark. She heard the clink of metal.

"Tomba," she whispered, "it is me, Ama."

She heard him sit up. He could not move without rattling his chains. She knelt by his side and let him feel first the bunch of keys and then the gun. She heard the surprise in his grunt.

After what seemed an age, matching keys to locks, he was free. He massaged his ankles and his wrists and she heard him wince.

"*Kòse*," she sympathised, knowing how raw his skin was.

He took her hands in his and squeezed them.

"Thank you," he said in his language.

She thought of Kwaku. She would need to wake him to use as an interpreter. She tried to lead Tomba to where the boys were sleeping. He resisted and she was aware of the vigorous shaking of his head. He led her to the bottom of the stairs and told her to wait. Then he groped his way along the wall to the sick bay. When he came back, there were two men with him. They whispered excitedly amongst themselves.

At the top of the stairs, she took Tomba's hand and signed to him to tuck the gun into his waist-cloth and use his other hand to hold his companion's. So they made a chain and followed her, step by step, across the floor of sleeping women. Ama set a slow pace. *If any of them were to wake,* she thought, *that might be the end.*

After what seemed to her an age they emerged into the narrow strip of moon shade under the edge of the quarter-deck.

The moon was higher now, and smaller.

Ama pointed out the guards sleeping on the hatch covers and showed Tomba the bunch of keys. She pointed up to the quarter-deck and raised three spread fingers. He held up three fingers of each hand. In the moon light she could see that he was asking whether there were only six guards. She nodded.

She said, "The others," and pointed to the shore.

He nodded, thought for a moment, and then whispered to his companions, indicating the guards on the hatches as he did so. Ama thought, *it is too dangerous, the others will wake up.* She grabbed his arm and shook her head. She tried to tell him by signs that it would be better to capture Williams and use him as a hostage; but the message was too complicated and she could not make him understand. Now he was impatient. If they were to act they must do so without delay. He signed to her that she should give him the keys and go inside the female hold. She protested vigorously. She had started this thing and she would see it through to the end. Tomba whispered to his accomplices and they removed their waist-cloths. He took one and demonstrated what he wanted them to do, wrapping the cloth around the neck of one and twisting it.

The men shook hands. Tomba took Ama's hand and squeezed it.

"Good luck," she whispered. "May the ancestors protect you."

As they tiptoed across the moonlit deck on their bare feet, Ama mouthed a silent prayer.

"Itsho," she said, "be with them. Guard them. Bring them success."

They paused at the first guard. Tomba left one of his men there. They went on to the second and he left the other. Alone, he went on to the hatch which gave access to the forward hold. Signals passed between them. Ama dug her nails into her sweating palms. Tomba raised the pistol high in the air and drove it down onto the temple of the sleeping guard. Ama closed her eyes. When she opened them, Tomba was rolling his victim over and taking his pistol. But the other two victims refused to die without a struggle. Waking to find themselves being strangled, they kicked and fought. Tomba ran across to help.

Suddenly there was a cry from the forecastle, "Wake up! Wake up! Guards, wake up!"

Ama broke out in a cold sweat. It was Knaggs. She had completely forgotten him. It was her fault: they were undone!

Tomba hesitated. He too had forgotten about Knaggs. He turned back to deal with him. Then it struck him that Knaggs was chained to the deck and could do no more harm than he had already done. He changed his mind and turned again, intending to help his co-conspirators.

"Tomba! Unlock the hatch," Ama shouted at him but, if he heard, he did not understand.

The three guards on the quarter-deck had run to the barricade. Shots rang out. The slaves might have taken their victims' pistols from them and fired back, but Knaggs' screams from forward and the firing from aft confused them. One of their victims was already dead; the other, free of his assassin's attentions but half dead from the attempted strangulation, rolled off his hatch cover and lay low. Now it was three against three, but the guards on the quarter-deck had the protection of the barricade and the advantage of elevation. Ama huddled beside the open door of the female hold, shivering from fear and the chill of the night air.

Tomba took refuge behind the main mast. At best he could fire a single shot with William's pistol. Then Ama saw the guard who had survived rise to his knees, take his pistol from where it had fallen and creep up behind Tomba.

"Tomba, Tomba," she cried, but it was already too late.

The revolt had failed. It was all over.

*****

Williams stumbled around the cabin in the dark, searching without success for his flint box and a candle. Finding his desk, he opened the drawer and felt for his pistol. It was not there. There was another gun-shot. He moved his hands over the table, exploring, and succeeded only in knocking the rum bottle to the floor. He went to the door; it was locked but there was no sign of the key. He got down onto his knees and searched for it.

Now his befuddled mind began to function. *The fucking bitch has taken my gun, left me in darkness and locked me in.* Stumbling back he stubbed a toe on the corner of the desk and cursed. Finding the chair, he stretched out for the bottle. Then he remembered. Again he got down on his knees, swearing as he searched. The floor was wet. By the time he found the bottle, he had rum all over his hands and legs. Swearing at himself for not replacing the cork, he raised the bottle and drained the dregs.

Yet another gunshot. He would have to do something. He could not just sit there drinking. But what if the girl had succeeded in unlocking the holds and freeing the slaves? The decks might be full of naked slaves, all thirsting for his blood. He would have to hold out alone in his cabin until the long boat arrived in the morning. But by that time the slaves would have broken open the armoury.

It struck him that Pamela must have his key. Could he rely on her to hide it in order to protect him from the anger of the rabble? Hardly likely. She would be the first to rip his guts open.

But suppose there was some other explanation for the gun-fire? The guards might have killed her. That must be it: six guards against one female. She was surely dead. Her nefarious plan had failed.

But if that were true, why so many gun-shots? There must have been three or four since he had woken. He dropped his head into his hands. There was nothing for it. He would have to take a chance. If fate decreed that he should die, he would do so courageously, like an English gentleman.

He went to the door, took three steps back and charged. The door stood firm. He collapsed, certain that he had broken his shoulder.

When the pain subsided, he began to bang on the door and shout.

"Open, open. Let me out."

*****

Ama, Tomba and their two co-conspirators lay on the main deck.

The guards had bent their legs back and threaded their handcuffs over their ankle-fetters. Ama's shoulders ached, but when she tried to move it was worse. She recalled her journey on Damba's horse. Then, at least, hope had borne her up. Now there was none. There would be no escape. Williams would surely hang them on the Chippy's gallows and let the sharks eat them, feet first, slowly.

The two men whom Tomba had taken from the sick bay groaned. Tomba whispered words of solace.

"No talking," said Joe Knox nervously and flicked his cat at Tomba.

Ama longed for death. *Itsho, I am coming,* she whispered. And then she wondered whether he would be there to meet her. She had had to bury him without the rites which custom demanded. Perhaps his spirit was still roaming abroad, unsettled. And her own? What would happen to her spirit after dying such a terrible death, eaten alive by sharks?

The other two guards came back from their inspection of the ship. On the forecastle Knaggs was screaming. He sounded delirious.

"Everythin in order?" asked Knox.

"Yeah, cept fer George an Arry. They's dead. An Fred. Sounds like e's gone crazy."

"Yeah, I 'eard. Ow's Bill?"

The report on the condition of the half-strangled Bill was interrupted by the sound of banging from the captain's cabin.

"Eh, the Cappin! I forgot all about im."

"Not much elp e was."

"Probably in is cups. We'd better go an see what's up."

*****

"Open, open. Open the door and let me out," Williams was still screaming as they descended the stairs.

"Coomin, Cappin, coomin," called Joe. "Ere, bring that lamp."

He found the key in the lock where Ama had left it. The door opened outwards. Williams was leaning against it and when it opened suddenly, he almost fell on Knox.

"Why, Cappin, where's yer clothes?" Knox asked when he recovered his balance.

The old man's gone off is rocker, he thought, *loik Freddie Knaggs.*

Williams came to himself. He felt the blood rush to his head. How could he have failed to realise that he was naked? What a humiliation!

"What do you mean by rushing in on me like that?" he demanded. "Here, give me that lamp."

Minutes later he appeared on deck, full clothed.

"Now what's been going on up here?" he asked.

"We ad a spot o trouble, sir," Knox reported. "Cappin Tomba, beg yer pardon, sir, the slave Tomba, got out wiv two others. Tomba killed George Atcher wiv a blow to is ed while e was sleepin. Is haccomplice strangled Arry - I dunno is other name, sir, but e's dead too. But me an the lads we managed ter hoverpower them fore they could do any more arm. Only Bill got isself alf strangulated and Fred Knaggs as gone off is ed."

"Where are the scoundrels?"

"We put em all in hi-rons, sir. They's a'lying on the main deck, Tomba, is two haccomplices an the girl, the one they calls Pamela, wot spiks Hinglish."

Williams went down on to the deck. He took one look at the captives, but said nothing.

"What weapons did they have?"

"Just this pistol, sir. Can't think where they got their ands on hit. Tis not one of hours."

"I'll have that," Williams interrupted him, "and those of the two dead men, too."

"Cappin, Cappin."

It was Knaggs. Williams made his way to the forecastle.

"Cappin," said Knaggs, "I seed hit all, I did."

"What did you see, Knaggs?"

"The guards was all asleep, they was. Soon as they took their rum. But no rum for Fred Knaggs so I was awake, watchin the moon rise."

He dropped his voice. He had a secret to share.

"I seed you unlock the door of the black wenches' room an I eard you call out. 'Pamela,' you called; and when the hussy comes out I sees you . . ."

"Never mind about that," Williams interrupted him hastily. "Did you see the insurrection?"

"Yessir, Fred Knaggs seed the srecshun. I seed hit all. If hit weren't fer Fred Knaggs we'd all be dead by now."

"What happened exactly?"

"I must ave bin dozin. Then I woke sudden and I seed this big nigger man bringin is and down on the guard which was sleepin on the first atch cover there. An two more is strugglin with the other two guards wot was on the atches.

"Then I gives the alarm. 'Wake up! Wake up, guards, wake up!' I ollers and they wakes up. Then the big feller ears me an panics an e starts ter come fer me.

"But jus then the girl, the same ussie, your Miss Pamela, beg yer pardon, Cappin, calls im.

"'Tomba! Tomba!' she ollers, 'Unlock the atch,' but I guess e doesna hunnerstand Hinglish cos e eads back ter elp is mates what is tryin ter strangle the guards wot was sleepin on t'other atches.

"Then the fellers on the quarter-deck starts shootin at im. E takes cover behind the main mast. Then I sees e as a pistol in is and. Is mates drops to the deck. Then one o the guards wot was bein strangled, rolls over and gets on is feet and sticks is pistol in Tomba's back. That were the hend of the srecshun, Cappin. The guards rounds hup the srecshunists, the girl too, an claps the hi-rons on em."

Williams was silent. He walked over to the gunwale and looked out towards the Danish castle, all moonlit white walls and shadows. He was thinking.

"Cappin," said Knaggs, his irons clinking as he moved.

"What?"

"If hit hadna bin fer Fred Knaggs givin the halarm, we'd a all bin dead by now. Twere a close shave, hit were."

"Knaggs, I am a fair man. You did well. I shall have you released. But on two conditions. The first is that I want no more trouble from you during this voyage. Do you understand?"

"Yessir. Fred Knaggs as larned is lesson, Cappin."

"The second condition is that not a word, not a single word, of what you have just told me is to reach the ears of anyone else on board. If I have any suspicion that you have opened your big mouth, I shall quickly find a good reason not only to clap you back in irons but perhaps to lose you overboard. Now will you swear that you will be silent?"

"Cappin, thank you, sir. I swear by God Imself. Fred Knaggs gives you is word uv honour, sir.

"An sir . . ."

"What is it?"

"If there be any way Fred Knaggs cin be of service, sir, speshul service, I mean . . ."

"Thank you, Knaggs. I shall remember that."

On his way back to his cabin he stopped for a moment and stood over Ama's prostrate form.

"You ungrateful hussy," he hissed.

*****

When Williams had finished addressing the crew he had the overseers and some of the women brought out.

The bodies of the two white men were laid on tables. The four captives were partly unshackled and made to stand before them.

"Before we consign the mortal remains of the unfortunate Hatcher and Baker to the deep," Williams told the crew, Dr. Butcher will make two incisions in their bodies and extract from each the heart and the liver. Two hearts, two livers. Each of the four criminals will be made to eat one organ."

He paused, waiting for the buzz of conversation amongst the crew to subside. The slaves, understanding nothing, were silent.

"The good doctor tells me," he continued, "that this punishment does not conform to the norms of civilised society. I have explained to him that this is not a civilised society. These people are barbarians, devil-worshippers, cannibals no doubt. It might well be that consumption of a white man's organs will have some beneficial effect upon them. I have said my say. Mister Butcher, please proceed."

In her worst nightmares, Ama had never expected this. To be subjected to torture; to be shot or hanged; to be fed alive to the sharks, perhaps. But to be forced to eat human flesh! From where she stood she could see George Hatcher's face, no longer red, grey now. She was sorry that fate had decreed that it was he who should be one of their victims. He was a good man, drawn into all this, as she had been, by forces beyond his, and her, comprehension. She was consumed with a terrible anger at the injustice of life.

"Williams," she screamed, "it is you who are the barbarian, the cannibal. It is you whites who eat the body and drink the blood of your god. It is you who buy human beings and sell them, sell us, as if we were sheep or cattle. It is you . . ."

William's face turned a livid purple.

"Gag her. Gag her," he screamed.

Ama's words were cut off in mid-sentence as a cloth was stuffed into her mouth.

Butcher finished his post-mortem operation. Then the two coffins were brought up. The bodies were put in them and ballast added. The Chippy nailed the lids down.

"Go ahead," Williams told Butcher.

Butcher looked up at him, appealing. Even at this stage he hoped that the captain would change his mind.

"Do what I say."

The bloody excisions lay on the table. At least the dead in their boxes would not witness the consumption of their own mutilated parts, thought Butcher.

"I cannot do it," he said, shaking his head sadly.

He was close to tears.

Williams looked at him with contempt.

"Knaggs," he called, "come forward."

"You are to feed each of these criminals with one of those organs lying on the table. Do you understand?"

"Yessir. Will they take em ole or shall I cut em up in pieces?"

"I leave that to you."

"I think we'll start with Missis Plum Duff. What'll it be miss, liver or 'eart?"

Ama said nothing. This was her second clash with this man. She had been lucky to win the first. Now she was at his mercy. He was clearly revelling in his power over her. There was nothing she could do. Her feet were fettered. Her hands were manacled before her. A man had threaded an arm between her elbows and her back. Another held her head immobile. Knaggs cut one of the livers into slices. He held up a piece of the meat between finger and thumb displaying it to the assembly.

"Let's 'ave no trouble now, miss. Open yer mouth."

Ama clenched her teeth. Knaggs put the meat down and tried to force her mouth open. He failed.

"She won' open er mouth, sir," he told Williams.

"Butcher," said the captain, "give him your speculum."

With a wan look, the surgeon opened his instrument case and took out the speculum oris.

"Do you know how to use it, Knaggs?" asked Williams.

"Yessir," replied Fred Knaggs.

He turned the thumb screw, bringing the two steel prongs together.

" Old er 'ead firm, now," he told his assistant as he forced the pointed ends between her teeth.

There was a murmur of protest from the watching slaves. It was silenced by a threatening flick of the cats. Ama strained every muscle in her body to resist but her strength was no match for the three men who now held her. Knaggs turned the thumb screw. The prongs forced her jaws open.

"Old hit now," said Knaggs, turning to the table.

Ama had been clenching her muscles tightly against the irresistible force of the speculum. With Knaggs' back turned, she relaxed; then she opened her mouth wide. The speculum fell to the floor. She clenched her teeth again.

There was a cheer from the slaves.

"Knaggs, you idiot," said Williams, "I thought you said you knew how to use the cursed thing."

Knaggs unscrewed the speculum and tried again.

"Go easy, man," said Butcher, "you'll break her jaw."

Ama closed her eyes. She was on the point of losing consciousness. Her head was forced back and she felt the raw meat slither down her throat. Involuntarily she retched. The piece of liver shot out of her mouth and hit Knaggs in the face. The seamen laughed at his discomfiture. Ama's body sagged and Knaggs' assistants had to hold her up.

"Lay er on the deck an I'll ave hanother go," said Knaggs.

"Captain Williams, sir," protested Butcher, "surely that is enough?"

*****

When Ama regained her senses, she was propped up against the main mast with her hands manacled behind it.

Tomba lay on the deck before her. The slaves had turned and were gazing upwards. She followed their line of sight.

Tomba's accomplices had been trussed, and now they were being hoisted to the lowest yard on the foremast. From the women there came a dreadful lament. Tears came to Ama's eyes and she closed them. *Such unimaginable cruelty*, she thought, *and it is my fault.* She opened her eyes. Determined not to watch the show, she looked straight ahead, blinking the tears away. As her vision cleared, she saw a line of seamen standing behind the barricade on the quarter-deck, each with a musket raised to his shoulder.

"Aim at their hearts," she heard Williams' voice, "I want no bullets in their heads."

A cry came from the men at the foremast, "Ready, Cappin."

"Hold tight," cried Williams. "Now men, ready, take your aim, fire!"

Fire and smoke emerged from the barrels of the guns. The crew cheered. The bodies of the victims slumped in their harnesses. From the watching slaves there rose an awful groan. Ama thought she heard an echo of the lament from the holds.

The trussed bodies were brought down and laid on the tables, blood dripping from their wounds.

"Firing squad, you may retire," said Williams.

Ama thought she saw a glint of madness in his eye, but his orders were short and precise.

"Knaggs, another job for you. Take the cutlass and decapitate the corpses."

"Sir?"

"Decapitate. Cut off their heads."

Even Knaggs was beginning to think that Williams was a trifle touched. He nevertheless prepared to do as he was ordered. Holding the cutlass in both hands he raised it above his head. Waiting a moment in order to achieve the maximum theatrical effect, he brought the knife down, severing the corpse's neck at a single blow. The head fell to the deck, rolled a short distance and came to a stop. Blood issued from each part of the severed neck. Again a groan of bottomless despair issued from the throats of the slaves.

"Good," said Williams. "They are beginning to get the message. And now the other one."

"Well done, Knaggs," he continued when the second head lay on the deck. "Now I need another volunteer. You, Knox; you have volunteered. Step forward now."

"Yessir," said Knox, stepping forward.

"Men," said Williams, addressing his crew, "I should like you all to be quite clear as to my reasons for staging this performance today. We have a job to do. We now have a full cargo. Our job is to get these slaves to their destination in marketable condition. During our voyage down the coast I have spoken to them many times, explaining that if they were peaceful and obedient, I would be just and merciful. Last night, not for the first time, my trust was betrayed. It is clear to me that these people do not have any concept of right and wrong as we do. I was consequently left this morning with no alternative but to display to them the power that lies within my hands. My intention is to cow them into good behaviour. There will be no more kindness on this voyage, only the strictest discipline.

He turned to Knaggs and Knox.

"You will each take one head. Hold it between your palms like this."

He demonstrated. Each man picked up a head.

"Now, Knaggs, you will start from the port side and you, Knox, from starboard. Present your head to each slave in turn and make them kiss the lips. If force is necessary to achieve this, it will be used. Now proceed."

As Knaggs pressed his head against the face of the first slave, forcing him to kiss his lips, Ama shouted, "No, no. Do not do it. Do not let them force you."

"That woman is incorrigible. Knox, take your head to her. Now make her kiss it."

Ama shook her head from side to side, struggling desperately to avoid the dripping head.

"Knox," called Williams, "Just press the bloody end of the neck into her face."

*****

When the kissing was over, Knaggs challenged Knox. Their mates wagered their rum allowances.

At a count of one-two-three the two men ran to the gunwale and simultaneously threw the heads far out to sea. Ama, sobbing still, her face covered with drying blood, remembered a nightmare she had had in Yendi, all that time ago. It was as if it were coming true now. Time seemed to have stopped. The heads appeared to float in the air, spinning, so that one moment they saw the face, the next the unkempt hair.

Knox was the winner: his head struck the water further from the ship; Knaggs, understandably, was in poor condition after the weeks he had spent in irons on the forecastle.

The two headless bodies were unceremoniously dumped overboard for the sharks.

Now Tomba was bound to the foremast. Williams descended to the main deck and swung the cat at his naked back. He inflicted the same punishment on Ama. Then he returned to the quarter-deck and watched as each member of the crew took a turn at lashing each of the two rebels. Only Butcher was exempt: his job was to count the lashes, making a tick in his record book for each. They took their time. Sometimes five minutes elapsed from one lash to the next. The first lash hurt Ama most. Some of the knotted ends of the whip drew blood from her back; some wrapped themselves around her and struck her naked belly and breasts. While she waited for the next she closed her eyes and tried to discipline her mind, forcing herself to concentrate on Itsho, numbing herself to all else. Then Knaggs threw a bucketful of sea water over her. She had not seen it coming and she screamed at the sting of the salt.

At every stroke, the watching slaves raised their voices in unison, sharing the agony of the victims. A moment later there came an echo from the holds, whose inhabitants could only imagine what horror was being played out above their heads.

While this beating was in progress, the long boat was swung out and the two coffins were lowered into it. It was rowed some distance out to sea. The ship's flag was lowered to half mast, Bruce blew a tuneless blast on a trumpet and one of his mates beat a monotonous boom-boom-boom on a drum. At a signal from the chief mate, in command of the long boat, Williams read from the Book of Common Prayer and Arbuthnot, a quarter mile to seaward, did the same. *The Love of Liberty* fired its guns in salute twenty times at half minute intervals, one blast for each year of the life of Harry Baker, the age of George Hatcher being unknown. During the homage, the long boat crew tipped each casket in turn into the water.

After the burial at sea, the time between the lashes became shorter. Ama tried to keep count. She was telling herself, *fifty, fifty, fifty* when Knaggs' turn came round again. He twirled the cat around and swung high, aiming at her head. One knot tore at her left ear. A bunch struck the back of her head. The knot on the longest strand took out her right eye.

Butcher ticked his chart. Then he put it down and went to examine her.

"Captain Williams," he called up, trying to contain his anger, "any more and I shall not be responsible for this woman's life."

"Surely it does not make sense," he begged, "to destroy merchandise of such potential value?"

Williams said nothing. He just indicated with a swing of his index finger that the victims should be carried away. Then he retired to his cabin.

CHAPTER 29

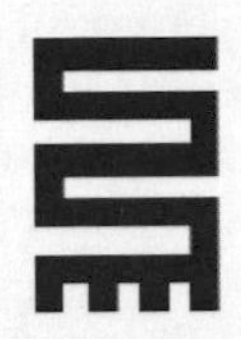

"Well, Nephew, what did you think of today's show?"

The nephew put down his knife and fork.

"A little too gruesome for my taste, Uncle, if you don't mind me saying so; but, then, I don't carry your responsibilities."

"Believe me, I find the gore as distasteful as you do. If I have said it once, I have said it a thousand times: the slave trade is no business for a gentleman. But you see, these blacks are capable of the utmost barbarity. It is a case of them or us. I had to frighten them, to ensure our own survival. *'And if ye will not hearken unto me, but walk contrary unto me then I will walk contrary unto you also in fury; and I will chastise you seven times for your sins.'*"

The nephew was reluctant to contradict an argument for which his uncle claimed the sanction of scripture.

"What happens next?" he asked.

"As far as the slaves are concerned, I intend to keep them penned up in their holds and on short rations for a few days, just to drive the lesson home. I shall drum this into their little brains: that their comfort, indeed their lives, are totally dependent upon my goodwill.

"Tomorrow at first light, you will see us get up the yards and topmasts, reeve the rigging and bend the sails. By mid-morning this accursed continent will be out of sight."

"How long will it take us to Barbados?"

"Two months, three months. It's all in the lap of the gods."

"Uncle . . ."

"Yes?"

"May I ask you a question?"

"Of course. What is it?"

". . . The woman . . . "

The senior Williams' face darkened.

"Which woman?" he asked.

"Oh, you know. The one who was whipped today. I believe she is called Pamela."

"Well, what of her?"

"I spoke to her the other day. Just a few words, I admit, but . . . Astonishing, quite astonishing. I mean to say . . . She speaks the most excellent English. Slightly accented, of course, but grammatical. Better, I would have to say than my Irish cousin Clarissa . . . Where on earth did you find her?"

The Captain's eyes narrowed. He wondered whether the boy was having him on. But no, his remarks seemed quite innocent.

"Would you like her?" he asked.

"Like her?"

"Yes, like her. To have and to hold, to love and to cherish, your very own chattel; to fuck or to beat according to your fancy. Your very own personal maid-servant in Barbados, your private piece of black arse, as I believe you put it."

The younger Williams was taken aback. His late father's brother had never used such coarse language in his presence before. He blushed. His uncle must be a mind-reader. He had indeed felt a strong physical attraction to the girl. He didn't know what to say.

"I'll sell her to you. I reckon I could get all of fifty pounds for her in Barbados. I know a Methodist preacher there who would snap her up at that price; use her to teach the slave children in his school. But I would let you have her for forty. Well?"

"I would need some time to think it over, Uncle."

The Captain grunted and drained his glass. There was an uneasy silence.

"Uncle, if you'll excuse me," said the nephew, " I think I'll make a few circuits of the deck and then turn in. I'm rather tired."

*****

"Let me take you up on deck. The fresh air will do you good," the doctor told her.

He had used up his stocks of ointment on her back and Tomba's. Their wounds had healed. The scabs had come off. *Their backs are a mass of scar tissue, but they have survived*, he told himself. *That is my job as surgeon. What more can I do? I cannot change the world.*

He helped Ama up the steps to the quarter-deck. She had not spoken to him since the beating. Indeed he had not seen or heard her speak to any one at all. She seemed to have shut herself off entirely from the outside world. That was not surprising. Such a lashing as Williams had inflicted upon her was a traumatic experience of the first order. As a doctor he could manage the physical recovery; but the healing of the psychic wounds was beyond the compass of his skills. *Does she know that she has lost an eye*? he wondered, as he settled her under the shade of the awning.

The young girl who was her constant companion sat by her side. Butcher put his foot on the gunwale.

"That's the Portuguese island of São Tomé or Saint Thomas as we call it," he told her. "We are now on the equator. Do you know what the equator is? I learned in school that it is an imaginary line drawn round the earth, 'like the belt about my middle', my teacher told us."

He mimicked his old teacher's large belly, but either she did not understand his joke or she was just not amused by it.

"I always wondered how it was possible to draw an imaginary line," he mused. "We are already a few hundred miles into the Atlantic Ocean. Tomorrow, so I am told, we shall sail for the Americas."

He knelt, lifted her chin and looked her straight in the eye. She looked back, but as if she did not see him.

"Is there anything I can get you?"

Sometimes Mijn Heer would use just those same words. Ama shook her head. As she lay in the hold recovering, she had made a resolution that no word of English would ever again pass her lips; and she would not co-operate with any of the whites in any way whatsoever.

She had mixed feelings about Butcher. She knew that he was not a bad man. If it weren't for him she might have died after the beating. But it was also true that he was white and that put him squarely in the camp of the oppressors, whether he liked it or not. She resolved her ambivalence by acknowledging his questions with a nod or a shake of her head, but without speaking. He seemed to accept this, which only served to compound her dilemma. It would be easier to maintain her resolution if the whites were uniformly cruel and insensitive.

Ama looked around. There had been a change in lifestyle on board during the period of her convalescence. The boys now spent the whole day on the quarter-deck with the women, much to the joy of Kwaku's mother. The men were allowed up on to the main deck for several hours each day, in shifts. They had been freed of their irons which were now used only for punishment.

Williams junior, William Williams, the nephew, Bill to his friends, was a bit of a dandy. In order to maintain a proper distance from the common seamen, he paid close attention to his dress. He kept his trunk in the captain's cabin and as soon as Williams senior made his appearance on deck in the morning Bill would nip down for a change of clothes. He spent part of his day circumnavigating the main deck. A clear path had to be kept for him along the gunwales on either side. He would examine the faces of the slaves with interest, nodding to himself as if confirming some private theory. He shared his uncle's love of books and had the Chippy fashion a deck chair for him which he placed in a corner of the quarter-deck in the shade of the awning. In the late afternoon Butcher would join him in a game of chess. Bill seldom lost. At the end of each game he would cry out in triumph, "Check-mate," and from this he acquired his nickname from the slaves.

"Check-mate, Check-mate," they would call as he perambulated and he would graciously tip the peak of his hat in acknowledgement.

He never entered the holds. However he did interrogate Butcher closely on the condition of his wards. He asked particularly after the two surviving rebels, the man called Tomba and the woman known as Pamela.

When Ama re-appeared on the quarter-deck, he moved his chair to where she was sitting. He was shocked at her appearance. During his year at Anomabu he had learned to distinguish one black face from another. He rather fancied himself as a connoisseur of African beauty. This girl had been quite pretty. Now her appearance was grotesque.

He tried to engage her in conversation.

"Well, miss, I am pleased to see that you have recovered sufficiently to be coming up for fresh air again," he said.

Surprised at being spoken to, Ama looked at him. Then she averted her eye. *Now what can this one's business be with me again?* she thought wearily. *These white men have given me more than enough problems. I will have nothing to do with him.* She moved so that her back was turned towards him.

"Well, now, that's not a particularly polite reply to my expression of goodwill," said Williams junior, "but I suppose, in the circumstances . . . "

He settled down to read his book. Ama looked out at the little town which lay between the beach and the forested hills behind. The only islands she had seen before were in rivers, in the Oti and the Daka. This one was enormous by comparison, with its own mountains, forests, rivers and towns. And all alone, isolated in the middle of the great ocean. *Just as we are alone and isolated, with no one to turn to for help. While we were close to the mainland, there was still some small hope: to rebel, to drive the ship onto the shore, to escape and hide; perhaps, perhaps to return to one's family without being captured. A slim hope, but still hope. Now there is none. Or is there some indeed? The men are now allowed out on deck and without their shackles. If they could overpower the guards and somehow run the ship aground on the island, we might all disappear into the forest and make a new life there for ourselves.* She interrupted her own daydream. *Ama, Ama,* she told herself, *haven't you caused yourself enough trouble? There must be four hundred black men on this ship. Men! Let one of them take the lead.*

Williams junior suddenly laughed out loud. Startled, Ama turned to look at him. He was slapping his thigh.

"Oh, marvellous stuff!" he exclaimed. "Marvellous stuff! Have you read it?"

He held the frontispiece and title page up for her to see. Ama looked away. It seemed an age since she had idled her time away in Mijn Heer's apartment reading novels.

"Do you read as well as you speak?" he asked.

There was no reply. All he saw was the ugly geography of lacerations on Ama's tortured back, welts criss-crossed with weals.

"Tell you what," he continued, "shall I read aloud to you? I'll start again at the beginning if you like. I've only read a few pages so far. Shall I? No answer? Well, they say that silence means consent."

And so he started. He read well. Ama considered moving away so that she would not hear him. But what would that achieve? She felt her good resolutions dissolving. She quickly became absorbed in the story, escaping from the harsh reality of the present into a different world. She looked out towards the island but what she saw was something else.

When he came to the end of the fourth chapter he said, "Well, I think that is enough for the present."

She looked around and for a fleeting moment he caught her eye. She turned away quickly. *This fiendish fellow has discovered a weakness in my armour,* she thought. *I was so immersed in the story that I completely forgot myself. Yet . . . What, after all, will I achieve by depriving myself of this small pleasure? At least it provides an hour's escape from dwelling upon the filth and smell of the holds and the hopelessness of our predicament.*

*****

He came and read again in the afternoon. When he had been reading for an hour and his voice was beginning to show signs of hoarseness, Butcher appeared, his day's work finished.

He observed the reader and the listener but said nothing.

"Just a few more paragraphs, Doctor. Please don't go away," Williams junior told him.

Ama turned and silently acknowledged the doctor's nod.

Butcher brought two stools, sat on one and placed the board on the other. Then he poured the pieces out of a velvet bag. He shifted black and white pawns from fist to fist behind his back and held them out for the other man to make his choice. Then they arranged the pieces. *It is only your own stubborn pride,* Ama told herself, *that dissuades you from indulgence in the small pleasures on offer. So what if the others brand you a collaborator? Haven't you suffered enough already on this accursed ship?* She shifted her position to give her a view of the game.

"So," Williams junior asked her as he made the first move, "you are a chess player too?"

Ama said nothing and concentrated her attention on the board.

"Awuraa Ama," a young male voice addressed her.

She turned.

"Kwaku," she replied in Asante, "how are you?"

Butcher looked up. Kwaku bowed his head in greeting.

"I am well. My mother says to greet you. She will come herself when you are less busy."

"Busy?" Ama asked. "What do we have to keep us busy?"

Ama noticed that he found it difficult to look at her directly. She fingered her face. It must be her missing eye. She must really look a sight. Resolutely, she redirected her thoughts.

"Have you ever seen this game before?" she asked him.

"The board looks like a draughts board, only smaller," he replied, "and the pieces are different."

"The white men call it chess. Would you like to learn to play? Do you know oware? Of course you do. Well, if you can play oware, you can learn chess too."

"But the white men . . . ?" Kwaku asked.

She laughed.

"Do you think they can do worse than they have done already? Now the first thing to learn is the names of the pieces. There are two armies, do you see, one black, one white."

He looked at her to see if she was serious, but she went on, translating the name of each piece into Asante. The king was *ohene* and the queen *ohemmaa*; the bishop was *okomfo* and the horse *oponko*; the castle was *aban* and a pawn *akoa*.

Butcher looked up from time to time, pleased that his patient was talking again. He wondered what she could be telling the boy.

"Do you think the wench knows how to play chess?" Bill Williams asked him, knowing full well that she would understand.

She looked at him with contempt. She had played chess with Mijn Heer practically every evening. She was not impressed with what she had seen so far of this young man's game, though Butcher seemed even less competent. He had just made an unnecessary sacrifice of a knight. Ama picked up the discarded piece and showed the boy the moves it was allowed to make.

"Two steps forward, one step sideways; or one step forward and two steps sideways. And it can jump over the other pieces. Have you ever seen a real horse before, Kwaku, one with four legs?"

Kwaku shook his head. Horses were rare beasts in Asante.

"My father told me that the Dagomba soldiers ride on them. My father fought in the Dagomba War," he volunteered with pride.

The Dagomba War. The Asante, Kwaku's father amongst them, defeated the Dagomba. The victors demanded an annual delivery of slaves. So the Dagomba went hunting. And that is how I come to be here on this ship.

Ama was lost in thought. She was tempted to ask Kwaku how he and his mother came to be slaves, too. Perhaps, like Esi, they had been pawned. She decided it would not be proper: his mother might be offended.

"Now the castle," she told him, "can only travel in straight lines and it cannot jump. It must capture any enemy piece that comes in its way and take possession of its square. Do you see?"

Kwaku nodded. Butcher lifted his remaining bishop. Before he could put it down, Ama stretched out her hand, caught his hand in mid-air and forced him to put the piece back on the square it had come from. The doctor turned to her, astonished at her action. Somewhat abashed, without saying a word, Ama explained with signs. That move would leave the doctor's single knight defenceless. Bill Williams would be able to announce his customary "check mate!" in not more than three moves if he were to make that move with his bishop. Butcher understood. However he lacked Bill Williams' will to win; he was too tired or too lazy to try to figure out his opponent's future tactics.

"Well, miss," he asked her, "what would you do?"

She leaned over and castled, moving Butcher's threatened king two squares sideways and bringing his rook into a position in which Williams' queen was in danger of attack. The two white men looked at the board; then they looked at each other; then, together they turned to look at Ama.

"Please, what did you do?" Kwaku asked her.

"That is a special, secret, magic move. You are only allowed to make it once in every game. But before you learn it you must learn all the others."

"Sister Ama," he asked, "can real horses jump?"

*****

Williams picked up the south-east trades. With a full head of sail, he made steady progress.

But he continued to sleep badly and his waking hours were afflicted with disabling headaches. Butcher bled him but the relief was transient. His temper was unpredictable and even his nephew steered clear of him. Williams senior consoled himself with rum and daydreams of a quick sale of his cargo and an early return to England.

In spite of herself, Ama was exhilarated by the speed of the small ship. She lay on her back, watching the great, taut, sweeps of canvas and the clouds scudding across the sky. Sharks were their constant, sinister companions but there were also grampuses, dolphins, whales. The boys would wait for the flying fish to break the surface of the water and then cry out in a single chorused breath, lifting the tone of their voices as the creatures rose to the zenith of their trajectory and then letting it fall as they re-entered the water with a splash; and they would laugh in delight.

Then the wind dropped and the sails drooped limply from the yards. The long flag which only a few days before had danced from the very top of the queen gallant mast, now hung lifeless. One day followed another. Even in the shade of the awnings the heat was oppressive. The crew began to fight among themselves and Williams had to threaten Knaggs that he would put him in irons again. They fashioned large fans from scraps of old canvas and at night had the slave boys stand over them, fanning the air to make a feeble breeze while they tried to sleep.

The male slaves became increasingly irritable. Fights were common. The Asante fought amongst themselves, but if one of them became involved in a quarrel with one of Tomba's people, they would stand together. Now that they were no longer manacled, small incidents could flare up rapidly into brawls, drawing in more and more of the despairing men. The crew kept constant watch, brutally suppressing any incident, treating violence with violence. The heat and humidity and smell in the holds became unbearable. During the day they might manage to doze. But awake in the darkness, the nights seemed interminable. Even the daily intervals on deck gave them little relief since, unlike the women and the boys, they were not provided with a canopy to protect them from the overhead sun.

The drinking water in the butts began to taste peculiar. Stocks dropped to danger levels and Williams reduced the ration. The crew were worse off than the slaves. Williams kept their container sealed so that it was only possible to suck water from it through the barrel of an old musket inserted through the bung hole. This straw was kept in the crow's nest and any sailor wanting a drink had to climb the mainmast, retrieve the straw and, when he had finished with it, return it to its place.

The bloody flux spread amongst the slaves and from them to the crew.

There was little to distinguish one day from the next. Williams appeared on deck from time to time and scanned the horizon for evidence of a change in the weather, but there was none. He cut the crew's weekly food ration to three pounds of bread and three pounds of meat, mostly fat and bones. He could not afford to starve the slaves by reducing their miserable allocation of corn mush, or even the twice weekly supplement of salt beef or pork. The hungry seamen swallowed their pride and begged rations from the Africans.

The incidence of the bloody flux increased. Butcher was overworked looking after his patients. He thought of asking the captain's permission to add Pamela to his small team of auxiliaries but he feared the violence of the man's language. Hardly a day went by without a couple of corpses being unceremoniously splashed overboard. Sometimes they would float beside the ship for hours before the sharks arrived for their obscene meal. The Chippy began to run out of wood and the white men were no longer accorded the dignity of burial at sea in a coffin. Now the English corpses had to make do with sailcloth.

The Love of Liberty floated idly in mid-Atlantic. Every day at noon, the captain brought out his chronometer and sextant and took a sight on the sun.

"We have not moved half a degree from the equator during the past two weeks," he told his nephew, "and we're just thirty degrees west of Greenwich. That puts us two thousand five hundred miles from Barbados."

Ama borrowed the chess board and pieces and taught Kwaku to play. Bill Williams' challenge she rejected. She also refused his offer, his request, that she should read to him. But he continued to read to her. Chess and stories apart, she had plenty of time to think. She stood at the gunwale and looked all around her. *The Love of Liberty* lay at the centre of a perfect circle. She recalled Mijn Heer's telling her that the earth was a sphere. She had wondered whether he was pulling her leg. Now she could see the evidence, the proof.

She explained it all to Kwaku, but he was unconvinced. If the earth is like an orange thrown up into the air, why does it not come down, as the orange does? And why does the water, the sea, not fall off the bottom? It was too difficult. She could see that it might require an act of faith to accept Mijn Heer's theory. She decided to try something less complicated. She would teach Kwaku and Mara the elements of English. Life in Barbados might be easier for them if they could understand the language of their masters. So the time passed: on the one hand the death and pain and suffering, the ever present humiliation, the longing for home, the fearful speculation about an unknown future; on the other the peaceful, idyllic ocean all around them, the beautiful sunsets, wonder at the enormity of the whales and the wanton play of the grampuses, the surprises of literature, the challenge of chess and the rewards of teaching.

Weeks stretched into a month, and then another. Now the slaves' rations, too, were reduced. The muster of corpses increased every day. Amongst them Ama noticed the proud Asante overseer with the bulging eyes. The bloody flux had taken him. She had never learned his name, she thought with regret. Back home, however humble his status, there would have been some ceremony to mark his transition to the world of the ancestors. She began to wonder whether it made any difference.

In the morning, the floor of the female hold, too, was filthy with the foul, liquid excrement of the sufferers. Ama wondered what it was that protected her from the vomiting and fever and dysentery. Only the bleeding of her gums disturbed her, and intermittent pain from the empty socket of her right eye.

*****

At first light the watch climbed to the maintop platform and scanned the horizon.

Excitedly, he reported a small black cloud. Arbuthnot summoned Williams, who had fallen asleep only an hour before. The Captain was in a foul mood; but when he saw the darkening sky the challenge of imminent danger quickened his pulse and purged his wrath. He sprang to action.

"Mr. Smith," he instructed Arbuthnot, "get the cook to feed the slaves at once; tell him to double their ration. It might be days before they get another meal."

"While they are on deck, have the carpenter fasten a web of ropes to the floor of each hold. I don't want a repetition of Anomabu."

"Once that is done, get the slaves back into their kennels. Batten down all the hatches."

"Then rig sails to make a catchment and bring up the empty barrels."

While they waited for their food, Ama watched the sails being reefed. The storm came nearer and nearer, the shifting dark clouds illuminated by the lightning. The women who had weathered the storm at Anomabu muttered amongst themselves, shaking their heads in alarm.

"Today our lives are in the hands of our worst enemy. The ancestors have surely forgotten us," one said.

A crack of thunder drowned the dreary murmur of agreement. They shuddered and huddled closer, without hope. Ama looked at the restless sea and thought for a moment that she saw Nana Esi's corpse riding the heavy swell. *That woman saw her own future. Did she also see ours?* she wondered.

Then, their hold was ready and they were herded into the darkness.

The first inside tripped and shouted back a warning. In her usual place Ama found that the Chippy had made a rope fast along the junction of the platform and the hull. She tested it. It gave her a sense of security: it would be easier to weather this storm with something to hold on to. Reluctantly she conceded to herself that for all Williams' faults as a human being, he knew his business as a mariner and slave-trader.

Up on deck, the captain turned over his options in his mind as he inspected his sails and rigging. Caution suggested that he heave to and ride out the heavy weather. The trouble with that plan was that once the storm had passed, they might be left becalmed as before.

The gale was blowing from the south. If he let *The Love of Liberty* scud before it, they might be blown right up to the latitude of Barbados. There he could pick up the north east trades and be in Bridgetown in no more than a week or two. It was risky, but tempting.

"Set the course sail on the foremast, Mr. Smith," he yelled into Arbuthnot's ear. "We'll run before her."

The first icy sheet of rain soaked the crew, every man jack of them but the captain, who owned a suit of oilskins. Day had turned into night. It was as if a malevolent heaven had descended upon them. An enormous wave towered above the fragile ship, took hold of it and pushed it forward. It swung this way and that, pitching, rolling. One moment they were in the depths of a trough; next they balanced on the crest. The wheel strained against its lashing. Communication became difficult. Arbuthnot, returning to Williams' side, slipped on the wet deck and grazed his knee.

In the hold, Ama hooked her elbows about the rope. The woman on her left had already vomited; now the one on the right did the same. Ama gripped her arm in attempt to comfort her but she was completely distraught with fear. She shat herself where she lay. Ama closed her eyes in despair. Soon the floor of the hold would be a uniform slimy mess of filth. Already the smell was overpowering. She squeezed her eyes, trying to shut out the world. The ship rolled away from her; the remains of her breakfast poured out onto her neighbour.

Williams realised that he had underestimated the force of the gale. In all his years at sea, he had never seen such a storm before. He shook his head. He would have to swallow his pride and turn the bow into the wind.

Before he could act, lightning struck the ship, splintering the foremast and the foreyard and setting fire to the small sail, wet as it was. For a moment there was an overwhelming smell of burning; then the rain put out the fire and the wind swept away the smell of it.

*****

Three sleepless days and nights later the storm began to blow over.

In the late morning the sun appeared and Williams was able to establish his position. Arbuthnot stood by him as he squinted through the sextant.

"Now," he said as the chronometer showed noon.

"We're off the coast of Brazil," he told the mate. "Bahia must be just over that eastern horizon.

"Open the hatches. Mr. Butcher, I want a report on the condition of our cargo. Cook, see if you can get a fire going. We could all do with a hot meal. Mr. Smith, rig what jury sails you can muster and set a course for the Portuguese port. And run up the Union Jack if you will. Give me a call as soon as you sight land. I'm going to take a nap."

Ama came out on deck, starved, dehydrated, filthy. The light of the sun blinded her and she shut her eye. *The Love of Liberty* was a floating wreck. Only one mast was intact. Another lay across the deck, broken. Pieces of sail, torn to shreds, lay everywhere. The other slaves looked like living corpses. The crew's condition was not much better. She drank deeply. The water was sweet and there was plenty of it.

"We filled every barrel with rain water," Butcher told her. "You can even use it to take a bath. We are close to land, now."

"Barbados?" she asked him, forgetting her vow of silence.

"No," he replied. "The storm blew us far off course. We are heading for Bahia in Brazil. We should be there by tomorrow at the latest."

*****

"Land ahoy!" came a shout from the watch high up on their sole remaining mast.

Bill Williams rushed down to summon his uncle. When he returned, he had a chart.

"Can you see it yet?" he asked Ama.

She shook her head. Then there came a cheer from the forecastle and a rush to the forward gunwales.

"There it is. Land ahoy!" shouted the young Williams in great excitement. "Do you see it now? Now, if I am not mistaken that must be Cape St. Anthony. Brazil! Robinson Crusoe country!"

"Have you read Robinson Crusoe?" he asked her.

She nodded. But Brazil? She couldn't remember any mention of it.

"I wonder where he had his plantation?" Bill Williams mused.

Late in the afternoon they rounded the Cape and entered a broad bay.

Williams savoured the sound of the words, "Bahia de Todos os Santos. The Bay of All the Saints."

Blue waters, a forest of tall masts, green islands; small sailing boats flying for refuge in the last hour before dusk. Some passed close by. Ama noticed again the curiosity of their crewmen. She could understand: *The Love of Liberty* was a floating wreck.

The sun picked out a row of gleaming white buildings on the top of the promontory, painting them a deepening orange as it sank.

"Cidade do Salvador, the city of our saviour," Williams told her, scanning the city with his uncle's telescope.

"Slaves to the holds," ordered Arbuthnot. "Let go the anchor."

AMERICA

At the end of the twentieth century, the population of Brazil stood at some 165 million. Of every ten Brazilians, six are descended wholly or in part from African men and women who were transported across the Atlantic against their will during the sixteenth, seventeenth, eighteenth and nineteenth centuries.

CHAPTER 30

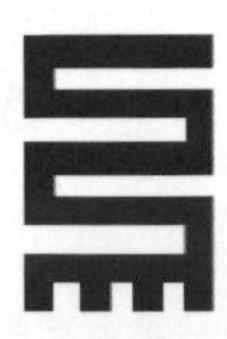

Coming out of the hold at dawn, Ama gasped. The upper city, the Cidade Alta, silhouetted against a crimson sunrise, seemed to have taken on a completely new character, ominous, threatening, somehow sinister. Then, rubbing the sleep from her eye, she discovered the straggling lower city, the Cidade Baixa, emerging from the early morning shadows at the foot of the cliff.

The bay was already filled with sails. One of the small boats approached *The Love of Liberty*. An impressive figure of a man stood at its bow, his gloved hands resting on a polished brass railing. He was dressed in a spotless white uniform with gold buttons and golden braid at the shoulders, and two rows of medals decorated his chest. Over his wig he wore a black tricorn hat with a red cockade. His uniform reminded Ama of Jensen, Esi's pig-god, the first time she had seen him. She leaned over the gunwale and spat into the water. Then she looked again. Of course it couldn't be Jensen. It was only the uniform.

The chief mate was overawed by this imminent manifestation of foreign officialdom. He sent Knox scuttling for the captain, who was enjoying his first good night's sleep in months.

The four black men who manned the official's boat were stripped to the waist. One of them threw a rope to the waiting Bruce and shouted something up to him with a broad grin.

"An the same to you, mate," Bruce called back.

The man asked him a question. Bruce shook his head and spread his palms.

"No savvy," he replied.

The official was struggling up the rope ladder, which seemed to have taken on a life of its own. He looked down and swore at the slave below. Arbuthnot helped him and his sword over the gunwale. He was adjusting his uniform when Williams appeared.

"David Williams, Master of *The Love of Liberty*, Liverpool, England," he said, holding out his hand. "Whom do I have the honour to address?"

"Christovam da Rocha Barbosa," Ama heard the man sing out his name. She thought she heard him announce that he was the director of the port of Salvador, but the rest was lost to her.

Williams resorted to sign language and a change of accent.

"Eengleesh sheep," she heard him say, pointing to the Union Jack, but then her attention was drawn elsewhere.

"My brothers," she addressed the slaves who were lolling idly in the boat below her, "do any of you hear Asante?"

One of them stood up and cupped his hand to his ear. She repeated what she had said but now that she could see his face and the unfamiliar incisions on his cheeks, she knew he would not understand.

The man identified himself with a flourish and a bow.

"Domingos Cabinda," he said and then pointed to the others, who laughed at their friend's fine manners.

Each waved an acknowledgement as he was introduced: "Santos Gêge, Bernado das Minas, Policarpo Nagô."

"Ama," she replied. "Asante, Kumase, Elmina. And you?" to his implied question.

"Costa das Minas," he said, indicating his companions; and then, pointing to himself, "Cabinda."

He put a finger to his eye and pointing at her empty socket, inclined his head, opened his palms and raised his eyebrows.

Ama couldn't help laughing: the man was a clown. She flicked her wrist several times, trying to mimic a beating. Domingos Cabinda twisted his lips and nodded gravely.

This conversation was brought to an abrupt conclusion as Christovam da Rocha Barbosa descended into his vessel, followed by Captain Williams. The long boat was lowered, sending the younger Williams in pursuit.

"They are going to look for the English consul," said Butcher. "We shouldn't be here at all: the Portuguese don't allow foreign ships to trade in their ports."

There was an awkward pause.

"Well, Pamela," he said at last, "or Ama, is it? I have heard you called that so I suppose that it is your real name."

He was searching for words.

"This might be the last chance I have to talk to you alone. Williams hopes to sell you all here in Salvador to pay for the repair of the ship. I have no idea what fate awaits you in Bahia, though I cannot imagine that it could be worse than what you have been through on this vessel.

"There is something that I want to say to you. I shall carry with me for the rest of my life a sorely troubled conscience. There are many evils in my own country: the English poor are little better off than you slaves, many of them. Yet it is the suffering that you have endured, and your disfigurement, that will haunt me. And that is because I have played a part in inflicting it upon you. For that I can only beg your forgiveness. I know that my apologies will do you no good but I want to ask you to hear me out all the same. I am deeply sorry for what we have done to you, to all of you. I know now that the slave trade is an evil business. I shall make my views known when I return to England, though I have few illusions as to what I might achieve by doing so.

"The engine of this trade is greed and as long as the merchants of Liverpool and Bristol, London and Glasgow can profit from it, it will continue. At least if I were to tell my story, and yours, it might be more difficult for those who rule us to plead ignorance. And I might feel a little better. Now, I have said my say. Will you shake my hand at least and say a word to me before we part?"

Ama turned to look at him. There was a tear in her good eye.

She gave him her hand and said, "Goodbye, doctor."

*****

The slaves noticed the sudden improvement in the quality of their food: fresh meat and vegetables: even fruit.

Bruce took on the job of chief barber and shaved the men's heads and beards. A bath house was set up on deck. Soap was distributed and there was a water, fresh water, hot water. They were given palm oil to rub into their skin. Butcher paid particular attention to the sick, trying to bring them to saleable condition.

Their old clothes, confiscated when they came on board, had been laundered and pressed with a hot iron while they were anchored off St. Thomas. These were now distributed. Ama retired to her place on the quarter-deck and cried quietly as she examined her ragged cloth inch by inch. It was all she had from home, her only memento of Tabitsha, of Nowu, of Itsho. She wrapped the cloth around her and tucked it in above her breast. It seemed to her a hundred years had passed since the day she was captured.

There was laughter on deck.

"I feel I am a human being again, dressed in my old cloth," Kwaku's mother told Ama. "Even the men! Look how vain they are, strutting around, throwing their torn cloths over their shoulders as if they were wearing royal kente! It is like the yam festival, with everyone dressed in his best."

Except, Ama thought ruefully, *that for most of us our best is much the worse for wear.*

"Mr. Williams," she called to the nephew, who was passing.

The English consul had been aboard and she was disturbed by something she had heard him tell the captain.

"Yes, Pamela, what is it?" he asked with a smile.

She had suspended her boycott of the whites. What purpose did it serve when it was clear that they would soon part company, never ever to meet again?

"What is a 'scramble?'" she asked him.

She saw his face darken. His explanation was confused. She knew he was dissembling. And he knew that she knew.

"Mr. Williams, sir. I think you know why I ask. I heard the Englishman who came from the town advising the captain to sell us in a 'scramble.' I just want to know what that means."

He shook his head sadly.

"Pamela. Pamela. Why do you always look for trouble? I am beginning to think that your command of English is a curse on you."

"Just tell me. What does it mean?"

"I am sorry, but I am not at liberty to do that. Now you must forgive me."

And he resumed his constitutional.

*****

The Bosun guided the long boat through the hundreds of canoes and small craft which crowded the approaches to the wharves. Many were piled high with baskets of fruit and vegetables, on their way from the islands and outlying farms to the city markets. There was a shouting and a screaming in strange languages as the vessels were poled in. Most of the sailors were black or mulatto. The few whites looked as poor as their darker fellows.

Can they all be slaves? Ama wondered. *Whites and mulattos too?*

The Bosun threw a line to Alsop who was waiting for them at the bottom of a wide flight of steps set into the stone wall. Bruce was there too. He helped them as they stepped out. Ama's bare feet splashed in the water and she nearly lost her footing on the wet step. She felt dizzy. The land seemed to roll away from her.

"Careful as she goes, Miss Desdimony," Bruce laughed. "You'll get yer land legs soon enough."

"Over there," he commanded them, as they came to the top of the steps.

The first load, all men, sat on the stone flags, waiting.

"Pini do. Pini do," one of the men teased Bruce as they approached.

Another got up and performed a fair imitation of Bruce's dancing. Bruce flicked his whip in mock anger. The laughter was relaxed and good-humoured. Strangers together now, in a strange land, slaves and crew had this at least in common, that they had shared a hazardous voyage and survived.

How quick we are to forgive and forget, Ama mused. *Now that our paths are about to diverge for ever, we begin to see human beings on the other side. But what is that to us now? It is too late. Soon we will be crawling on our hands and knees in the 'scramble' and the crew will return to their own country and then back to Africa for another cargo of misery.*

She looked about her. The bustle and scurry of the scene drove out her melancholy thoughts. Gangs of African men, barefooted and bare-chested, pairs, fours, sixes, eights, carried sacks and barrels suspended by ropes from heavy poles which rested on their shoulders. Some sang or chanted as they went. None paid any attention to the newly arrived slaves.

"What a strange way to carry things," said Kwaku's mother. "Why don't they just put the loads on their heads as we do back home?"

She was anxiously scanning the sea for *The Love of Liberty*'s long boat, hoping that Kwaku might be in it. Ama followed her gaze.

"So many ships," Ama said, running out of fingers to count them with. "Do you think that all of them have come from Africa? No wonder this place is so full of black people. It is almost like being at home."

A hawker with a headload of oranges approached them. He began to rattle off his sales patter in one language after another. The first Ama recognised from its sound as Portuguese; she laughed as he said a few words of Asante. He spoke Hausa too; and Dagomba.

"More languages than ships," she said to Kwaku's mother.

"Master of oranges," one Asante man said to him, "we would like to buy your wares, but we have only just arrived in this your country and we have no money yet. Won't you let us have some on credit?"

But the man ignored him and continued on his way.

"Look at that fellow," said Kwaku's mother. "I think he must be mad."

The man in question was dressed in a waistcoat, no more. He stood at the edge of the wharf directing a stream of invective out over the water, barely pausing to take a breath.

"What an enormous thing," giggled one of the younger girls, causing general merriment.

Men and women had not been allowed to mix on board. Now, sitting in close proximity, old drives were re-awakened.

"That's nothing," said one of the young men. "You should see mine."

The orange seller returned as the laughter subsided.

"Santo Antonio de Padua," he said; and then dropping into fluent Asante, "He thinks he is Saint Anthony of Padua, one of the gods of the white man's religion. He is talking to the fish in the sea, telling them to behave. Quite mad! The life of a slave has driven him crazy."

And he passed on, describing circles in the air around his temple with his index finger.

"Mama, look," cried Kwaku.

An ornately curtained sedan chair passed close by, born on the shoulders of four men, all dressed in rich matching livery down to their ankles and bare feet. A gloved hand pulled a curtain a little to one side and Ama caught a glimpse of a pale female face peering out from the gloom within.

The cliff behind them had been in the shadow. Now as the sun climbed, they could see more clearly the steep paths which were the only connection between the *Cidade Baixa* and the *Cidade Alta*. At the lower end of each, several sedan chairs were lined up. Small boys employed as touts, harried potential customers with the call, "*cadeira, cadeira senhor*," running after them and quarrelling amongst themselves.

"Sister Ama, look, a horse, a horse!" cried Kwaku. "Now I have seen a real horse. At last."

The rider was a white man, dressed in uniform and with a sword hanging by his side. He reined in his mount and ran his eye over the seated slaves. He summoned Alsop and asked him a question in Portuguese.

Alsop opened his arms wide, palms up.

"No savvy Portugeez," he said. "Spick Eengleesh?"

Butcher had the crew marshal the slaves into a line, four abreast. Then he walked slowly from one end to the other, ticking off each four with his forefinger and counting under his breath. As he completed his second count, a sedan chair came to a halt opposite where Ama stood with Kwaku and his mother. The bearers, poorly dressed these, lowered the conveyance to the ground. With a flourish, two of them drew aside the grubby curtains and out stepped Horatio Cooper, the British consul.

"Ah, Mr. Butcher is it?" he said, as he paid his fare.

"I have sent my own *cadeira* for refitting," he explained, "so I had to hire one by the roadside. Now where is your captain?"

He took out a pocket watch and looked at it.

"Ah, I see him approaching now. Good morning, Captain Williams. Precisely on time. It is such a pleasure to deal with one's own countrymen, I must tell you. The Portuguese have little enough concept of time; but even that their Brazilian offspring have lost. Are you ready to move off?"

"Butcher, everything in order?" Williams asked.

On hearing his affirmative reply, Cooper hailed a passing *cadeira*.

"Is it far?" Williams asked. "Shall we not walk?"

"Walk? No sir. Unheard of. No person of quality in Bahia walks. It would be the cause of gossip. This is a small town, you understand. The governor would be sure to make a butt of me at his next soiree. After you, Captain. We will take the lead and show the way."

They passed first along one edge of a vast market. It looked much like the markets Ama had seen in Africa, a forest of temporary tables displaying a great variety of goods, both buyers and sellers mostly black; but the scale, the scale was much greater; there were just so many people, so much traffic, such animated bustle and noise. Everywhere there seemed to be bales of goods, crates, baskets and barrels; and sweating black men. At the entrance porters and hawkers crowded around those who approached, singing out the praises of their wares or offering their services.

Only the filth was worse. The ground was carpeted with muck, decaying vegetables, and other rubbish. Coming from a slave ship they had some special experience of bad smells, but this was really something.

"That must be the fish market," said Kwaku's mother, holding her nose.

Ahead of them the curtained sedan chair bobbed up and down.

As they entered a winding, narrow street, Ama saw a sign on the corner of the first building.

"Ru-a De-rei-ta," she mouthed silently.

It's not much different from English, she thought. *I already know the letters, so it shouldn't be too difficult to learn.*

The stone buildings which flanked the street were built hard up against each other. Most had shops or workshops or warehouses on the ground floor; many had small balconies overhanging the roadway. Here and there there was a small untidy garden tucked in between the buildings, planted with fruit trees. On one balcony several high spirited young girls, whites, flowers in their hair, chains around their necks, long earrings glinting in the sun, giggled and screamed. One leaned over the ornate iron railing, looked down at Ama and her fellows and said something to her friends. They all burst out laughing.

"Ru-a São Ped-ro," Ama read, as they turned off into another narrow street, recalling that she had seen the word Rua before and guessing what it meant.

"Rua, rua, rua," she repeated to herself, to impress the word upon her memory.

Here the buildings were old and the paint on the walls peeling. The paving stones were uneven and irregular. Her eyes on her surroundings, Ama stepped into the shallow gutter which ran along the centre of the street. She slipped and almost lost her balance.

"Shit!"

"Ama!" said Kwaku's mother.

"Sorry. The word escaped me. But just look at that!" she replied, struggling to keep up as she scraped the excrement off her foot.

The street of Saint Peter was still in the shade of the cliff which loomed above. It was lined with small workshops. The wares of the iron smiths and copper workers, hatters and makers of guitars and drums were hung outside on display. In the dim spaces within Ama could see people at work.

Peddlers and bearers with all sorts of sacks or boxes born on heads or shoulders met and passed them. Others overtook them. All in a hurry. None paid the slightest attention to the procession of slaves.

At the end of the street there was a solid stone building, its great wooden double doors wide open.

Williams and Cooper stepped out of their *cadeira*. A uniformed official conducted them into the building. Then the slaves were marched straight through the doors and into a spacious hall. As the last of them marched in, the doors closed behind them with a resounding bang.

*****

Ama clapped her hands to her ears.

Feeling confused and giddy, she closed her eye. Someone pushed her and spoke harshly. It was a black man. She noticed that he was wearing boots; and that he wasn't averse to using them.

She had been so intrigued by the passing show of the *Cidade Baixa* that she had completely forgotten her apprehension about the coming 'scramble' whatever that might be; now it returned.

The man herded them like sheep, pushing and pulling and abusing them loudly in a language none of them understood. Ama looked around, trying to get her bearings. The hall was square in shape. Massive columns rose to support a high, ornately plastered dome, unlike anything she had seen before. High clerestories lit the centre of the hall. Beyond the columns there was an aisle with a lower ceiling.

Temporary wooden barriers had been erected between the columns. The ushers shepherded the slaves into the central arena and forced them to sit down, facing outwards. Williams and Butcher, the consul Horatio Cooper and two other white men whom Ama had never seen before watched from a raised platform on one side. When they were satisfied with the arrangements, the two strangers led Williams and Butcher on an inspection, with the consul in attendance as interpreter. Jointly, they took an inventory of the slaves. As each was counted, an usher hung a wooden board with a number around his neck.

Ama was confused and afraid. The mysterious word 'scramble' obsessed her. Soon, it seemed to her, its terrible meaning would be revealed. Then, gradually, old habits prevailed. *Pull yourself together. If something is going to happen here today you might have to react quickly,* she told herself. She twisted her board round and read the number, "117."

She had become separated from Kwaku and his mother. On her right sat one of Tomba's womenfolk, a stranger. Though it was hot the woman was shivering. Ama took her hand and spoke to her.

"My sister," she told her, trying to comfort herself as much as the other, "everything will be all right."

The woman squeezed her hand tightly in acknowledgement.

She looked to her left. Sitting two slaves away was Tomba himself. He had been watching her. He smiled and waved. Then he showed her a clenched fist. It was their first communication since the rebellion.

He put his finger to an eye and shook his head sadly.

She mouthed a silent reply, knowing he would understand.

"It is nothing. It was not your fault."

The bells of a nearby church rang out the hour. As the last echo died away, a band of black musicians began to play, guitars and drums. Then the doors were opened once more. A crowd of men, mainly white, but with a sprinkling of mulattos and blacks, poured into the room.

A large sign board showed the day's asking price, 120 Milréis. The purchasers strolled round the outside of the barrier, viewing the goods on offer and making notes. The ushers stood behind the slaves, alert.

"Seventy three," a customer called out in Portuguese, pointing to a man sitting behind Ama. An usher prodded the said number seventy-three to his feet and pushed him to the barrier to allow the gentleman to take a closer look at him.

The music stopped. Outside a man's loud sing-song voice repeated the same phrase over and over again, accompanied by the jingling of a small bell.

The crowd of buyers and casual spectators thickened. The hall began to fill with the noxious smoke of many pipes.

An old white man with a walking stick and two personal slaves in attendance, stopped in front of Ama. He wore a white beard and moustache and in one eye, a monocle. He stared down at Ama, evidently intrigued by her missing eye. Then he removed the pipe from his lips and silently crooked a finger to summon an usher. The usher forced Ama to her feet. Tomba protested but two more ushers came up at once to suppress any trouble.

"Tomba, it is all right," Ama told him.

The old man stretched out over the barrier and, putting his hand under her chin, drew Ama's head forward. When he had examined her eyeless socket to his satisfaction, he turned aside and moved on. Ama felt totally crushed. Not for a moment had the old man looked into her seeing eye. Neither had he spoken. He had treated her as if she were no more than a tethered one-eyed goat up for sale in Yendi market.

The usher pushed Ama down to the floor. Now it was Tomba's turn. He refused to rise and the two ushers had to force him to his feet. They held him, one at each arm.

"Tomba, Tomba," said Ama, "it is no use fighting here. You cannot win."

The old man extended his stick and tapped the muscles of Tomba's arm. He turned and nodded his approval to one of the slaves who accompanied him, a grey bearded black man, as old as he, neatly dressed, but bare footed. Then he pointed with his stick to the cloth which Tomba wore around his waist. Before Tomba knew what was happening, one of the ushers had grabbed the cloth, leaving him naked. Tomba swore violently and struggled to free himself, but the ushers knew their job. Calmly the old man extended his stick and used it to lift Tomba's penis, adjusting his monocle with his free hand. Then, without another look at Tomba or the ushers, he passed on to the next slave.

Tomba recovered his cloth and turned on the ushers with a look of hatred and contempt. They paid no attention. This was all in a day's work for them. He sank to his knees, elbows and forehead on the floor, his head grasped in his hands.

Ama hesitated.

"Tomba," she called, "bear up. It is all right. We are all in this together."

*****

Once they had completed their inspection, the purchasers made their payments to the clerks.

The clerks issued a numbered token for each hundred and twenty Milréis paid. The total number of tokens sold was marked up on a chalk board. When the number of tokens sold equalled the number of slaves on offer, the 'scramble' would start. Some wandered back to take another look at the slaves, pointing out their preferences to their agents or employees. Others sat and drank the free rum and *mate* which were on offer and chatted quietly amongst themselves or just listened to the music.

At last an announcement was made. The ushers forced the slaves to their feet and drove them to the centre of the hall. Some marched around them, threatening any who were stupid or brave enough to step out of line. Others removed the barriers. The slaves huddled together, murmuring apprehensively. The purchasers or their agents took up positions on a line which had been painted on the floor from column to column.

Ama saw them fiddling with lengths of ribbon and handkerchiefs knotted end to end. She felt that something momentous was about to happen. Was this the 'scramble' she dreaded?

Kwaku pushed his way through the crowd to greet her.

"Kwaku," she told him urgently, "go straight back to your mother and stay with her. Hold her tight. Do not let go of her."

As she was saying this the trumpet player blew a fanfare. In the ensuing silence the master of ceremonies spoke a few words in Portuguese. Ama saw the surrounding host stiffen. Then there came a short count followed by the single shrill blast of a whistle.

At that signal, the eager horde of buyers rushed at the slaves. Some of the men stood firm, ready to fight. There was pandemonium. The band blasted out on its kettle drums and brass; buyers shouted and screamed. And the women and children shrieked in terror

Then the enemy was upon them, grabbing at their arms, their cloths, pulling them to one side, throwing them down to the ground, tying them with their ribbons and handkerchiefs.

Suddenly, almost as suddenly as it had started, it was all over. Only the few stragglers who had paid for five and only managed to capture four were heard to complain as they sought to identify those who grabbed more than their entitlement.

The band played soothing music, strings. One of the musicians sang a plaintive song.

"Kwaku, Kwaku," came a desperate cry.

Ama found herself in a group of ten, some of whom she knew by sight, but none well. Tomba was not amongst them. Her good eye searched the little groups of slaves but she could see no sign of him.

Their herder, a black man, fussed over them. Apprehensive that they might try to run off, he forced them to sit on the floor. The two of them who were women were sobbing. A man sunk his head between his knees.

Then the white master appeared and spoke to his black minion.

"Roberto," Ama heard him call.

Roberto ordered the slaves to stand. First he spoke Portuguese but it was clear that none understood.

"*Mónsoré-o*, get up, get up," he tried in Asante.

Uncertain, a man rose. Ama and the other Akans did so too and the rest followed their example.

"Brother, you speak Asante?" Ama asked Roberto.

"Don't call me brother, woman. I am not an unseasoned guiney bird like you," he replied. "Now stand in a line so that master can look at you properly."

The master examined and counted them. He seemed satisfied with his prize.

"*Vamos. Mma yeñkô*. Let's go," Roberto told them.

At the door they paused. A clerk checked them off against the tokens which the slaves' new owner returned to him.

Ama caught a glimpse of Captain Williams, glass in one hand, cigar in the other, in earnest conversation with Butcher and Cooper. And then she was blinded by the bright sunlight.

*****

Ama found a place and sat down with her back against the wall.

Suddenly she was very tired. She closed her eyes, the good one and the empty socket.

When will this humiliation cease? she wondered.

She tried to conjure up a vision of Itsho.

Itsho. She concentrated fiercely. *Itsho, I have crossed the great water. Today I set foot in another country. They call it Bahia. There are many of our people, black people, here. They are all slaves of the whites. Itsho, I pour libation to you and the other ancestors. I have nothing, only my one cloth from home. I have no drink to give you, but I know you will understand. I don't know what will happen to me. I am tired and hungry and thirsty. Itsho, come to me, help me.*

But Itsho did not come.

Perhaps he has forsaken me, she thought. *Perhaps the ancestors have no power in this country. Perhaps they cannot speak to us here.*

She tried again, forcing all other thoughts out of her mind and summoning up Itsho's image. At first she could not recall what he looked like. Then, all at once, he was there, a careless smile on his handsome face, just as he had looked when they were young lovers so many years, it seemed, so many years ago.

She opened her eye and looked around. The master was still recording details of the new arrivals in his book. Morose slaves lounged against the walls. A woman lay next to her, her head hidden in her cloth. On the wall opposite there was a gaudy coloured poster of Mary the mother of Jesus Christ. Ama recognised the word Madonna, spelled out in ornate letters. Next to it there was a picture of a black man with his arms raised. He wore white robes and there was a shining golden ring floating over his head. To one side there hovered two black cherubim with white wings growing out of their shoulders. At the man's feet sat two smaller black men in attitudes of Christian prayer. Ama read the title. The words were not all that different from English. She thought they meant 'The miraculous Saint Benidito, Protector of Angola.' She wondered why Van Schalkwyk had never mentioned this black saint to her.

*****

It was dark and cold when she awoke.

Roberto came in, clapping his hands to wake up late sleepers. Ama went out to the back and stood in the queue that had formed outside the latrine. When she returned to the hall, a young girl was sitting in her place.

"Good morning," Ama greeted her.

The girl was examining her reflection in a small mirror. Her reply lacked the customary courtesy.

"Fanti, eh?" was all she said.

"Fanti, Asante, I hear both," Ama replied patiently.

"They call me Ama."

"Luiza Fernandez," the girl replied casually.

Cardozo, the master, came in at the front door. He paused to genuflect and cross himself in front of the picture of the Madonna; then he went to his desk, opened a ledger and prepared a quill. Luiza got up and went to stand before him. Others fell in behind her.

Luiza untied a knot in one corner of her cloth and poured coins out onto the desk. One fell to the floor. She retrieved it. The master counted the coins. Then he spoke to her brusquely in Portuguese. She pouted her lips, untied another knot and added two coins. He made an entry in his ledger and dismissed her with a curt nod.

When she returned to Ama's side, she poured a heap of silver and copper coins onto the floor before her, arranged them in heaps and counted them, murmuring the numbers as she did so.

Ama was curious.

"May I look?" she asked.

Silently Luiza gave her a silver coin and one of copper. Ama examined them. On each there was a picture of a man's head and some writing around the edge. She spelled out the words.

"You can read Portuguese?" Luiza asked in astonishment.

"No," Ama replied, "only English. I can make out the letters on the coin but I don't understand the meaning."

"You must be bluffing. I don't believe you. I have never met an African who can read. Certainly not a woman. A few mulattos, yes. An occasional black Creole, Bahia-born, perhaps. But a black African woman?"

She shook her head and used tongue and teeth to make a sound of disbelief. Ama turned the coin over.

Luiza just shook her head again. Ama returned the coins to her.

"Where did you get the money? Are you not a slave, too?"

"Of course. Everyone here is a slave, even that scum Roberto. The master sends some of us out to work. Every day I have to give him one Milréis. Whatever else I earn he lets me keep. If I can save two hundred Milréis, I might be able to buy my freedom."

"And how much have you saved?"

Luiza shook her head and sighed.

"Only five. I have too many expenses. At this rate it will take me ten years."

"How come you work at night? What work do you do?" Ama asked, wondering if she, too, would be given a chance to work to buy her freedom.

Luiza looked at her, astonished at her naïveté; but she saw that the question had been innocently put.

"I am a prostitute," she said.

She used the Portuguese word.

"A prostitute?" Ama asked, repeating the word. "What is that?"

"A whore," Luiza explained, using another Portuguese word.

Then seeing that Ama still did not understand, she tried again.

"I sell my body to men. I let them fuck me and they pay me for it."

Ama turned to her, baffled.

"What kind of men?" she asked.

"What kind of men? What do you mean: what kind of men? Black men, white men, mulattos, Indians. They are all the same. Any man with some money in his pocket and a standing prick between his legs."

Ama turned the situation over in her mind.

"Is that what he will do with me?"

Luiza took her pocket mirror and gave it to Ama.

"Look at yourself," she said. "You are lucky. No man would look at you. You couldn't earn one Milréis in a week, let alone a day."

Ama hesitated. She hadn't seen her face since losing her eye. Then she clenched her teeth and raised the mirror. She took one look and put it down again. Sitting quite still, she closed her eye. Luiza was watching her.

"I'm sorry . . . I didn't mean. . . . "

Ama pulled herself together and wiped her face with a corner of her cloth. Then she raised the mirror again.

"It's nothing. It's not your fault. Only this is the first time. . . . ," she said and broke down again.

"Tell me," she asked when she had recovered. "How long have your been doing this?"

"Oh, three, four years now."

"But," Ama looked at her, "you can't be more than seventeen?"

"I think I'm sixteen, but I'm not sure. I came with my mother. She was already sick when we got off the ship. She died soon after the master bought us. He said he had been cheated; that he had wasted his money and that he would make me pay back every Milréis he had spent on her. He used to take everything from me. It is only since last month that he has let me keep anything I earn above six Milréis a week. Now I am saving up to buy my freedom."

*****

During the week there was a constant coming and going of customers. Again and again she was examined and inspected. She dealt with the humiliation by blanking her mind or focusing her thoughts on something far away and pleasant.

The customers made their notes. Afterwards they sat and talked with Cardozo, drinking rum or coffee. Sometimes money changed hands.

On Friday morning when Ama woke up, Luiza was huddled by her side, her head under her cloth as usual, fast asleep.

Roberto summoned her. She rose and went to the master's table, expecting to be inspected by an early morning customer. Cardozo identified her from her number. He found her name and number and ticked if off in his ledger.

There were six of them. She was the only woman. A stranger was waiting for them, a black man, a slave judging by his bare feet, but dressed in neat, clean working clothes, trousers and shirt.

Cardozo wrote a waybill and the man made his mark at the bottom.

"You have been sold," Roberto announced. "This is Josef Vellozo. He will take you to your new master."

Then he spoke to Ama.

"You are lucky. He is a Fanti man. He will look after you."

*****

Every step required an effort. When Ama put a foot down, the heavy clay seemed to embrace it; when she tried to lift it the clay sucked it down; when she pulled it free it carried a sticky load. From time to time she found a small patch of grass and stopped. Balancing on one foot, she used the other to scrape off some of the accretion.

Josef slowed down to let her catch up.

"Massapé," he said.

"Massapé?" she asked.

"That's what we call this clay. It's good for the cane, but the devil to walk through when it's wet; and worse still for carts."

Massapé. Ama concentrated on the word.

"Sister Ama," Josef called back, disturbing her reverie, "do you know what this is?"

He was pointing to the plants on either side. They grew thick and green, twice as tall as a man. It was like walking through a green tunnel.

"Sugar cane?" she guessed.

She had interrogated Josef relentlessly during the journey across the bay.

"Clever! Right first time. You must have seen it before."

"No, never. This is the first time. It looks so beautiful, swaying in the breeze."

"Beautiful? Yes, perhaps, but you will soon learn to hate the sight of it. You see these, with the purple flowers and the seeds just beginning to form on top? That is the sign that it is ready for cutting. If they leave it much longer it will start to dry up and the juice will turn sour. That's why the *safra* is about to start. The big rains are over and the cane is ripe.

"Once the cane is cut they must take it to the mill and crush it without delay or it will spoil. That is why you will learn to hate it. Our lives are ruled by this beautiful cane: clear the land for it; hoe the massapé for it; plant it; weed it; cut it; send it to the mill; mill it; boil the juice; turn it into sugar; pack it; send it to Salvador and from Salvador to Portugal. And then start all over again. Day in day out; week in week out; year in year out. Sugar cane and sugar until the day you die."

*****

An ox cart blocked their passage.

It had overturned, depositing its load of firewood in the road. Josef stopped and he and his five men helped the carter and his mate to tip the vehicle back on to its wheels. They gave it a push to help the four oxen on their way. The carter cracked his whip.

Ahead of them three more carts, their axles creaking, lumbered slowly through the mud. The wheels were crudely fashioned out of solid wood. The oxen seemed to be fighting an unequal battle. Ama gave them a wide berth. She feared them but she pitied them too.

They look as if their hearts will break, she thought.

The drivers greeted them with a crack of their whips.

"They are from one of our outgrower plantations," Josef explained.

A white man approached them down the track, followed by an emaciated, mangy dog. Ama had never seen a white man like him before. He was dressed in ragged pants and a dirty shirt open at the front. He carried a half empty bottle and from his gait appeared drunk. Josef's party stepped aside to let him pass.

"Good afternoon, senhor," Josef greeted him politely, but he paid no attention.

"Who is he?" Ama asked when he was out of earshot.

"I've never seen him before, but I know his kind. He probably owns a small engenho but has run it so badly that he has had to sell all his slaves. Now he has none left. He is too lazy and, like all the whites, too proud to do any physical labour himself. God knows how he lives. He probably begs from his neighbours or steals from the vegetable plots of the slaves on nearby plantations. But he has a white skin; so we must call him senhor."

As the sun went down the track took them right through the yard of a ruined engenho. The buildings were dilapidated. The front wall of one had collapsed, bringing down the roof. An emaciated dog barked at them. Josef picked up a stone and it retreated. A scrawny hen scratched at the ground, surrounded by miserable chicks.

Josef saw Ama surveying the premises and laughed at her dismay.

"No," he told her, "this is not our place. This is the Engenho do Meio. It's a *fogo morto*, a dead estate."

Small black children, naked, with swollen bellies, came out of a shed and watched them shyly. A pot boiled on an open fire, unattended.

The door hung on fragile hinges. Josef pushed it open and, announcing himself, went inside.

"Ama, come," he said.

She bent low to let the basket pass.

In the gloom a woman and several children of various ages were sitting around a pile of cassava tubers, scraping away the poisonous skin.

A man came out of the darkness. Josef greeted him as he helped Ama to put the basket down.

"I brought you some fish," he said in Fanti as he selected two. "I am sorry that is all I can spare."

The woman rose, wiping her hands on her torn cloth. She bent a knee and bowed her head. Then she took the fish.

"My brother, I don't know how to thank you," the man said. "You never forget us. If it weren't for you . . ."

Josef stopped him.

"If I were in your place and you in mine, would you not do the same? Indeed it is little enough. How is the baby?"

The woman turned away. The man just shook his head.

"There was nothing we could do," he said. "We buried him this morning."

Josef put a hand on his arm.

"Perhaps it was for the best," he said. "Now we must go. It is already dark. Please give us a torch to light our way."

"There's not far to go now," Josef told Ama as they made their way out the yard.

He waved to his friend who had come to see them off.

"Fifi and I were captured together. When we first came here, this was a rich farm. I was happy to have a friend so close by. Then his master died. He had many mulatto children but only one son by his white wife. The boy is a spoiled good-for-nothing. The first thing he did was to sell his own half brothers. Then, one by one, he sold the livestock and equipment and the other slaves. Now none remain except Fifi, whom he left to guard the place until he can sell the land and the buildings. They say that in Salvador he lives a grand life. Who knows what he will do when he has sold the plantation itself and finished spending the proceeds?

"What I fear most is that they will sell the woman and the children first, leaving Fifi alone. I know my friend. That would drive him mad."

CHAPTER 31

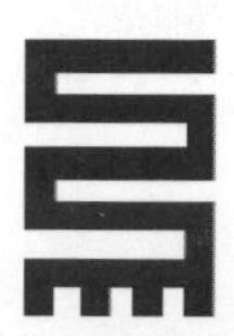

Two dark bundles came hurtling out of the night and almost bowled Josef over.

"Papa, Papa," Ama heard, but the rest of their talk was in Portuguese and beyond her.

"My boys," Josef told her proudly. "They were lying in wait for me."

She heard him speak her name. The two small boys came shyly to shake her hand and then to greet the other newcomers. Then they led their father, one at each hand, through the gate and into the yard.

"Well, here we are at last," Josef told Ama. "I will take you to greet the Senhor and then we'll see if we can find something to eat."

They had left the sticky massapé and were walking on sand. Ama paused to wipe away some of the mud. Somewhere in the darkness, dogs barked. There was no moon but she could see the outline of the double storied building silhouetted against the milky way. The rooms upstairs were dimly lit. By contrast, the downstairs veranda was ablaze with light.

Josef led them to the bottom of the steps and had them stand in line.

"Senhor, good evening," he said and then helped Ama to set the basket down.

The Senhor was a large, untidy man. On his forehead his white hair was receding, but at the back and sides it was long, uncut and unkempt. His shirt was open at the front, exposing a large belly, fat breasts and a hairy chest. He sat in a rocking chair which he kept constantly in motion. On a table before him there was a chess board with a game half played. The player who sat opposite him in an upright chair was much younger. He was dressed in a severe soutane and his dark hair was sleeked back. A chandelier bathed them in candle light.

A mulatto boy sat on a stool behind the table. He had been watching the game but now he rose, took the three steps in a single jump and shook Josef's hand.

At the Senhor's feet three small children, two black and one mulatto, played with discarded chess pieces. In the gloom behind the circle of light Ama glimpsed a young black woman in a long skirt, apron and cap.

"My move," Ama understood the Senhor to tell the priest before he gave his attention to Josef.

Josef made his report.

"Narciza," called the Senhor.

"Senhor?"

The maid stepped forward. She was barefooted.

The smallest child, the mulatto, intercepted her at the top of the stairs.

"Mama," he said and embraced her leg.

She lifted him to her hip. He grasped her ample breast and groped for her nipple; but before she had reached the bottom of the short flight of steps, he had fallen asleep. She shifted him onto her back and took the two largest fish from Josef. She held them by their tails and showed them to the Senhor. He grunted his approval without looking. His attention was back on the game. Ama craned her neck and saw him triumphantly capture a pawn with his white bishop. He picked up a glass and took a deep draught of the brown liquid.

Josef asked for permission to leave. The Senhor grunted again. The audience was over.

*****

Ama was woken by a loud continuous clanging.

She heard people moving nearby but it was still dark and she could see nothing. She had no idea where she was. She rubbed her eye and sat up. It was chilly. She pulled the cloth around her shoulders. Now she had a dim recollection of the previous evening. She had already been half asleep as she ate the bowl of corn porridge which Josef had given her. He had put her in the care of an old woman who had led her into a room and spread a sleeping mat on the earth floor for her.

She rose and found her way to the door. Fires had been lit. Several small boys sat around the nearest, hugging themselves and shivering. The old woman was nowhere to be seen. In the first light of dawn Ama saw that the hut she had slept in was the last of a row built on the side of a hill. There was a bustle of activity on the rough roadway. Beneath them, on a lower terrace, there was another row of huts, and beneath that a third.

A harsh male voice shouted orders. Ama wondered what to do. She was relieved when Josef appeared.

"Where is the old woman?" he asked directly.

"I haven't seen her this morning," Ama replied.

"Do you want to go somewhere?"

She nodded.

"I'll get one of the girls to take you."

When she returned, Josef was waiting for her.

"Good morning," he greeted her, "did you sleep all right? Good. This morning you can take your time. The field workers are going off now but there will be no work for you today. I've spoken to the General Manager and he's allowed me to take the morning off to show you over the plantation."

Ama squatted by the fire. The small boys stared at her empty socket and whispered amongst themselves. Josef spoke a single word to them and they got to their feet and ran off.

"Ah, there's the old lady now," he said.

Ama rose to her feet.

"Her name is Esperança," Josef explained. "She was born in this country and she has seen many generations come and go. She was retired long before I got here. You will sleep in her *senzala* at least for the time being. She speaks only Portuguese but since she lost the last of her teeth many years ago no one can understand much of what she says anyway."

"Maame Esperança," he shouted into her ear, "this is the new woman who has come. Her name is Ama. She will be staying with you."

Ama bent a knee and shook the old woman's knarled hand. She was rewarded with a toothless smile.

"She is deaf. You will have to shout at her."

Esperança's white hair was cropped close to her skull.

"How old is she?" Ama asked.

"Maybe eighty, maybe more."

"And she was born here?"

Josef nodded.

Then he said, "I think I can read your thoughts.

"But that is nothing. One evening, when you have picked up enough Portuguese, one of the old hands will tell you the story of the great *quilombo* of Palmares. They always tell that story to the new arrivals, to keep the memory alive. They say that Palmares kept its freedom for a hundred years and that it is nearly a hundred years since it succumbed. That means that it is at least two hundred years since the first slaves were brought here from Africa."

Ama shook her head slowly.

Then she asked, "Has Maame Esperança no family? Did she never have children?"

"They say she had three husbands, five children and many grand-children and great-grand-children; but they are all either dead or were sold long ago. Now she is all alone. She shares her cabin with Jacinta. Have you met Jacinta yet? She must still be sleeping."

"Maame Esperança, where is Jacinta?" he shouted.

He bent first one and then the other lower arm. Each time he touched his elbow. The old woman bent her head to one side and put her hands, palms together, to her cheek.

"Wake her then. She can't sleep all day. It is not good for her."

Esperança went to call Jacinta. Josef dropped his voice.

"Jacinta is from Kongo," he said. "She had a terrible accident; she was still new and young and inexperienced. They put her to feeding cane at the mill. One of her hands got drawn between the rollers. In trying to free herself, she put her other hand in too. By the time they were able to stop the oxen. . . . Well, you will see for yourself. Esperança helps her. When you see how difficult things are for her you realise how much we depend on our hands. She can't wash or dress herself. She has to be helped to eat. I hope you will be patient with her. She doesn't endure her fate with resignation."

"Ah, Sister Jacinta," he greeted her in Portuguese, "this is your new cabin mate. She is called Ama. She had just arrived from Africa."

Jacinta emerged from the cabin. She wore a simple shift which hung from her shoulders by two straps. Ama smiled a greeting, studiously avoiding looking at the stumps of Jacinta's lower arms. But Jacinta held up her stumps for inspection as if to say, "Here, take a good look." Then she saw the hollow which had once held Ama's right eye. Ama thought she sensed a softening in her expression. She held the right stump out for Ama to shake.

"Esperança," she shouted at the old woman, lifting her stumps to her mouth, "where is my food?"

*****

The accountant was a mulatto called Vicente Texeira.

"Be careful how you answer his questions," Josef warned her as they approached his office. "He is the Senhor's creature."

Texeira was a small wiry man. He had inherited his broad nose and fleshy lips from his African forebears, but his skin was as pale as the Senhor's.

"Name?" he asked, looking at the waybill which Josef had brought from Cardozo.

"They gave her the name Ana das Minas," Josef said.

Texeira made a tick against the name.

"We already have one Ana das Minas," he said. "We can't have two of the same name: it will confuse the records. I will enter her as 'One-eye' for the time being. When she is baptised she will be given a proper Christian name."

Josef was silent.

"Tell her what I said."

"Senhor Texeira says I am to tell you that until you are baptised with a proper Christian name, you will be called 'One-eye.' I am sorry. The man is like that."

"It is nothing," Ama replied.

"What does she say?"

"She says she understands."

"Ask her what happened to her eye."

Josef translated.

"Tell him it was an accident."

Texeira wrote a chit authorising the store-man to issue Ama with a length of coarse homespun cloth.

As they came out of the store, they met a tall, muscular white man. *A giant*, Ama thought, *like an executioner*.

"Who is this?" he asked Josef.

"The new woman I spoke to you about this morning, Senhor. You told me to take the morning off to show her around the engenho."

"Don' you tell me what I told you, boy," Senhor Vasconcellos replied. "You didn't tell me that she is missing one eye."

Josef said nothing.

"We celebrate the start of the *safra* tomorrow. The day after she will join the cane gang. Today you can keep her with you. You may spend the morning showing her around. In the afternoon I want you in the mill. Bring her with you. The sooner she gets to work the better. Do you understand?"

"Yes, Senhor."

"Who is he?" Ama asked when they were out of hearing.

"Jesus," replied Josef.

"How?"

"His name is Jesus Vasconcellos. He is the *feitor-mor*, the general manager. We say that on this engenho the Senhor is God. Senhor Vasconcellos, who sits by his right hand, is Jesus. I am talking about his power, mind you, not his compassion or his mercy. It is he who runs this place and he does so with an iron fist. If you want to live a peaceful life keep on the right side of him. If he takes a dislike to you, for whatever reason, he will make your life a misery. What Senhor Jesus demands is subservience. If you grovel before him, you will have no trouble.

"They say that once, before I came here, he was seen to smile. I can't imagine what might make him do that. The truth is, I believe that he hates all slaves, and particularly those of us from Africa. I thank the gods and our ancestors that my work takes me away from this place so often. But today we should be grateful to the man. He has allowed us the morning off to let me show you around the *engenho* and introduce you to some of our people."

*****

It was dark when the bell rang.

Still exhausted from the previous day's labour, Ama slept on. Old Esperança, who had risen earlier, prodded her awake. She washed her face and drank a mug of the mate which the old woman had prepared. At the assembly ground Benedito, the old Crioulo catechist, led them in a brief prayer to the Virgin Mary. Then they trooped down the familiar path through the swirling mist.

At the yard they formed into their gangs.

By the light of an oil lamp Texeira took the roll call. Then Vasconcellos assigned the day's tasks. Ama wondered whether the General Manager could read. It seemed not.

The carters inspanned the oxen in pairs and the cane field gangs climbed onto the carts. A crack of the whip set the oxen lumbering out of the yard and onto the rutted track. Mounted white and mulatto overseers followed, their dogs snapping at the horses' hooves. As they entered the copse at the bend before the cane fields, the birds in the trees began to serenade the approaching dawn. The clearing gang fell out first; soon afterwards the planters and the weeders also jumped down from their carts. The cutters were last.

When they reached their field the women made a fire and put a kettle on to boil. One man unsaddled the overseer's mount while the carters offloaded the carts and drew the first two up into position. The men passed a stone from hand to hand and honed their blades

The oxen settled down to graze in the firebreaks which divided the cane fields into *tarefas*, each seventy paces square. The cane from one *tarefa* could keep the mill working for twenty-four hours.

The men flexed their muscles and swung their scythes. The overseer assigned work partners: a man to cut, a woman to bundle and load; and staked out each pair's task for the day. As soon as there was light enough to see by, he cracked his whip as a signal to start work. The first heavy scythe whistled through the mist: *swish*! Then *thunk*! as it struck home. The women moved in to gather the fallen canes. They bound them into bundles and loaded them onto the carts. The sun rose and drove the mist away. The overseer strolled up and down, watching, playing with his whip. Time passed. The cutters established a rhythm. There was nothing for the overseer to do. Bored, he lay down, rested his head on his saddle, drew his hat over his face and slept.

Swish! *Thunk*! *Swish*! *Thunk*!

Ama's partner quickened his pace, building up a stockpile of canes. She knew what he was about and made no effort to work any faster. Then he paused, untied his headband and wiped the sweat from his face. He walked across to the barrel, dipped the mug into the water and took a deep draught. Then he poured a mugful over his head. As Ama lifted the last cane, he was at it again.

Swish! *Thunk*! *Swish*! *Thunk*!

Now Ama quickened her own pace, struggling to discipline the recalcitrant canes. When she had cleared her backlog, she went to attend to the fire. The lid of the kettle was bouncing.

"Water's boiling," she called in Portuguese.

The overseer lifted his hat and stood up. He wiped his eyes, stretched and yawned.

"Right," he called. "Breakfast."

Ama ladled water from the butt into a basin and carried it across to an empty cart. The women queued to wash their hands.

The men talked quietly amongst themselves.

"Speak Portuguese," the overseer insisted. "I want none of your pagan languages in my gang."

He watched them take their food, cold jerked beef, manioc meal and beans. When they had finished eating he handed over authority to his underdriver and ordered his horse saddled. As he mounted, the first two carts were turning off into the track on their way up to the mill.

"Good appetite," the wag of the gang shouted after him.

They went back to work. Ama started to chant.

"Twelve canes to a faggot, bind them tight."

The other women joined in the chorus, "How many canes to cut today?"

"Ten faggots a finger, five fingers a hand."

And then the chorus again, "How many canes to cut today?

Another woman offered a line, and then a third took her turn.

"One fifty faggots fill a cart;

"How many canes to cut today?

"Twenty four cart-loads feed the mill;

"How many canes to cut today?

"Send more canes, the mill must run;

"How many canes to cut today?"

"Ring the bell; crack the whip;

"How many canes to cut today?"

"The furnace burns, the kettles boil;

"How many canes to cut today?"

"Eight loads of firewood, stacked to burn;

"How many canes to cut today?"

At each line the scythes swung. Then the men began to improvise.

"Pity the downtrodden African slave;

"How many canes to cut today?"

"Curse the ships which brought us here;

"How many canes to cut today?"

"Senhorita Miranda, open your legs," sang the wag.

"How many canes to cut today?" came the automatic reply, but it was interrupted by laughter.

They all straightened up and took a short rest to applaud the man's impudence. The song was over.

"What did he say? Why are you laughing?" a woman asked Ama.

Warming to the applause, the wag spread his arms, looked beseechingly up at the heavens and mimed himself wooing the Senhor's precious daughter.

"Ah sweet, white, beautiful, innocent, virginal Miranda," he said, adding more emphasis to each successive hosanna, "I beg you. By Saint Gonçalo, I beg you. Let Luis dos Santos make you a fine mulatto baby!"

"Heh, enough of that," interrupted Pedro the underdriver, trying to suppress his own laughter, but scared that he might have some explaining to do if any of this reached the *casa grande*. "Back to work."

At midday they stopped to eat the food left over from breakfast. A returning cart brought enough *garapa* to give each man a swallow. They took off only just enough time to down the food; then they were back at work.

Swish! *Thunk*! *Swish*! *Thunk*!

Now the sun was hot; the sweat flowed; backs ached and the pace flagged.

Pedro flicked his whip. He had only recently been plucked from the ranks of the cane cutters and given a pair of leather boots, a whip and a bottle of *garapa* twice a week to mark his new status. But that was not all that had changed. His former mates now treated him with reserve. He sensed that an invisible barrier separated him from them.

He regretted the loss of companionship. Yet he certainly did not regret his release from the grinding hard labour. He was getting special food rations too; those frequent pangs of hunger were a thing of the past. But it was not selfishness, he persuaded himself, which had led him to accept promotion. His wife had a baby daughter. He had made a sacrifice; and it was for the child's sake. As if he had had a choice anyway! Yet he was ill at ease. He was drinking too much. Most nights now he got drunk. And he had started to beat the woman. Afterwards he would be sorry; yet a few days later he would do it again.

In the early afternoon they heard the approaching hoof beats of the overseer's horse. They saw him stagger as he dismounted and exchanged knowing glances. This was not the time to trifle with the man.

The first cutter completed his row and went to help the slowest member of the gang. No one would leave until the whole *tarefa* had been levelled. As the western sky turned crimson they regained a little energy and drove themselves to finish the work before sundown. As the men helped the women to load the last cart, their evening meal arrived. It was the same bland stuff they had eaten before.

They filed back to the yard in the dark, dragging their heavy legs, tripping over the ruts in the track, too weary even to talk. By the light of a brazier they handed their tools in at the store. Senhor Vasconcellos ordered them to report at the mill. Ama asked for permission to go and relieve herself. At the back of the kettle house, the furnaces roared, sending great orange flames flickering upwards, silhouetting the glistening naked bodies of the stokers. Ama stopped for a moment to watch the inferno. There was a terrible beauty about it. *Like the Christian hell*, she thought.

Her work was to collect the spent canes, the bagasse, and dump it outside the mill. Every muscle ached. Her eyelids drooped. The driver flicked a whip at her. By midnight all the cane had been milled. It would be morning again before the final ladle of sugar syrup had been decanted and the last of the sugar pots sent to the purging house.

Ama hardly remembered finding her way back to her cabin and collapsing onto her mat.

She dreamed. Fragments of an old Yendi nightmare. Decapitated heads boiling in a cauldron. Heads in a basket, still dripping blood, on the night of Osei

Kwadwo's death. Her work, to take the heads, one by one, and throw them into the furnace beneath the kettle house. They turned and grinned at her obscenely as they floated through the air. She woke up in a cold sweat, shivering, her bones aching.

It was dark when the bell rang. Still exhausted from the previous day's labour, Ama slept on. Old Esperança, who had risen earlier, prodded her awake.

So it continued, day after day, week after week, month after month, each barely distinguishable from the one before.

*****

On Sundays the bell was not rung until dawn.

Milling started again in the late afternoon and the first kettle was filled soon after dark; but the field slaves generally had the full day off.

Ama went to Mass.

The Bishop had chosen for the site of the chapel a place which had once been sacred to the former owners of this land, the Tupi. The building was modest: earth floor, whitewashed walls. The furnishings, too, were simple: a wooden pulpit with two steps and a canopy, carved by Bernardo in the carpenter's shop, a pair of silver candlesticks on a white tablecloth, two rows of benches and a curtained confessional.

The Senhor and his extended family sat on the front bench; paid employees sat on the second; the slaves stood behind.

The service was in Latin. The other slaves, Ama discovered, even the Crioulos, understood no more of the words than she did. But she enjoyed the incense and the bells and the sense of some special mystery. And unlike the interminable Dutch service at Elmina, this one didn't last too long. Even the sermon (this in Portuguese) was short. If ever the young padre forgot himself, the Senhor would rap his knuckles on the bench and Father Isaac would terminate his homily forthwith.

Now that she was beginning to master Portuguese Ama was expected to attend the Sunday school which Benedito the old catechist ran after Mass. There were a few adult African pagans like her; the rest were children. The Angolans left immediately after the Mass. They had all been baptised en masse before leaving the shores of their native land. Each carried a certificate of baptism in the form of an imprint of the royal crown of Portugal, burned into the skin of their breasts with a red hot iron. This brand, Jacinta told Ama bitterly, served also as a receipt for export duty paid to the Portuguese King.

The Senhor's mulatto son, Alexandre, always stayed on. He imbibed Christian doctrine with undiscriminating enthusiasm and planned to take holy orders when he grew up.

"This is the power which the Holy Church has given to our Priest," Benedito told them. "With a few words, the words of Jesus, 'Eat this bread: this is my body; drink this wine: this is my blood,' he can bring God Himself down into his hands. With a few more, saying, 'May almighty God have mercy on us, forgive us our sins, and bring us eternal life,' he can save us from the everlasting flames of perdition, shut tight the fearful gates of hell and open wide for us the glittering portals of heaven.

"In order to qualify for God's mercy you must first be baptised. Until you have been baptised you will remain a savage, little better than the wild beasts which live in the forest. Once you have received the sacrament of baptism you will become a proper member of Christian society. Then you will be permitted to confess your sins and to receive the blessed Eucharist.

"Serve our Senhor well. Bear the hardships of slavery with patience. God has sent these things to test us. He tells us 'be not slothful.' If we do His bidding we shall certainly have our reward. For it is written in the Holy Book, 'blessed are the meek: for they shall inherit the earth' and also 'blessed are they which are persecuted for righteousness' sake: for theirs is the kingdom of heaven.'"

The children who had been born at the Engenho de Cima and had been baptised at birth, yawned and looked at the familiar dusty pictures of Saint Benedict the Moor and Santa Efigenia which hung on the wall; and at the little brown-faced statue of Our Lady of the Rosary in its niche. And when they became bored with the images, they scratched lines on the earth floor and played furtive games of tic-tac-toe.

Ama's experience, first with Van Schalkwyk at Elmina and then with Williams on board *The Love of Liberty*, had cured her of any possible predilection for the white man's religion. But she suffered from an insatiable curiosity. This business of eating the body and drinking the blood of Jesus intrigued her. *There is some mystery in it*, she thought, *something concealed and unspoken. Perhaps the first Christians were cannibals and the Holy Communion is a secret commemoration of the Apostles' consumption of the physical remains of their leader? If not that, what can the strange ritual mean? Nana Esi must have heard something about this. Perhaps that was why she thought that the white man was going to cook her in his palm soup. Poor Nana Esi. Rather it was the sharks which ate her.*

Eating the body and drinking the blood of Jesus is really not that different, she reflected, *from the ceremony in which the Owner of the Earth would cut the throat of a white cockerel and let its blood flow onto the shrine. The Asante custom is similar, only they bring their sacrifices to the altar of Tano or another of their abosom. At bottom all religions seem to have common elements. And if that is so, why exchange your own customary beliefs for those of your oppressor?*

As for the priest's constant harping on sin, that is just so much hypocrisy. It is the whites who are the greatest sinners; yet the priest is always accusing us.

Ama was tempted to raise these matters with Benedito, but she decided against. *The old Crioulo's Christian faith is a crutch which helps him hobble through a difficult life*, she thought. *What purpose would be served by trying to sow seeds of doubt in his heart?*

She didn't discuss her private views with Alexandre either. The Senhor's bastard son was in the full flush of adolescent religiosity. Indeed, in his youthful enthusiasm, he regarded Ama as his first convert. Sometimes after Sunday School they would climb the forested hill behind the *senzalas* and find a quiet place to sit. Then, haltingly, she would read a chapter of Exodus or Ruth in the Portuguese bible which Alexandre had stolen for her, and the boy would correct her pronunciation or explain the meaning of a difficult word. Soon she began to pick up whole passages by heart. She would make time pass in the fields, when she was bundling cane, by rehearsing in her head the familiar stories in the unfamiliar language. She swore Alexandre to secrecy: nobody must know that she could read, neither his father nor any of the slaves. She saw how he relished the conspiracy, though she had no illusions as to how far she could trust his discretion.

She soon discovered that the elegant classic language of the Portuguese Bible was of no practical use to her. The newcomers from Africa, arriving with so many different languages of their own, soon picked up what they needed of the basic utilitarian pidgin which had been developed by former generations of slaves. One step removed from pidgin was the dialect which all the Bahians spoke, both the white masters and the black and mulatto Crioulos. She discovered a higher level of Portuguese one day when she eavesdropped on the Senhor while he was conducting a distinguished visitor from Lisbon around the *engenho*. The Senhor struggled to express himself in an idiom in which he clearly lacked practice. The visitor's face was a book in which she read his contempt for his host's inadequate command of his own language.

When the time came for her to be baptised she had no trouble trotting off the ten commandments and the creed. Josef and Wono were her god-parents. By this time the previous owner of the name Ana das Minas had died, so she inherited it. But only the priest ever used it. Vasconcellos still called her "One-eye." To the slaves she remained Ama.

*****

Sunday was a day of rest; and yet it was not really a day of rest.

Truth to tell there was really no day of rest at the Engenho de Cima, at least not during the long months of the *safra*. But Sunday was different. On Sunday the slaves worked for themselves. Most of them worked on plots of land which the Senhor had allotted to them. This suited the Senhor, for the food crops they grew on their allotments supplemented their diet at no cost to him. Moreover, they offered him a cheap source of produce for the *casa grande's* kitchen: he could buy vegetables from his own slaves at half the price he would have had to pay in the nearest market.

After Mass and Sunday school (and sometimes a secret reading session with Alexandre) Ama would join Esperança and Jacinta at their allotment.

But first she had to do her week's laundry. She put on her spare cloth, the old one she had brought from home, from Africa, and threw the coarse homespun smock, which she wore all week, over her shoulder. The laundry was a natural stone pool on the side of the hill behind the *senzalas*. Water tumbled into it from a leaky wooden aqueduct fed from the *engenho's* stream. During the dry season the flow contracted to a trickle, but for most of the year it kept the basin full. At one corner, the overflow cascaded out over the rocks and found its way down into the forest below, where it disappeared into the ground.

On her way Ama plucked handfuls of leaves from one of the soap bushes which grew prolifically on the path up to the pool. It was at this private place that the women bathed on those rare occasions when they were not at work during the daylight hours. There were two small girls there now, singing as they rubbed away at sheets from the big house. They answered Ama's greeting shyly. Ama plunged her dirty smock into the pool. Then she crushed the leaves and worked them up into a lather, washed and rinsed her garment, wrung it out and hung it on a rock to dry. Then she took off the cloth she was wearing and jumped into the pool and soaped herself. The girls decided to join her and they splashed about together.

This is what children ought to be doing at their age, Ama thought, *rather than spending their time washing the Senhora's sheets and table cloths.*

But didn't you have to work when you were their age?

Of course I did, but that was for my own mother and it was like a game. When Tabitsha gave me a task, I was proud to help her. It was a recognition that I was old enough to accept the responsibility.

It is true that these girls are probably doing the Senhora's laundry so that their own mothers can work on their allotments, but they are still too young for such a heavy load. And they are both so thin, like wraiths.

When she arrived at the allotment she was still wet. *One day*, she thought, *I will save enough to buy myself a towel.* She spread her smock on a bush. Esperança was bent double, picking at the soil with her hoe. Jacinta stood by her, pointing at the weeds with her stumps. They were both waiting for Ama. There was little the two of them could achieve without her. The old Crioulo woman soon became tired. Jacinta's main contribution was to carry a bundle of firewood or a basket of vegetables back to the *senzala* on her head.

They needed little persuasion to sit down in the shade.

"Do you know what you can do for me, my mother?" Ama asked, raising her voice.

The old woman shook her head.

"Brew me a mug of *mate* on your fire, I beg you."

She wound her cloth around her waist and set to work, hoeing, weeding, nursing the seedlings, transplanting. She knew the value of manure from home and had set some of the small boys who worked with the oxen to collecting baskets of dung from the paddocks. There was joy in this work. She always grew excited as she approached the allotments after a week's absence, anxious to see just how much her corn plants had grown in the seven days. She grew red pepper and groundnuts and some of the European vegetables which she knew she could sell at the Senhor's kitchen. She recalled the guinea corn and millet which grew on the flat plain around Tigen's hamlet and the rice and groundnuts and yams which they cultivated on the low hills nearby. She hummed the old prayers, begging the ancestors to bring rain and control the fierce unpredictable force of the wind, which could destroy a year's work in less time than it took to eat a meal. Itsho had cultivated her own little groundnut farm for her. She had sold some of the crop and used the proceeds to buy this very cloth she was wearing. *Itsho.* She felt guilty. She had forsaken his memory. She would borrow some *garapa* and use it to pour libation to his spirit that very evening. And when this corn was ready for harvest she would brew beer from it and pour libation again with the fruit of her own labour.

All along the contours below the forest there were similar allotments. This was the only activity in which the Senhor granted the slaves some independence, some little control over their own lives. On Sunday afternoon there was singing in the hills, not the measured worksongs of the cane fields, but songs remembered from home, songs of love, lullabies, poetry put to music.

Sometimes Ama would straighten up to rest for a moment and just listen.

*****

Alexandre lost interest in religion.

Now he was crazy about sailing. The Senhor would not let him use the boat alone so Josef had to spend his Sundays on the water. Sometimes he took his own two boys along with him.

One Sunday afternoon when she returned from the allotments, Ama collected her bible from its hiding place and headed up into the forest to the outcrop of rock which was their secret place. Alexandre, ever the willing thief, had brought her a pencil and some sheets of paper. She was working her way slowly but systematically through the Old Testament. When she came upon a word she didn't understand, she would write it down. Later she would ask Alexandre its meaning and if he couldn't explain he would ask the padre, who was his teacher. Father Isaac's conviction that Alexandre would be an acquisition for the Church grew and he lost no opportunity to tell his patron so. He little guessed the source of the boy's inquiries.

Ama settled down with her back against a rock and made herself comfortable. She decided to read the story of Abraham and Lot and the cities of Sodom and Gomorrah which she remembered from the English bible. Perhaps in the Portuguese she would find a clue as to why God had destroyed the two cities. She struggled with unfamiliar words and read and reread the passages aloud to try to make sense of them.

She came again to the verse which says: "And when the sun was going down, a deep sleep fell upon Abram; and, lo, an horror of great darkness fell upon him." She shut her eyes, the good one and the blind one, to rest them for a moment. The sun was pleasantly warm; a gentle breeze blew up from the valley below; and Ama dozed.

She dreamed and in her dream she saw the Owner of the Earth speaking to her father, Tigen, at the Earth Shrine. The Owner of the Earth had cut the throats of a young female goat and a young cow. He raised his bloody hands and said, "Your descendants will become strangers in a land far away and will serve the people of that land; and those people will persecute them for four hundred years."

She was awoken by a gentle shaking of her shoulder.

"Sister Ama, what are you doing here? It will be dark soon. This is no place to spend the night all on your own."

It was Olukoya, Josef's Yoruba *malungo*, slave driver by day and *babalorisha*, so it was said, by night.

"And what's this you have here?"

He picked up the Bible; the paper and pencil fell out from between the pages. He looked at her with astonishment. Then he sat down next to her.

"Read," he ordered her.

Ama looked back at him wondering what all this could mean. She rubbed her good eye.

"In the beginning," she read, "God created the heaven and the earth. And the earth was without form, and void; and darkness was upon the face of the deep. And the Spirit of God moved upon the face of the waters."

"Now write something on the paper."

"What shall I write?"

"Write what you have just read."

She started to do so, struggling with the blunt pencil and the special

Portuguese letters which she still found difficult to form. Olukoya watched her in silence. He was trying to impose some discipline on the thoughts which raced through his mind.

"Are you a Christian?" he asked her.

She detected a note of suspicion in his voice. She shook her head.

"No," she said. "I have been baptised but I am not a Christian."

"Why not?" he asked.

She looked up at him. He seemed to be testing her; yet she felt no resentment: Bra Olukoya was no threat to her. She felt comfortable with him and could tell him the truth.

"Christianity is the religion of the white man; it is the religion of slavery. If I were to accept it, I would be acquiescing in my own enslavement. I will never do that. Not until the day I die."

"Well said, my sister," he replied. "But if you are not a Christian, what are you then?"

Ama was puzzled. This was a question she had never considered.

"What am I?" she asked slowly, groping for an answer. "Well. If you had asked me that question when I was young, I might have said only, 'I am a human being, a female human being, a girl, daughter of my father Tigen and my mother Tabitsha.'"

She was carried back to the long discussions she had had with Itsho; but this was not something they had talked about.

"What am I?' she mused. "Sometimes I saw other people in the market, Hausa, Mossi, Yoruba; but it was not until I was captured by Dagomba marauders that I became conscious that my people, we call ourselves Bekpokpam, were different from others.

"I was taken to Kumase, you know, the Asante capital. The queen mother changed my name. She it was who gave me my Asante name, Ama. I had been torn from my family. Part of me longed to go home to my mother; but part of me became Asante. Sometimes I still speak to my ancestors in my own language; but mostly now I think in Asante."

"So you are Asante now?"

"No. I cannot be Asante. To be Asante you must be born into an Asante family; you must have an Asante mother. I had no family there. And it was the Asante who sent me to be sold to the Dutch. Yet I don't hate them. I was their slave, but they treated me like a human being."

She paused to think. *Koranten Péte bore me no malice. He sent me away because he saw me as a danger, a threat to the Asante state; because of his boy king's mad love for me, because Osei Kwame wanted to make me his first wife.*

"I will tell you something that nobody else here knows, not even Josef."

Again she paused, collecting her thoughts.

"In Elmina Castle, the Director-General, a Dutchman, took me from the dungeon to use me for his pleasure. By chance, as they write in this book, I found favour in his eyes. He taught me the language of the English and to read and write. He taught me that the world is like an orange floating in space; that there are six continents and that one of them is Africa. Have you ever seen a map, Bra Olukoya? Do you know what Africa is like? Let me draw it for you. This is Africa. This is the sea, all around it. And here is Elmina."

Olukoya looked at her crude map and nodded. He suppressed the question which was on his lips and let her go on without interruption.

"You ask me what I am. It is a difficult question. When they put me on the ship, there were already many slaves in the holds. They spoke a language I had never heard. To this day I don't know the name of their country. We called them Tomba's people, because that was the name of their leader. But they were black, like us. Then I realised that Africa is the continent of black people; and I understood for the first time that we black people are all Africans.

"So I think that the answer to your question is that I am a human being; I am a woman; I am a black woman; I am an African. Once I was free; then I was captured and became a slave; but inside me, I have never been a slave; even today, inside me, here, and here, I am still a free woman."

"Well spoken, Ama. You are wise beyond your years. Why have we never talked before? And why have you kept this gift a secret?" he asked, pointing to the Bible and the paper on which she had written the opening words of Genesis.

"What use would it be? Our people would think me a witch."

"Some, maybe, but not me. That is the greatest gift that their God gave to the whites, greater than their ships, greater than their guns. Until we learn to read and write, we will never be able to defeat them and regain our freedom. But tell me, where did you get the book?"

"Alexandre."

"It was his? He gave it to you?"

"Not exactly. He stole it from the priest."

Olukoya laughed.

"That boy, he is incorrigible. One day, when he grows up, he will be invaluable to us. But now you should not put too much trust in him. He is only a boy. And the Senhor is his father. He could easily talk out of turn."

He looked up at the sky.

"It looks like rain. And it will soon be dark," he said. "We should be going. We can talk some more on the way."

"If I were to give you a message," he asked her as they clambered down the rocks, "could you write it down on paper?"

"In Portuguese?" she asked.

"It would have to be," he replied.

"I could try. Who is the message for?"

"You must swear that you will tell this to no one else. It could be dangerous. It could even cost us our lives."

"I swear."

He looked back to make sure that there was no one following them.

"We keep in touch with our brothers at the other *engenhos*, in the towns and in Salvador itself. We send them news and they send us news. Josef is one of our couriers. Since none of us knows how to read or write, all our messages are sent by word of mouth. But in Salvador, some of the Crioulos are with us and some of them can read and write. If we could send and receive written messages . . . do you understand?"

*****

The Senhora needed a new maid.

This time she was determined not to recruit another candidate for the bed of her ageing and ailing husband, who had so often in the past been the agent of her shame.

"Bring me," she instructed Vasconcellos, "the six ugliest wenches you have."

Of course the news got round: there were few secrets at the Engenho de Cima. When Ama learned that her name was on the short list of the ugly, she felt crushed. She ran to her cabin, buried her head under her blanket and cried until she could cry no more.

Jacinta tried to console her.

"Look at me," she said, holding up her stumps.

But that only set Ama off on a fresh fit of sobbing.

Then Benedito took up his Christian duty and came to visit her, misquoting Ecclesiastes on vanity. She bit her tongue. *You really are a stupid illiterate old man,* she thought, *with your scraps of ill-digested quotations from the Bible.* Immediately regretting her harsh thoughts, she thanked him with the humility and respect due to his years and sent him on his way.

It was Wono, Josef's wife, who at last brought her to her senses.

"Don't be stupid, sister Ama," she told her. "After all, who cares about what Vasconcellos or the other whites think? In a way you are lucky - at least Senhor Jesus may keep his hands off you if that is what he thinks. And if the Senhora selects you, just think. You will be better fed and better clothed and you won't have to work so hard. What is more, you will keep us informed about what is going on up there."

*****

The house slaves gathered in the kitchen yard.

Father Isaac read a passage from the Bible and delivered a brief homily. Ama was to discover that he found in the Holy Book a seemingly inexhaustible stock of verses relevant to their condition and behaviour.

"Let him that stole, steal no more: but rather let him labour," he advised them and then, skipping over a few verses, "Let all bitterness, and wrath, and anger, and clamour, and evil speaking, be put away from you."

"The Epistle to the Ephesians," he told them.

Ama made a mental note to look for the passage in her stolen Bible.

Alexandre was there of course. For the Senhora he had once been just one more dark-skinned reminder of her shame; but he had long since won her heart. It was Alexandre, Ama was to learn later, who had been instrumental in swinging the Senhora in her favour. The Senhora was easily led and Ama was the only candidate who had such an influential advocate.

The Senhor was there too, unshaven, bleary eyed, in a dressing gown.

At the end of the short service, a young mulatto boy stepped forward.

"Senhor," he said, "I beseech your blessing in the name of our Lord and Saviour Jesus Christ."

"Jesus Christ bless you forever," the Senhor mumbled.

CHAPTER 32

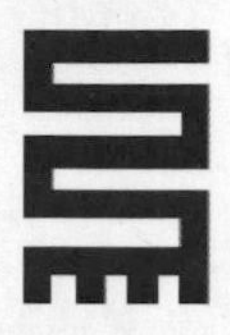

When Ama returned from the cane fields the following Saturday it was already dark.

She strapped their rolled up sleeping mats onto Jacinta's back. Esperança helped her to raise her basket to her head.

"We will be back tomorrow evening," Jacinta told the old woman.

The others were waiting at the edge of the forest, shadowy shapes in the dark, murmuring quietly. Josef was going from group to group, peering into faces, making sure that they had no uninvited guests. Ama heard the bleating of a sheep. Soon they moved off into the trees, following the path up the hill, past the allotments.

"Keep close behind me," Jacinta told her.

When they were over the brow, out of sight of the *engenho*, they paused while torches were lit. Then they pushed on through the light undergrowth. There were no paths here. Each followed the one before, trusting Olukoya, at their head, to lead them to the place. The torches cast grotesque shadows on the canopy above. The smell and feel of decaying leaves brought back memories of other journeys.

This is so like the African forest, Ama thought. *Yet why is it,* she pondered, *that the trees and the wild animals are all different from ours?*

*****

Ama was near the back of the file. When she entered the clearing, torches had been tied to the trunks of young trees and the men were lighting a fire. The women gathered on one side, spreading their mats and arranging their bundles and baskets. Ama unloaded Jacinta.

Every one talked in subdued tones; this forest, like all others, was full of spirits.

Ama looked around and counted. There were about thirty in the party, mostly adults, but one or two infants too. Ignacio Gomes, the *cabra* leather worker, a free man, half Tupi, half Kongo, was there. The rest were slaves and all of them were Africans; no other free men, no Crioulos, no mulattos, only blacks. Some *boçal,* mostly *ladino,* but all black.

Josef and Bernardo emerged from the enveloping darkness, bearing drums. Olukoya clapped his hands for silence.

"My brothers and sisters," he said, "we have all had a long, hard day. We need to sleep so that we can awake refreshed in the morning. But before we retire for the night, let us first go and announce our arrival."

There were calls of assent. They fell in at once behind the torch bearers and the three drummers. The shrine was close by, in another clearing. A stream wound its way past both. The sound of water tumbling over the stones would accompany their oblations.

An enormous tree, buttressed by its spreading roots, stood near the centre, dominating the cleared space. They arranged themselves in a half circle around it.

"In our country," Jacinta whispered to her, "our god Tempo lives in the tree we call *nsanda*. There are no *nsanda* trees in this place, so those who came before us made a home for Tempo in this one which is its brother. They call it *gameleira branca*. The white flag is the way we dress *nsanda*. The ribbon around the trunk is for the Yorubas."

The *bata* drums called for silence. Olukoya stood before the tree, barefooted and bare from the waist up. Gazing up into the dark canopy and then down into the space behind the roots he spoke a few sentences in Yoruba. Then, to Ama's surprise, Jacinta stepped forward, and raising her two stumps, addressed Tempo briefly in Ki-Kongo. Next to speak was Josef and this time Ama understood.

"Onyankopon Kwame, creator of all things, lord of the universe; Asase Yaa, spirit of the earth," he intoned. "Your children greet you. We have come to tell you that we are here. Before dawn tomorrow we shall return to praise your name and to honour the spirits of our ancestors. Tonight we beg you to protect us as we sleep. Protect us from *sasabonsam* and all malevolent spirits which may live in this forest. Now we beg your permission to take leave of you. We shall go and come again tomorrow."

*****

It was still dark when Josef gently shook Ama awake.

"Ama, come, we need your help. Sister Jacinta, it is time."

As they walked towards the shrine, he explained, "We have only one sheep and two cockerels. That is not enough to allow all of us to make a sacrifice to our own gods. So each nation has selected one person to follow its own custom. Olukoya wants you to represent your people, even though you are only one."

"What will I have to do?"

"If you like, say a prayer to your own gods and ancestors. Otherwise just watch and listen."

In the flickering torch light Ama saw several objects which she had not noticed the night before. One was a solid clay cone, about waist high, with a small flattened top on which lay two pieces of iron. Another was the familiar Asante *Onyame-dua*, God's tree, supporting a basin in its arms. Around the base of the *gameleira*, under its roots, was an array of pots and calabashes, some upright, some inverted.

The last object was a crude ladder-like framework of trimmed branches. A goatskin had been stretched across it to make a table top. On the skin lay cow horns, shells, a seed rosary, the red spurs and comb of a cockerel, an earthen dish full of clay with feathers and teeth protruding from it, stones, and cracked fragments of glazed pottery and mirror glass.

"That is Tempo's altar," Jacinta whispered. "Ama, pluck some leaves from this bush and lay them on it for me."

Seven iron stakes had been driven into the earth around the altar.

"Mind the lances," Jacinta warned.

There were six in their party.

Olukoya was their acknowledged leader. He had earned this status by virtue of his personal qualities; but there was more to it than that. As a young man he had been a novice in a shrine devoted to the performance of sacred rites in the service of Shango, deified fourth king of Oyo. While he was in Oyo, Abiodun, the Alafin, had decided it was time to reassert the dwindling authority of his office by crushing the forces of his own military commander. Olukoya had become an innocent victim of the resulting civil war, ending up a slave upon a Portuguese ship.

There were only a few Yorubas at the *engenho* and even those were recent arrivals on the Bahian scene. But the power of their gods (four hundred and one in all, Olukoya said) was known far and wide. And Olukoya knew how to invoke that power. It was this knowledge which gave him such authority.

He lifted one of the pots and poured water from it onto the ground as he spoke.

"Eshu,
"gate-keeper of the gods, intercessor for mankind,
"we come to you in peace, to greet you at this cross-roads,
"where the spirits of Africa meet those of this country, this Brazil,
"and the fierce god of the white man, Jesus-Mary-Joseph.
"We cool your brows with this fresh water from the river."

Unseen drummers accompanied him, quietly, so as not to drown out his words.

"Take our humble messages, we beseech you,
"to almighty Olodumare, supreme amongst the gods,
"who gives the breath of life to man
"and seals our destiny;
"to Obatala, creator, god of the overarching skies,
"whose purity of spirit, goodness and kindness know no bounds;
"to Shango, lord of fire and tempest, essence of courage and of justice;
"and to his wives;
"to Oshun, river goddess of Oshogbo,
"goddess of love,
"who sustained us during the terrible journey across the great sea
"and brought us safely to these shores; and
"to Oya, mistress of lightning and the tornado and of sudden death.
"Take our words to Oshumare, serpent of the rainbow, messenger of Shango;
"to Ogun, his brother, fearless god of iron and war;
"to Obaluaye, who with his broom can sweep the sesame seeds of pestilence
"over the face of the earth;
"to Orunmila, leopard, messenger of the gods, who knows all things,
"to whom there is no secret;
"Orunmila, who sat watching Olodumare as he made the universe;
"and knows the secrets of his laws."

He paused to finger the beads of Orunmila's necklace of divination which hung at his neck.

"Let our words fly to Yemoja, most fruitful of goddesses, mistress of the seas;
"and of chaste love between men and women.
"Yemoja, giver of children,
"we tie this ribbon about the trunk of this tree to ask you to bind us to you,
"as a mother straps her child upon her back."
"We pour the blood of this black cockerel,
"to honour the spirits of our ancestors."

Josef handed the squawking cockerel to him. He held it over the altar while Josef drew a sharp knife across its throat. The blood spurted onto the altar. Josef held up a bowl to catch the last drops.

The sheep which they had stolen for the sacrifice had been scrubbed clean and its hair combed. It had a broad sash about its waist, the knotted end tied into a bow. Olukoya gripped its body between his knees, held its mouth shut and pulled its head back towards him, stretching its neck.

The drums fell quiet. All knelt and prayed. The clear tones of a struck bell rippled across the clearing. A calabash rattle joined. The sheep struggled. Ama wondered whether a sheep could foresee its own end as humans can.

The knife did its work and the sheep's blood spurted into the bowl. The drums rolled, celebrating the sacrifice. Olukoya raised the bowl and poured some of the blood upon the clay altar.

Then Jacinta stepped forward. She spoke for the BaKongo; and for the others who had been brought to Bahia from the barracoons of Luanda and Loango and Benguela in Angola. Their ancestors from the ancient states of Tio and Loango and Ndongo had been crossing the Atlantic to Bahia, though not by choice, for the past two hundred and fifty years. The Angolans asked Jacinta to speak for them because they knew that since she had lost her hands, Tempo had frequently entered her body and taken possession of her spirit.

She pulled Ama forward with her right stump. Kneeling before an open bowl she drew Ama down after her. She pressed her stump into the bowl, charging it with powdery dry white clay. She tried to draw on the ground but failed. She signed to Ama to help her. Ama took a handful of the powder, watching Jacinta's eyes. Jacinta mimed to her to sprinkle the powder on the ground in a circle and then to draw a cross within the circle in the same way. She nodded her approval and then showed Ama that she should draw two circles on her face, one around each eye.

Ama stood up and stepped back. Jacinta slowly lowered her head towards the circle on the ground.

"Oh Tempo," she chanted,
"let this circle become a mirror.
"In it show us the faces of the *pretos velhos*,
"of the spirits of all who have come this way before us.
"Invest the power of our ancestors in us.
"Let it shine forth from us with a blinding radiance.
"Here at this cross roads,
"where this great tree sinks its roots into the ground,
"where the clearing meets the forest,
"where the darkness of night meet the dawn of a new day,

"give us the vision to see into your world."
"In the evening the sun descends into the underworld of darkness.
"Yet every day it rises again,
"in a new dawn.
"The cycle is without end.
"So it is with our lives.
"When we die we too enter the world of night,
"Where the sparks of departed souls light up the sky.
"And yet we too are reborn.
"So it is with all living things:
"birth, maturity, death and rebirth."

A breath of wind lifted the ribbon of white cloth which hung from the tree and it fluttered, rising and falling. Ama followed the eyes of the crippled woman. Jacinta's shoulders were trembling as if the force which had lifted the bunting, had taken possession of her too.

"Oh, Tempo,
"I see your spirit moving in your flag.
"I know that you have heard me.
"Move us, as you, too, move.
"Take us with you on your road.
"Intercede for us with Nzambi Mpungu,
"Lord of all Creation.
"Heal the shattered edges of our souls; restore our injured bodies;
"Make our spirits round as the sun is round.
"Help us to stand tall and straight and whole as this tree which guards your spirit."

She rose and signing to Ama to follow with the bowl, went to one corner of the clearing. With the stump of her right arm she drew a circle in the soft topsoil, and divided it into four quadrants. In each she drew a different symbol. Ama took a handful of the white powder and dribbled it into the shallow grooves. Jacinta stepped back, then dropped to her knees again and bowed before the symbol.

"Oh, Tempo
"With this sacred white clay,
"I make the sign of the dawn
"And the seal of your world."

Then they repeated the performance three more times, defining the corners of the clearing. Josef stepped forward and dribbled blood on Tempo's altar.

Gregório, he who had run away from the *engenho* and been recaptured, spoke for the Ewe, neighbours of the Akan and the Yoruba, known in Bahia as Gêge. Gregório had fought for the Anlo in a war against the Ge. He had been captured and sold. Now, too late, he brooded on the futility of Ewe fighting Ewe, African fighting African. Only the white men benefited from those wars.

Josef spoke for the Akan, the Fanti of the coast and the Asante of the hinterland, known in Bahia as Minas. He poured libation with rum, invoking the spirits of the ancestors. Then three times he lifted the bowl from the tree of god and placed it on Ama's head.

Ignacio Gomes, the leather worker, a free man, half Tupi, half Kongo, was next.

Ignacio was a man of few words. To both the slaves and their masters he was an enigma.

The Senhor recognised and valued his consummate skill as a craftsman. He feared that a misplaced word might drive the man from his employment; and so he ordered Vasconcellos and his white and mulatto minions to treat Ignacio with the greatest circumspection.

The slaves found it difficult to understand why he stayed on at the *engenho*, poorly paid and poorly housed as he was. After all he was a free man. He could leave at any time. In Salvador, with his skills, he would surely prosper as an independent artisan.

The answer to the riddle lay in the roots which bound Ignacio to the soil. His father's ancestors had worshipped at a forest shrine at the very site where the Christian chapel now stood. Through him flowed the ancient spirits of this land, the *caboclos*; and in him they merged with the spirits which his mother had brought from Africa. He was the curator, the custodian, of these lands.

Portuguese rule, he knew, was no more than a brief episode. In time the ancient spirits of the place would reassert their power and swallow up the white man and his religion.

Ignacio wore only a loin cloth. He had painted patterns on his body with the dark blue dye of the *jenipapo* fruit. He spoke quietly. Though the drums were silent, the others had to strain their ears to hear him.

"Great Tupi gods,

"spirits of the forest,

"spirits of Ai the sloth and Tatu the armadillo;

"of Capibara the water hog and Tamandua the anteater of the night;

"of spotted Paca;

"of Macahuba the macaw, Seriema the crane and Tucano the toucan.

"Great Tupi gods,

"Welcome the gods of Africa who have come to live amongst us;

"Welcome Oxóssi, armed with his bow and arrow, protector of the hunter;

"Welcome Tempo the tempest, the storm which plants its seed in woman.

"Tustáo and Flecha Negro, Pai Joaquin and Mãe Maria.

"ancient *caboclos*,

"in your honour we dress the neck of this pot in feathers.

"Free of our bodies.

"Lend us the power of birds to soar above the earth.

"Make us invincible.

"Return our land to us."

He made obeisance before the tree and withdrew quietly.

Now it was Ama's turn. She had been considering nervously what contribution she might make. Back home it was the Owner of the Earth who poured to the earth and the oldest man, the senior elder, who held the people, held the earth. Their prayers were always concerned with the fertility of the soil, good rains, freedom from destructive winds; the fertility of women; or the success of the hunt. She would certainly not pray for the success of the sugar harvest and it seemed trivial, after the powerful invocations she had heard, to petition the ancestors for blessings on their tiny allotments. As to praying for the fertility of women, it would be nonsensical: they would only be making more slaves for the Senhor. Moreover, the animals which were the totems of the clans, leopard, crocodile, cobra, hyena, did not live in this country. She could speak to Itsho, but her relationship with his spirit was too private, too personal, too intense to display amongst these strangers.

Olukoya looked at her. She shook her head. He nodded. It seemed that he understood.

*****

When they returned to the other clearing the pots were already simmering.

The sheep was gutted, skinned and butchered. Luis dos Santos the wag, who was here too, praised the Senhor for what he called his "gifts." While the food was cooking, the men busied themselves with weeding the clearings.

"Josef, Ama, please come," Bernardo called. "Bring a bowl of *garapa*."

He led them some way into the bush. He put down the axe he was carrying and indicated a tree.

"What do you think?" he asked. "This part at the bottom I will hollow out for a great war drum. From the part above I will be able to make five or six *atabaques* or *batas*."

They approved his choice.

"Be my witnesses," he told them.

He raised the bowl.

"Hear my voice, spirit of this noble tree. I bring you this drink. I water your roots."

He poured some liquor from the bowl.

"I beg your forgiveness for destroying your abode. Enter, I beg you, into the drums which I will carve from the wood of your tree. Teach the hands of the drummer. Let no harm come from anything I do today."

He put the bowl down and slowly lifted the axe. Josef and Ama retired to a safe distance to watch.

*****

Olukoya led the procession. The drummers beat out a quiet slow rhythm with their hands.

At the entrance to the shrine they halted. Olukoya genuflected briefly. Then he went forward and laid a plate of chicken stew before the altar. Speaking Portuguese, he invoked the spirit of Eshu and gave notice of his offering. One by one the others followed. Each man removed the cloth from his shoulder and wrapped it round his waist; the women removed their head-ties. Each bore a gift; for Obatala a plate of white rice or the fermented corn called eko, wrapped in plantain leaves; for Oshun, chicken and honey; for Yemoja, wild orchids; for Tempo, a pair of cow horns; and fresh greens and coconut for the other gods. Shango's plate, with a hot red peppered mutton stew, was made of wood, for his spirit is too hot for fragile pottery.

Instead of food some laid personal gifts which they had brought: a precious cowrie, smuggled from Africa; a ball of soap; for Oshun the treasured feather of a parrot, a brass trinket or smooth stones from the bed of the tumbling stream which ran behind the clearing.

Finally, when all had delivered their offerings, Olukoya stepped forward again.

"Eshu,

"great god of vengeance, intercessor for mankind,
"we come again in peace, to greet you.
"We cool your brows with this fresh water from the river."

"Great gods of Africa and Brazil, and all our ancestors," he called, "we greet you again. May your spirits descend upon us."

He gave a signal and in an sudden explosion of violent rhythm three drummers struck the taut skin of their drums with short *baquetas*, making them speak now with a voice so loud that it would heard back at the *engenho*; *agogo* was beaten with its iron rod; *xaque-xaque* and *chocalho* shook; and in the background the sweet tones of the *marimba* rose and fell. At this signal, the worshippers began to dance. Counter-clockwise they shuffled round before the spirit-laden fig tree, rotating their hips, slapping thighs and chest, circling, snapping fingers in a miscellany of dancing styles.

Olukoya led a dance in honour of each Yoruba *orisha* in turn. As always, the virile Eshu, keeper of the gate, was first. The rhythm was new to Ama. She was shy at first, watching the movements of the others for a clue. Some mimicked Olukoya, learning; others, immersing themselves in the spirit of the drums, improvised, some gracefully, some with furious gyrations and stamping. For was there one of them who had not learned to dance, strapped to his mother's back, before he could walk? This was the first time Ama had danced since landing on the soil of Bahia. She relaxed and lost herself in the music. Beneath the soles of her feet she felt the crushed dry leaves of the forest floor.

Obatala was next. Olukoya put on a brilliant white cloth to honour the god of spotless repute. Obatala's dance was gentle and graceful. As he danced, Olukoya sang a poem of praise to the transparent honesty of the incorruptible judge and prayed for the perfect peace and tranquillity which only this paragon of gods can grant. He called Jacinta into the circle to dance with him for Obatala is the protector of the handicapped. And he made her laugh; he made them all laugh with joy.

Shango's dance, by contrast, was violent in the extreme. Olukoya swung Bernardo's axes in wild arcs which threatened the lives and limbs of the circle of dancers, who fled in terror. In the dance he seemed to take on the god's identity, to become Lord Shango himself, Shango the dangerous, Shango the leopard who leaps down to earth like a bolt of lightning. (The drummers made a drum speak in the voice of a leopard.) Shango, father of twins. Shango, who rewards moral courage in the face of great danger and temptation. Olukoya's eyes bulged. Shango, who sends thunder from a cloudless sky. (The drums thundered.) Shango, who made the first bata drums, and taught them to play with the flash and roar of the squall which turns into a tempest. Shango who breathes out fire and smoke, the flash of whose lightning is like a sharp knife drawn across the eye of the liar; Shango, whose fire consumes those who dare to transgress custom and morality. Shango who throws us his thunder stones from heaven. Shango: fire and water in the heavens. Shango on his horse Erinla.

Olukoya was exhausted. He went and lay down on the cool earth. His wife, Ayodele, danced for Shango's wife Oshun, beautiful goddess of sweet water and love, a gentle, graceful dance. She mimed the stalking female leopard, she danced the dance of Oshun the coquette and epicure, carrying the narrow-necked pot with smooth river stones and cool river water in it, like the water from the river at Oshogbo which bears her name. She danced with a flash of fire in her eyes. She was transformed into the river Oshun. She mimed sexual ecstasy in a way that made it chaste and pure.

Olukoya joined her. Together they placed two horns upon the altar in tribute to Oya, wife of Ogun and mother of Shango's twins. Then they danced. The swirling river Niger, Oya's home, was in their dance; the whirlwind; the zigzag of lightning; sudden conflagration; night; and sudden death, for Oya is mistress of the shades, mother of the faceless, of the masked Egungun.

Olukoya struck the horns together.

"Oya, I summon your presence," he sang. "Destroyer of worlds. You alone amongst the gods can still the charging buffalo, seizing its horns and conquering its fierce anger. Mother of nine children, mother of nine colours. Oya spare us. Oya guide us. Oya protect us."

Ayodele joined him again. Separately and intertwined, they danced for Oshumare, an undulating, flowing dance, sinuous, spiralling, looping, serpentine, ambiguous, at once both male and female.

Olukoya danced alone for Ogun, supergod amongst the gods, immune to swords, immune to bullets. He placed two knives upon the altar and Ayodele poured oil on them to invoke the spirit of the god. Ogun, master of iron and steel, red-handed, fierce and unshrinking, Ogun, god of war, who fears only defeat.

This was a dance full of savage energy, extravagant flourishes, terrifying war cries. Ama thought she saw Olukoya miming a struggle for freedom, a war against their masters.

"Ogun, sustain us in the battles to come," he called out as if to confirm her instinct.

"Ogun, sustain us in the battles to come," the others chorused.

When he had finished dancing for Ogun, Olukoya sank to his knees before the altar. Then he stretched out, face down, upon the ground, arms extended. The drums were silent. No one spoke. The only sounds were those of the water on the stones and the wind rustling the branches of the trees. After an immeasurable time he rose and washed his hands and face. Then he called those who danced with him closer and in a low voice, explained.

"I was praying to the most dangerous of all *orishas*," he told them, "he whose name must not be spoken aloud. I was captured and sent into slavery before I was able to master the secret of his dance. I know only that a single wrong step can arouse his anger and bring his wrath down upon the whole community."

He jabbed his face repeatedly with his index finger, miming the dreaded smallpox.

"You understand? So I prayed only for forgiveness for not honouring him this day, because of my own ignorance."

"And now I have one last duty to be done for which I need your help. Please take a bowl or calabash each, empty it onto the ground and follow me. We are not going far."

He led them into the knee deep river. Its bed was full of rounded stones, which the current lifted slightly and then put down again. The sun penetrated the forest canopy here, sparkled on the surface, and lit up the stones in the bed with a rippling light.

"We have come to honour Yemoja, who lives in the Ogun river but also in all living waters. If you stand quite still, you will hear her speaking to you."

It was difficult to keep one's balance: the bed was loose and irregular and the current swift. Ama almost fell. Then there was a splash behind her and a scream. One of the other women had fallen into the water. Those by her pulled her to her feet. Her cloth was dripping.

"Yemoja has selected her favourite daughter from amongst us," Olukoya told them when the laughing stopped.

"Now bend and pick a stone or two and put it in your vessel. Be careful now. We want no more accidents. Then fill your vessel with water and go and put it under the roots of the fig tree."

*****

While the drummers and the dancers rested and refreshed themselves with mate, Ama, after asking permission, took up a drum.

At home this was not woman's work, but here things were different. She experimented. First something Itsho used to play for her. Then she tried her hand at *adowa,* which Esi had taught her to dance in Kumase. The drummers listened, at first amused by the thought of a woman invading their territory, then intrigued by a rhythm they had not heard before. Tentatively, quietly, they fell in with her beat. Ama was excited. She knew the music in her head. Now, without any training, she found that she could make the drum speak. After a fashion. Imperfectly. But well enough for someone to dance to.

The dancers were drifting back. The third drummer came to reclaim his drum. He, too, took up the rhythm.

"Show us," he commanded with a nod of his head.

Ama hesitated. The man had a strip of cloth wound around his forehead to keep the sweat from running into his eyes.

"May I?" she asked him.

Then, alone in the centre of the ring of watchers, she danced *adowa,* slightly bent at the waist, the cloth stretched taut to keep her hands a palm's width apart, one hand above and then below the other, the movements of her feet controlled, deliberate, turning her head this way and that, looking first upwards and then down at her feet, stooping, bending at the knee, circling, straightening up, lost in the flowing beat. Then others came to join her, mimicking the elegance and refinement of her movements, as if to make fun of her, but learning. When the drummers stopped at last, the dancers clapped their hands for Ama and she, in turn, applauded them and then the drummers, too.

Jacinta danced for Tempo in the centre of the circle. She started slowly but then a change seemed to come over her. Ama noticed her open stare: she saw nothing around her. Her eyes were blank, unfocussed, looking inwards. She seemed to be overtaken by some sort of ecstasy, beyond herself. The spirit of Tempo possessed her and she began to chant in a language none understood and none heard her speak on ordinary days. It seemed that she was Tempo's vehicle, that he spoke through her. She seemed to have become Tempo. She was Tempo.

Ama wondered whether she was mad. She had seen a similar performance several times in Kumase. The *akomfo* in their grass skirts and whitened faces also spoke in tongues. An assistant would translate for the benefit of those who did not understand the language of the spirit world.

Behind her hand Esi had laughed.

"Charlatans. Crooks. Confidence tricksters," she had said. "They take your gold. If you pay them enough they will say anything you ask of them. But beware, if you persuade them to say something that offends the Asantehene, or his interests, and he comes to hear of it, he will deal with the offending *okomfo* summarily. Do you understand?"

Esi had drawn a finger across her throat.

Jacinta's nose began to bleed. First a trickle. She paid no attention. Olukoya signalled to the drummers and they slowed their tempo. Now her nose was bleeding badly. She seemed unaware. The drumming stopped. Jacinta sank to the ground. Her eyes opened. Ama rushed to her with a cloth and squeezed her nostrils.

"Breathe through your mouth," she told her.

*****

Olukoya brought his bowl and came to sit by her.

"Well, sister Ama," he asked, "how did you find it?"

"I'm glad I came," she answered. "Thank you for asking me."

"I am sorry we didn't ask you earlier. We have to be careful, though. I think you understand that?"

Lost in her own thoughts, she ignored his question.

"I feel free," she said. "It was as if I was carrying some great burden, like a hunchback's hump upon my back. Now, suddenly, it's gone."

He smiled.

"That's what this is all about."

"One day," he continued, "this country will be ours. Orunmila tells me so and my own intelligence confirms it. We are many; they are few. In the course of time our numbers will tell. In the meantime, we must prepare. We must get to know one another, to build up trust amongst us. We must learn whatever there is to learn from the whites. I mean useful things, like reading and writing, making sugar, building ships. We must make plans. But above all, we must preserve ourselves, our own beliefs and customs. We must restore our self respect. If we begin to believe that Africans are natural slaves, the first battle will be lost and we might never recover. Do you understand what I am saying? What we do here is part of all this.

"Our brothers and sisters in Salvador are the key. Salvador is like the hub of one of Bernardo's cart wheels. Every *engenho* has links with the city. Those links are kept alive by the carters and the boatmen, by brothers like Josef. Here in the Recôncavo we have the numbers, but it is difficult for us to organise ourselves. It is the slaves in Salvador that must mobilise our Crioulo and mulatto brothers. It is they that must do the planning and give us the leadership. When they are ready and give the signal, every *engenho* in the Recôncavo will rise up. And when that happens, the country will be ours, just as Palmares was ours.

"Our greatest enemy is not the whites. It is our own disunity. They know that, of course, and they encourage it. Their Christian religion is one the weapons they use to divide us. That, by the way, was why I was disturbed when you told me the book you were reading was their Bible."

"Bra Olukoya," Ama interrupted, "I told you I am not a Christian. If I were to tell you the story of how I came to be here you would know that I will never become a Christian. But the Bible is a wonderful book all the same. It is full of marvellous stories. And it is the only book I have."

"I do not doubt your word," he replied. "You must tell us some of these stories.

Perhaps we can learn something useful from them. What I hate about the Christians is their arrogance. They tell us that we are pagans, that we worship many gods. They tell us that there is only one god, the one they worship; but they are hypocrites. They themselves have many gods. They worship Jesus and Mary and they have hundreds of saints whom they worship too. How does that differ from us, I ask you? We also have one supreme god, Olodumare. We worship him through the many *orishas* who are all his children."

They were silent for a while.

"Bra Olukoya," she said hesitantly, "there is one thing that worries me."

"What is that my sister?"

"I felt the power of your gods today and of Tempo too. Our gods are not so strong. We ask them to bring us rain, good hunting and fishing and to preserve us from the winds that destroy our crops. And even in those small things they often fail. It is hardly surprising that they could not save us from being captured and sold into slavery. But you yourself, you were serving the gods. How is it that they could allow you to be captured by your enemies?"

"Sister Ama," he laughed, "at home if you had asked such a question you might have had your head cut off. I must admit that it has troubled me too, though I have never spoken to anyone else about it before. All I can say is that I do not know the answer. The ways of the gods are inscrutable. Sometimes they come to our aid; sometimes it as if they have not heard us or even. . . ."

"What?"

"Nothing," he replied, "just an idle unworthy thought which came unbidden into my head. Slavery does strange things to us, you know. I am not immune."

They were silent again.

"Bra Olukoya, you mentioned Palmares. I have heard the name before. Bra Josef mentioned it when I first came here. He said that once I knew Portuguese I would hear the story."

"Good idea," Olukoya replied. "We are all packed and ready to leave, but we mustn't go too early or we might be seen arriving. We can fill the time telling of Palmares. Like the knowledge of our gods, it is something we must nurture and pass on from generation to generation. It is a story that even we, who have come from Africa only recently, can be proud of."

He rose to his feet.

"Brothers and sisters. Please gather round. Sister Ama has asked for the story of Palmares. It can never be retold too often and it will fill the time until we are ready to return to the *engenho*."

*****

"How old is Esperança, do you think?"

"Maybe eighty," someone volunteered.

"Let's say she is eighty. This is a story of long ago. It started a hundred years before Esperança was born; and when it ended she was still not yet born."

"It has not ended," said Olukoya.

"My brother, you are right. It lives on in our memories. It is part of our present and of our future. One day we will honour the Palmarinos in public, not furtively, as we have to do today."

"The story, the story!"

"All right, all right. The story! Let me begin at the beginning. Even the very first slaves whom the Portuguese brought to these shores from Africa ran away into the bush. They ran away even before they had learned the Portuguese language. . . ."

And so he told the long story of the independent African state which flourished for a hundred years in the forests of Brazil, pausing only from time to time to wet his throat or to point a moral which the tale revealed.

"Do you know what the worst thing was that we lost when we were taken into slavery? Of course you do. It was our families. Suddenly we had no grandparents, no fathers or mothers, no uncles or aunts, no brothers or sisters, husbands or wives, no children; no one to bury us with proper ceremony when we died, to send us to join our ancestors. Now, in Palmares, they began to build new families. The slaves regained some of their humanity and their children and grandchildren became complete human beings again.

"But this was something that the whites could not accept. They did not go to all that trouble and risk to bring Africans across the ocean in order that we should be human beings, citizens, Brazilians, *senhores* even. No, they brought us here for one purpose and one purpose only: to work us to death making their accursed sugar, that useless rubbish. So they determined to crush Palmares."

He told them of the repeated attempts by the Portuguese and Dutch to conquer the twenty thousand Palmarinos and their king, the Ganga-zumba. He told them how the last Ganga-zumba negotiated secretly with the enemy and how his treachery was discovered and punished. He told them how the war continued under the leadership of their military commander, the Zumbi.

When he came to the end he said, "I have finished my story for today, but the story is not yet finished."

"You have spoken well, my brother," said Olukoya. "The struggle goes on even today. Soon after I was landed in Salvador, I heard about the heroic defence of the *quilombo* of Carlota in Matta Grosso and two years later news reached us that there was a war in progress in which an army of slaves had joined with our Tupi brothers to conquer a vast area in the state of San Jose de Maranhão."

"Bra Olukoya. . . ." asked Ama.

"My sister?"

"Why do we of the Engenho de Cima not plan and just slip away one dark night and find a place to set up a quilombo of our own? Even here?"

"That's a question I have often asked myself, my sister, ever since I first heard the Palmares story. I think the answer must be that times have changed. Over the years the Portuguese have destroyed more and more of the forest to open up land for sugar and tobacco. If you go to the top of next hill and then climb a tree, you can look out over a plain where there are only patches of forest with vast open spaces in between. Grassland that is good for cattle, but bad for quilombos. With their superior arms the militias would find us and wipe us out in days. There is no way we could hold out like the Palmarinos did. They are even growing sugar now on Palmares land.

"No, if we want our freedom, if want to destroy slavery in this country, we will have to be more ambitious. We will all have to rise up together, those in Salvador and those of us in the Recôncavo. When the time comes, the smoke from the burning cane fields will be our signal. It will not be long now, but we still have much to do."

CHAPTER 33

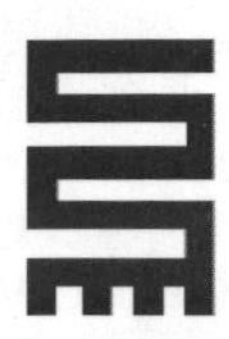

Josef returned from Salvador late one night.

He brought the mail to the kitchen the next morning and Ama took it out to the Senhor with his breakfast tray.

"Girl, what-is-your-name? Go and call Father Isaac and tell him that I want to speak to him," he told her when he had read the first letter. "Father Isaac, the priest. Do you understand?"

Ama said she understood.

"Sit down, Father," the Senhor said when the priest came. "Girl, pour the Father a cup of coffee."

"Father, do you know any English?"

"English? No, Senhor. Latin, yes. A little Spanish, but no English. If I may ask, Senhor, why?"

"Look at this. The English consul in Salvador wants to do me the honour of being my guest. The Governor has authorised the visit. There is no way I can refuse. Please draft a reply for me to sign. Tell them that he will be welcome but that there is no one here who understands the man's language. If he does not speak Portuguese he will have to bring an interpreter with him."

Please Senhor, Ama imagined herself saying, *there is no need. I know English well. I could act as the Consul's interpreter if you would permit me to do so.*

"What does it say? When will he be arriving?" the Senhor asked.

The English consul had come aboard *The Love of Liberty*. Ama tried to recall his face.

"Next Friday, subject to your agreement," Father Isaac replied.

"Make a list. We'll invite all our neighbours to a banquet on Saturday night. And their wives too. They can sleep over and attend Mass on Sunday. You would like that, wouldn't you?"

He rubbed his hands together.

"We'll show this Englishman the meaning of Brazilian hospitality."

*****

There was a great hustle and bustle in the *casa grande* of the Engenho de Cima.

Additional slaves were brought in to help with the preparations. The seamstresses worked long hours repairing the uniforms of those who would wait at table. The best plate and silver was washed and polished. Linen was aired and ironed. Bernardo made new beds. The excitement was felt even in the mill and in the cane fields. It was almost as if the expected visitor were Jesus Christ Himself, or at least the Governor of all Brazil.

Ama was kept busy in the kitchen. She hadn't seen so much food since Kumase. Wono was there too. And Josef would be serving at table.

The Senhora was flustered.

"We are short of one server," she said. "Ama, do you think you could manage?"

"Of course, Senhora. At least I shall do my best."

"I hope the guests won't be frightened by your bad eye; but there is no one else. Go to the seamstresses and get yourself fitted."

Wono took Ama's hands and they did a little dance together.

Ama was in the sewing room, trying on her new dress, when the English consul arrived. It was the fanciest garment she had worn since Mijn Heer's death.

*****

The dining room was ablaze with the light of a hundred candles and oil lamps.

On the brilliant white table cloth the silver and plate and glassware glittered and gleamed. Around the walls stood sixteen bare footed slaves, the men in smart livery and the women in full petticoats. Two Crioulos played fiddle and guitar.

The Senhor led in the beautiful young wife of a neighbouring senhor de engenho. She wore a dress of green damask and silk which took Ama's breath away. Slaves stepped forward to pull their chairs.

Ama turned to look at the next couple and suddenly felt faint. The Senhora was clutching the arm of none other than William Williams, the nephew of the captain of *The Love of Liberty*.

Can it really be him? she wondered. He was deep in conversation with the Senhora, Portuguese conversation. Ignoring the slave whose duty it was, he pulled back the Senhora's chair at the lower end of the table. Then Williams took his own seat, facing Ama, next to the beauty in green who sat in the place of honour beside the Senhor.

The Senhor's daughter Miranda came in last, on the arm of Father Isaac. She was wearing a modest white organdie dress which Ama had helped to make. The priest led her to her seat at her father's left, where he could keep a watchful eye on her. This was the first time Miranda had been permitted to attend an adult function. She smiled nervously as Ama drew her chair for her.

Father Isaac rose and said grace. When the guests had added their amens, the slaves stepped forward to serve them, one slave for each guest. The first course was a selection of local delicacies, spicy green *pamonha*, corn paste with coconut milk cooked in strips of banana leaves and *efo*, a pungent shrimp dish.

Ama poured red Portuguese wine into Miranda's glass. As she did so, Williams noticed her. He was struck first by her missing eye. Then he took another look and at once he knew her. He sat back in his chair and stared. Ama put down the bottle and retired to her position behind her young mistress. She raised her head proudly, returning his stare, but giving no indication that she recognised him as anything other than just another visiting white man.

"Just a sip, now," the Senhor admonished his daughter.

"Senhor Williams, this is my daughter, the apple of my eye."

Williams forced himself to pay attention to his host.

"Of course, Senhor, the good Father introduced us just a few moments ago.

Senhorita Miranda, if I am not mistaken? A young woman, if you will permit me to say so, Senhor, of remarkable beauty."

Miranda blushed and the Senhor smiled indulgently.

A silent signal sent Ama to the kitchen. When she returned with a tureen of steaming turtle soup Williams was deep in conversation with his host.

"Senhor," he asked, "how long has this *engenho* been in your family?"

"Twenty-five years," replied the old man. "It used to belong to the Jesuits. When they were sent packing from Brazil, the government sold it by auction. Mine was the best offer. Fortunately the great families decided not to bid."

"The great families?"

"Rocha Pitta, stand up if you please," the Senhor called to the husband of the beauty who sat beside him. "Our guest wants to know who our great families are."

Amidst laughter, Senhor Rocha Pitta stood up and bowed to left and right.

From his seat Williams returned Rocha Pitta's bow.

"Our great families, the Rocha Pittas amongst them, own the best estates and the largest, mainly on the shores of the bay."

One course followed another: first fish from the bay grilled over charcoal; next, *caruru*, a richly seasoned stew of seafood, okra and amaranths in palm oil; then *frango ao molho pardo*, chicken cooked in blood.

Ama wondered at the amount they were able to consume.

Two slaves brought in a spit-roast suckling pig on a great platter. There was general applause from the guests. The slaves carried it round the table for all to see and then took it aside to carve it.

The food these sixteen are eating in one sitting, even the left-overs on their plates, would last us all a week, Ama thought.

In between her trips to the kitchen, she caught snatches of conversation. The Senhor was flattered by Williams' questions and held forth at great length on the problems of the sugar trade; on the extortion practised by priests of the Santa Casa da Misericórdia, which, in the absence of a banking system was the only source of capital in Bahia; and on the corruption of government officials in Salvador. From time to time he called on Rocha Pitta or Father Isaac for support.

"Every one loveth gifts, and followeth after rewards," contributed the young priest who was beginning to show the effects of the wine.

Williams shook his head in sympathy and pencilled a note in the small book he kept by his side.

Miranda, Ama saw, was excruciatingly embarrassed by her father's harangue.

The Senhor paused to do justice to his *xim-xim.*

"This fowl is delicious," said Williams. "Senhora, please accept my compliments on your magnificent cuisine."

The Senhora blushed and bowed her head in acknowledgement. Miranda, too, blushed in sympathy with her mother's embarrassment. It struck Ama that none of the women had said a word.

*****

The men took one end of the veranda to drink their rum and smoke their cigars and pipes.

The ladies, at the other end, now talked freely over their sorbets.

In the kitchen the slaves were tucking in, but Ama had been told to stay on to serve the men.

"Senhor William," the Senhor said when they had settled, "I will hide nothing from you. When my grandfather of blessed memory arrived in this country he owned little more than a uniform and a musket. But he was a Portuguese, mind you, pure Portuguese, without the slightest taint of what we call - you will forgive me, Father Isaac - the infected races."

"The infected races, Senhor?"

"Moor, mulatto, Jew. Those are the infected races. The Marques de Pombal made a law twenty years ago. In order to preserve the purity of the race any Portuguese of pure white descent who is crazy or stupid enough to want to marry a woman of the infected races has first to obtain the consent of the King."

"I see. I heard a story in Salvador recently of a *senhor de engenho* in Inhambupe who freed one of his female Angolan slaves and married her."

"Manoel Dias Lima, the scoundrel, the madman."

He looked around to make sure that the ladies were out of earshot.

"Senhor William, there are some matters which we do not discuss before the ladies. This is one of them."

"I am sorry."

"No matter. They heard nothing. I mention it only for future notice."

"You were telling me about your grandfather."

"Soon after he came to Bahia he fought in the campaign which destroyed the notorious quilombo of Palmares. He was decorated and rewarded for his role in that war. He married my grandmother whose blood was as pure as his own. My father, of blessed memory, was born to them. By dint of his own efforts my grandfather managed to send his son to Lisbon for his education. When my father returned to Bahia, my grandfather sent him with twenty slaves to search for diamonds at Tejuco. He was fortunate. The diamonds bought my family's first *engenho* and paid for my own education in Portugal. I stayed there for four years during the reign of King João V.

"Today, after three generations, my family has reached the level of the nobility. Even the old families, like that of Rocha Pitta here, accept us. We are people of quality, what I believe you English call gentlemen."

Ama, standing by the wall, dozed.

"Girl, bring another bottle of rum," the Senhor commanded.

"Some are born into the nobility," said Father Isaac. "Others enter it through merit and the nobility of their nature."

Ama removed the cork and topped up the men's glasses.

Are you all not drunk enough already? she wondered.

"Thank you, Pamela," said Williams in English as she poured for him.

"I beg your pardon?" asked the Senhor.

"Nothing, nothing. Just an English phrase which escaped my lips."

The Senhor looked at him quizzically, then shook his head.

Josef appeared.

"Go and eat," he told Ama in Fanti. "I will take your place."

*****

The Senhor sat on his veranda. He had overslept and missed morning prayers again.

A full week had passed since the dinner party. His Brazilian guests had stayed just long enough to attend a late Mass in the little chapel.

Only the Englishman lingered on at the Engenho de Cima, riding the Senhor's fine stallions down to the cane fields; studying the processes in the mill; inspecting the *senzalas* and the allotments. And always asking questions and making copious notes in his little book.

Familiar sounds floated across from the mill. An overseer came galloping back from the cane fields. It was time for his breakfast. On the steps Alexandre whittled a piece of soft wood into the form of a horse. He was frustrated: just as he had seemed to be making some progress he had broken a fragile leg. Now he would have to start again from scratch. He peeped at the Senhor; but knew better than to attempt to talk to him at this time of the day.

Ama came out with the breakfast tray.

"Senhor," she said in a dull monotone, "I beseech your blessing in the name of our Lord and Saviour Jesus Christ."

The Senhor grunted what might have been a blessing but might just as well have been a curse. He was cool towards this new maid with the missing eye. He found it difficult to look her in the face. Vasconcellos called her "One-eye." He wondered whether "Evil-eye" might not be more appropriate. Every time she made an appearance, he was reminded, uncomfortably, of the story of the senhora who had gouged out the eyes of her husband's mulatto concubine and served them up to her victim's master for his dinner.

Apart from the unfortunate Narciza, he had never had an African as a house slave before. He preferred mulattos, or at least Crioulos. The Africans were not to be trusted; they were too proud and rebellious. He would have to ask his wife why she had brought this one into the *casa grande* as a replacement for Narciza; and why she had done so without consulting him beforehand. His authority was being undermined. Everyone seemed to be taking advantage of his advancing years.

Ama stole a sidelong glance at the Senhor as she put down the tray. He was usually in a bad temper at this time of the morning, particularly when he had drunk too much the night before. His face was unshaven. Strands of white hair lay untidily across his red pate. She wondered whether he was upset that Williams had defeated him at chess the previous day. She had noticed that Father Isaac took great pains never to beat the Senhor. Williams was the old man's guest. It was insensitive and undiplomatic of him to humiliate his host like that.

"Will there be anything more, Senhor?" she asked.

She took his grunt to mean "no" and retired to the back of the veranda, out of his sight but ready to react to his slightest gesture or command, as she had been taught. But she was tired. They had kept her up late several nights running. She let her back slide slowly down the wall until she was sitting on the stone floor. She hugged her knees to her chest and dozed.

"A very good morning to you, Senhor," she heard Williams say. "May I join you?"

Ama wondered whether she should get up to pour coffee for Williams but he was already helping himself.

"Thank you for the chess last night. I really did enjoy it."

Ama laughed inwardly at the Englishman's attempts to draw a reply out of the Senhor. She stretched forward so that she could see them.

"Senhor. There is an important matter which I should like to discuss with you. Could we talk now or would another time be more convenient?"

The Senhor adjusted his bulk in his chair and took a deep breath. No doubt more questions about the running of the *engenho*. The young man was too persistent. But then he was a guest and guests have certain rights which no *senhor de engenho* would deny.

"Speak, Senhor William. There is no time like the present."

There was an awkward pause. The Senhor turned to look at Williams. He was folding and refolding his handkerchief with meticulous care.

At last he summoned up his courage.

Looking straight ahead, he said quietly, "It is about your daughter, Senhorita Miranda."

Ama peeped out again. The Senhor was cutting himself a cigar. It was unusual for him to smoke so early in the morning.

One of the overseers trotted up on a horse.

"Later, later," the Senhor dismissed the man.

Then he saw his bastard son sitting on the steps.

"Alexandre," he said. "Shove off!"

"What about Miranda?" he asked when the boy had gone.

"It is no use beating about the bush," Williams replied. "She won my heart the moment I first set eyes on her. I want to ask your permission . . ."

He looked up. The Senhor was staring into the distance.

"Your permission . . . Senhor, I hope I haven't offended you."

"Have you spoken to her about this?"

"No, no, we have hardly exchanged half a dozen words all the time I have been your guest. And those were mere pleasantries; hardly even a conversation. Senhor, I hope I haven't stepped out of line in speaking to you as I have. I know that customs . . ."

"Senhor William, you are a Protestant."

"Oh, that would not present a problem. I could become a Catholic if that were your wish."

"You are an Englishman."

Williams had half expected this.

"And proud to be one too," he replied. "There is nothing I can do about that, I'm afraid."

"You would take my only daughter away from me."

"Not while you live, sir. Not while you or the Senhora is alive. That I promise. That I swear."

Ama's single eye was wide open and her ears too. She wanted to get away and tell someone the news, tell Miranda, tell anyone. But how could she escape without them noticing her? Williams, at least, would know that she had heard and understood. As for the Senhor, he thought that slaves' ears had no function beyond the receipt of commands.

"What are your means?"

"Well, sir, as you know, I am the Consul of His Majesty's government in Salvador. For that service I receive no more than a modest stipend. But the post gives me a status in the city which, as a foreigner, I could not otherwise hope for. Your daughter would join me in gracing His Excellency's table at least once or twice a year."

"Your means?"

"Yes, I was coming to that. You will have heard me mention my uncle of the same name, Captain Williams. He left the sea some few years ago and has established himself in a successful business as a manufacturer of cotton cloth. I act as his agent in Salvador. That brings me a satisfactory income. I have also made some successful investments in the gold mines and indeed I deal in the precious metal myself, exporting it to England."

"Means, Senhor William. You have not answered my question. Means, wealth, property. You are telling me about trade. It is not a profession we think of highly in this country. What land do you own, what buildings, what other property? I would not want to give my daughter to a man who immediately afterwards would become my dependent. Do you understand?"

"Yes sir, I think I do. At present my means are modest. I do have a moderate income but I admit that at present it depends upon my continuing labour. However, I am my uncle's only relative and I have some expectation of a very substantial inheritance in cash and property at some time in the future."

"How old is your uncle, Senhor William?"

"He must be fifty sir."

"He has no wife, no issue at all?"

"No, sir, not to my knowledge. I mean I believe he would have told me if he had married."

"You English are peculiar. A man of fifty and not yet married? Senhor William, what if he has indeed married during your absence from your country and has had children? And if he has forgotten to inform you that you are no longer a beneficiary of his will?"

"It is possible, sir, but unlikely. The old man is fond of me. I cannot imagine him treating me in that manner."

"Senhor, I will speak to my wife. I make no promises, no commitments. You should on no account discuss this matter with my daughter unless and until you have my consent to do so. Do you understand?"

"Of course."

"We will talk again presently. And tonight I will avenge my defeat on the board."

*****

When Ama reached the Senhora's quarters she found Alexandre swinging Miranda round and round at arm's length so that all the furniture was in danger of being toppled over.

Dearly beloved Miranda, his elder sister, his half sister, the apple of their father's eye.

"Senhora William, Senhora William, Senhora William. Say a mass for Saint Gonçalo for finding you a husband," he teased her.

Miranda screamed in mock fear, blissfully ignorant of what he was talking about.

"Alexandre, stop that this minute."

Ama spoke with authority. Alexandre let go of Miranda. She stumbled around drunkenly until the dizziness wore off. Then she collapsed in a heap on the floor.

"Alexandre," Ama reprimanded him, "you have been eavesdropping again."

"Eavesdropping? Me? Ama, I thought you were my friend. Why do you make false accusations which will get me into trouble? Eavesdropping on whom?"

"Why were you calling Senhorita Miranda Senhora Williams?"

"Oh that!" he replied dismissively.

"Yes, that! You were eavesdropping on the Senhor's conversation with Senhor Williams, weren't you?"

Alexandre pouted and said nothing.

"What is this all about, Ama?" Miranda asked.

"Senhorita Miranda, can you keep a secret?"

"Of course. Tell me, tell me. What is it all about?"

"If you give me away, the Senhor will send me back to the cane fields."

"I promise. Cross my heart and hope to die."

"This morning I took the Senhor's breakfast tray to him on the veranda. Then I waited in case he needed anything. I was tired and I sat down next to the cabinet. Senhor Williams came out to join your father. He asked for permission to discuss something very important with him."

"This doesn't sound very interesting. They are always talking business. Something about the *engenho*, no doubt. Why are you telling me this?"

"Young lady you are too impatient. The important matter Senhor Williams wanted to discuss with your father was you."

"Me?"

"Yes you."

"What have I done now? I have hardly spoken to the visitor."

"Can't you guess?" Alexandre chipped in.

"Alexandre be quiet," Ama scolded him. "This is serious. Now listen carefully, Senhorita, and brace yourself for a shock. Senhor Williams was asking your father for permission to court you."

"To court . . .?"

Miranda's eyes and mouth opened wide. Then she blushed deeply.

"He wants to marry you."

A tear descended from each of Miranda's eyes. Then she began to sob. Ama put her arm around her shoulder.

"Don't cry. It is nothing to cry about. He is a fine man. You should be flattered."

This only made things worse. Miranda bawled. She hugged Ama and sank her head into her breast. Ama did her best to comfort her.

The door opened and the Senhora entered.

"What's going on in here? The Senhor is complaining about the noise. He has a headache."

Then she saw her daughter crying.

"Miranda, my child, what is the matter? Why are you crying? Alexandre, have you been teasing her again?"

Miranda looked up, speechless, and shook her head. Ama moved aside. The Senhora took her daughter's hands.

"There now. Surely it can't be bad enough to make you cry like that?"

Miranda burst into tears again.

"Ama, what is it? Do you know?"

Ama was silent.

You should have kept your mouth shut you stupid slave. Now you are in real trouble, she thought.

Miranda looked up and wiped her face with her hand. Her mother helped her with a handkerchief.

"Tell her," Miranda ordered Ama.

"Senhorita, you promised."

"Tell her. I promise you on my honour that my father will not send you back to the cane fields."

"Well?" asked the Senhora, losing patience.

There is nothing for it, I shall have to tell her, Ama thought.

"Senhora, Senhor Williams, the Englishman . . ."

"Yes? What about him? Speak girl, or I'll have you given a good beating."

"He has asked the Senhor for permission to pay court to Senhorita Miranda."

CHAPTER 34

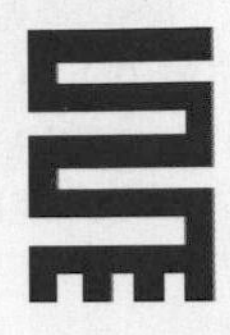

Overcoming his misgivings, the Senhor gave his consent to Williams' courtship of Miranda.

For practical reasons, he sent his wife and daughter to take up residence in the town house in Salvador. Miranda begged her father to join them, but the Senhor was wedded to the *engenho* and too lazy to make a move.

Ama had become the girl's favourite companion. Miranda wanted to take her as her personal maid. Ama was thrilled at the prospect. But the Senhor vetoed the plan. There was no way he would permit himself to be made a laughing stock in Salvador. Employing a one-eyed maid to serve his daughter! He would be the butt of malicious jokes. He had convinced himself that Williams would be a good match and had no intention of allowing the Englishman to slip through his fingers by presenting him with a scandal as a pretext for second thoughts. So Miranda gave in and Ama stayed behind.

Miranda had more success in persuading her father that Alexandre should go with them. The Senhor decided that it was time to send his mulatto son to the seminary in Salvador to prepare him to take holy orders.

Weeks passed. Josef brought regular news. Williams had been received into the Catholic Church. He dined regularly with the Senhora and her daughter. He showered Miranda with exquisite gifts. He escorted them to Mass every Sunday. He took them out driving in his coach.

It was still too early for him to make a formal proposal but the Senhora had sufficient confidence in his honourable intentions to start assembling her daughter's trousseau. Orders were sent to Lisbon.

Then the Engenho do Meio, the *fogo morto* which was the Senhor's neighbour, was sold. The new owner came to call on the Senhor. He brought in many new slaves. Fifi was made a senior driver by virtue of his local knowledge. Josef and Wono rejoiced for him and his family. They had been living in the direst poverty. Now things might be a little better.

Williams returned to the Engenho de Cima to make a formal proposal of marriage to the Senhor. He offered to forego his right to a dowry but the Senhor insisted. They compromised. The Senhor would make a generous settlement upon his daughter. A day in January was fixed for the wedding and Williams returned to Salvador. He bought a house in a quiet street in the *Cidade Alta* and his fiancée and prospective mother-in-law helped him to equip it.

The Senhor's two elder sons arrived at the Engenho de Cima, together with their wives and children, and began to make preparations for the wedding. The house was too small to accommodate all the guests who were expected. The neighbouring *senhores de engenho* would help, but tents would also be required; and a grand marquee for the reception. The sons arranged to borrow carriages and ox-carts and boats. They auditioned the slaves who could play musical instruments and sought out others in the neighbourhood. The Senhor decided to close down the mill for a month after Christmas. His sons needed the extra labour and it was not practical to keep the mill running with a skeleton staff. So a hundred slaves, men, women and children devoted all their energies for four weeks to the preparations for the festivities. There would be horse racing and cock fighting, hunting and cards to amuse the men. And eating and drinking, of course. On the night of the wedding there would be a great ball with an orchestra brought all the way from Salvador. The annual issue of clothes to the slaves was postponed until the eve of the wedding. Each male field hand would receive a pair of drawers that reached below the knee, a coarse homespun shirt and a bright head kerchief; each woman, a shift, a frock and an apron; and each child a shirt with long tails. And as a bonus, a new tin plate, a spoon and a mug.

The Senhor was beginning to receive subtle intimations of his own mortality. He was determined that no effort or expense should be spared on what might well be the last manifestation of his power and prestige.

*****

Miranda returned with her mother a week before the date set for the wedding.

Williams came with them and immediately went to stay as the guest of the new owner of the Engenho do Meio. He brought an educated black Crioulo with him as his valet. Every morning he rode over to take breakfast with the Senhor. The valet followed on foot.

This man was the subject of animated conversation amongst the slaves. He did not speak the pidgin Portuguese which was the lingua franca of both slaves and many of the whites; no, this one spoke with the accents of an educated man. Williams dressed him in the uniform of an English butler. He wore shoes, polished shoes, which was unheard of for a slave. It was rumoured that he had travelled to Portugal; someone said that he had also been to England. No, said another, he *is* English, a black Englishman, specially imported by the consul.

Only the Senhor was not impressed.

"A monkey dressed in silk is still a monkey," Ama heard him tell the priest.

As the big day approached the pace of work quickened. The glamour and excitement of it all affected the slaves, too. The Bishop arrived from Salvador, carried on a litter and surrounded by a retinue of his personal slaves. The slaves of the *engenho* lined up and watched the family and the guests kiss his ring. As each party of guests rode up the Senhor came out to welcome them formally. The yard was full of fine carriages, otherwise seldom used because of the condition of the roads. Strange horses raced up and down the paddocks. The estate was alive with strangers. They inspected the livestock and the mill. Some of them even toured the *senzalas*, poking their heads inside the cabins. The young men regarded the female slaves as fair game, squeezing breasts and pinching buttocks. Ama found her missing eye a valuable weapon. Assaulted in this way, she turned her remaining eye on the assailant with a fierce look and spat on the ground. Her victim warned his fellow rakes of her evil eye and they steered clear of her thereafter.

The unmarried sisters of these young men were kept in virtual purdah in the Senhora's quarters. Their time would come with the grand ball, an occasion to put their virtuous gifts on display for the benefit of prospective suitors.

The slaves had their own guests to accommodate and entertain, for every white family brought with it a retinue of servants.

"Maybe we can find you a husband, too, Ama," teased Wono.

*****

At ten o'clock precisely (more or less) on the big day, the bridegroom arrived.

A great cheer rose from the assembled slaves and the guests on the veranda as his carriage approached. It was drawn by four magnificent white mares and escorted by a mounted retinue of the younger male guests.

"Look," said Ama, clutching Wono's arm, "Fifi. Doesn't he look grand?"

"Who is that beside him?" Wono asked.

Fifi, dressed in a red uniform with gold braid, held the reins. Beside him, bolt upright, sat a stranger in similar attire.

"It must be one of the new slaves at Fifi's place," said Ama.

"Fifi, Fifi," cried Wono, as if it were he who was the centre of all this pomp, rather than his passenger.

Ama looked again at the new man.

"Wono," she said faintly, digging her nails into the flesh of her friend's arm.

"What?" asked Wono.

"I know him. I am sure I know him. He was on the ship with me. *The Love of Liberty.* He is my *malungo.*"

And then she fainted.

*****

When Ama came to she was lying in the shade of a tree.

Wono was kneeling by her side. They were surrounded by a crowd of anxious friends.

"Move away, move away," she heard Wono say. "Give her some air."

She opened her eye and blinked.

"What happened?" she asked.

"You fainted," Wono replied. "Are you all right now? Can you sit up? You wicked girl, you gave me a quite a start. For a moment I thought you were . . ."

"Dead? Me? Not yet, sister Wono."

"Ah, here they come," said Wono.

"Who?" asked Ama, sitting up.

"Fifi and Josef. And Fifi's friend, your *malungo.* I sent for them."

Ama felt her heart pumping. She struggled to get up but she was too weak.

"Wono, help me," she insisted.

Josef asked, "Wono, what is the matter? The lad you sent sounded anxious."

Ama said, "It is nothing, Bra Josef. We just wanted to greet Fifi in his fine new clothes."

Fifi greeted Ama in Fanti, "Sister Ama, *maakye.* How are you?" and shook hands.

When she had replied, he said, "As for these clothes, they dress us up like performing monkeys when it suits them. I would be happier in my working shirt, hot and itchy as it is. But I forget myself. I haven't introduced our new brother. João, this is Wono, Josef's wife. And this is Ama."

Wono was about to add, "Who is looking for a husband," but her friend's stern look shut her up.

Ama turned and looked Tomba straight in the eye. She would never let him forget the open-mouthed astonishment with which he recognised her. Recovering quickly, he took both her hands in his.

"Sister Ama and I," he said to his new friends in Portuguese, "have met before."

*****

Ama and Tomba saw little of the wedding celebrations.

There were so many other slaves on hand to serve the masters that it was easy for them to slip away unnoticed.

They spent the time talking. They talked from dawn to dusk and half way through the night. At first they talked at random about what had happened to them since they had last been together at the slave auction in the *Cidade Baixa*. No slave caught up in the harsh reality of life in sugar Bahia was immune from bouts of self-pity; but it was not in the nature of either to dwell upon their troubles. As they talked they grew to know one another, confirming the impressions each had formed on board ship. They shared reminiscences of their journey across the Atlantic.

Tomba reminded her how she had brought him water to drink soon after she had come on board.

"What made you do that?"

"Huh? I don't know. I didn't think. I just did it."

He took her hand.

"I never had a chance to say thank you. You cannot imagine how that simple act of courage and compassion sustained me through that voyage."

Shyly, Ama changed the subject.

She said, "We have one thing to thank our oppressors for."

"What is that?" he asked.

"They have given us a common language."

"Do you think that we have to give them credit for that?"

"Of course not. They are the masters; we are their slaves; it follows that we have to learn their language. But we arrived here speaking many different tongues. We didn't know one another. Had you ever heard of a place called Angola? Now we know that we are all Africans.

"Do you remember," she asked, "after I unlocked your chains, I tried to lead you to the boys?"

"Yes, but I knew that there were two of my own men in the sick-bay. They were stronger, in spite of their sickness. And there was another thing. I didn't want to involve the youngsters in what was, to me, an unknown and risky enterprise. As it turned out, I was right, wasn't I?"

"What I wanted to do was to get the boy Kwaku, to use as an interpreter, so that I could brief you properly on the situation up on deck."

"That makes sense. I didn't think of it. I was impatient, anxious to get on with what we had to do."

"A typical man," she smiled.

"If there is one thing that this country has taught me, apart from Portuguese, it is to force myself to allow time for thought before making important decisions. It has been hard. It is not in my nature."

"Do you remember, later, when we were standing together on the deck?"

"Of course."

"I tried to tell you that I had locked the captain in his cabin. He was drunk. My plan was that you would take him hostage before tackling the guards."

"You had locked the captain in his cabin?"

He slapped his forehead with an open palm.

"I didn't understand. If we had used the captain as a hostage we might just have succeeded in forcing the guards to leave at least one hatch cover long enough to let us unlock it. Oh, oh, oh. We were so close to success. If only I had understood and given more credit to that brilliant intelligence."

He pointed to her head.

"Can you ever forgive me? We might have won. You would still have had both your eyes. And that boy I killed, the best of the lot he was, might have survived."

"George Hatcher he was called," she mused. "He was a good lad, simple, not a scrap of malice in him."

She drew her thoughts together.

"Can I forgive you? There is nothing to forgive, bra Tomba. We were the victims of a cruel trade. We still are. We did our best to escape, but we never really had much of a chance. Even if you had gained control of the ship, what could you have done? Could you have sailed it, even with the captain and the six guards under your control? Where would you have taken us?"

"Some uninhabited stretch of the coast where we could have built a new society, where we could have lived in peace together," he replied, but without the strong conviction that his words suggested.

"A *quilombo* in Africa? Like Palmares. Have you been told the story of Palmares?"

"Yes, I know the story and of other *quilombos* too. Even today there are some that survive."

"And have they made any difference to our condition as slaves? No, my brother, that is not the way. You must talk to Olukoya. If we have a leader at this *engenho*, it is Olukoya. Olukoya will ask you, 'Is it not true that we are many and they are few?'"

"That is true."

"Then how is it that they find it so easy to control us?"

"It is because we are divided amongst ourselves. We are suspicious of one another, Akan of Angolan, Yoruba of Hausa."

"Ahaa! Yet there are some things that unite us all."

"That we are Africans; that we are black."

"More than that."

"That we are slaves, that we are treated as property to be bought and sold."

"Bra Tomba, you are a good pupil!"

"Sister Ama," he replied with a smile, "you are a good teacher. The more I listen to you the more I am astonished at the quality of your mind. It is unusual in a woman."

"You sound like a *senhor de engenho* talking about his slaves, all his slaves. Women can think as well as men if you would only give us half a chance. Anyway, you flatter me too much. It is true that these ideas were in my mind, but they were all mixed up, without proper form. It is Olukoya who has helped me to understand. Without his guidance I would still be confused."

"So what does this your Olukoya say we should do?"

Ama wondered whether she detected a note of jealousy in his voice.

"In one word, prepare."

"Prepare for what?"

"To take over this country; to make ourselves the masters. Or, rather, to do away with masters altogether."

"And how will we do that? It sounds wonderful but isn't it as farfetched as the dream of another Palmares?"

"Not if we do our work properly. Olukoya says we have two main tasks. One is to learn all the skills of the Portuguese that give them an advantage over us, particularly reading and writing, but also how to make sugar, since that is the life blood of this country."

"And the other?"

"Olukoya says he can describe it best if you picture a spider's web. The centre, where the spider sits, is Salvador. The points where the threads meet are *engenhos* like this one. The threads are messengers, men like our Josef, who travel in and out. When the web is complete, our people in Salvador will be able to reach every *engenho*, practically every slave in the country. When we are ready the messengers will spread the word and we will rise together, all at the same time. If we do that they can never defeat us."

"Hmm," said Tomba. "Exciting things are happening in this place. I must meet this Olukoya."

*****

The sound of music floated up from the *casa grande* and the smoke from cooking fires rose in the still air.

She had taken him to the rocky outcrop which was her reading place.

"Did you know that the bridegroom was on the ship with us?" she asked him.

"You are joking, surely? How?"

"His name is William Williams."

"I know that. I talked to the man he calls his valet."

"The captain of our ship was called David Williams. This man is his nephew. He used to work for a white man at Anomabu, a man called Richard Brew. Brew died, the night of that first terrible storm, if you remember. Williams senior collected his nephew. He was going to take him (and us) to a place called Barbados, but then the second storm struck us and damaged the ship. That was how we came to Bahia. Williams (the uncle) never intended it. He must have left his nephew behind here when he returned to his country. Now the nephew is an important person, the ambassador of his king in Salvador."

"When I first saw him a few days ago," Tomba replied, "I thought his face was vaguely familiar, but I put the thought aside. I find it difficult sometimes to distinguish between the faces of white men. Now that I come to think of it, he gave me a strange look when I opened the door of the carriage for him. It was the first time I had seen him at such close quarters."

He paused. There was a comfortable silence between them, as if they had known one another all their lives. From the *casa grande* there came the sound of cheering and hand clapping.

"Ama, tell me," he asked, "how do you know all these things? About the voyage, about the whites?"

"You don't know much about me, do you? Nor I about you, for that matter."

"Tell me, then," he asked her, "tell me the story of your life. From your earliest memories. Your parents. How you lived. Tell me how you became a slave. Leave nothing out. Nothing. I want to know everything about you."

"We will be here all night," she warned him.

"Never mind," he said.

He looked at her and she thought for a moment that he was going take her, but the moment passed and he lay back on the flat rock and closed his eyes.

"Well?" he asked, opening his eyes for a moment. "I am waiting."

*****

She told him all.

She told him about her happy childhood, when her name was still Nandzi; about her love for her mother Tabitsha; about Satila's extended courtship of the little girl that she then was; she told him about Nowu.

When it was time to tell him about Itsho, she hesitated and he noticed.

"Some things are difficult to speak of," he said. "I had no right to ask you. Tell me what you will. If there is anything you find too painful, pass over it. There will always be another time."

She closed her one eye and tried to summon up Itsho's spirit. To her surprise she saw his face before her almost at once. He was smiling. He moved his lips. No sounds came out but she knew what he was telling her.

"You have been faithful to me," she heard him say. "All these difficult years you have been faithful to me. Even when you lived with Mijn Heer, you were faithful to me. There was never a time when you didn't turn to me when you needed me. I shall watch over you until the end of your days on earth. This man Tomba loves you. Tell him everything."

"I am sorry," she told Tomba and wiped away a tear.

Then she told him about Itsho; about their long talks and their expeditions together; she told him about their love for one another; and about her fear of losing him when it was time for her to go to Satila.

She told him about that long ago morning when she had been left alone to look after Nowu.

"I saw a puff of dust on the horizon," she told him. "I looked at it but paid no attention. My thoughts were elsewhere. If I had not been daydreaming, I would have had time to take Nowu and run and hide. They would never have found me."

"And you would not be here today and I would never have met you."

She smiled at him and took his hand. He leaned forward and kissed her on the lips. She held him for a moment and then she pulled away.

"Not now," she said. "There will be plenty of time."

It was a strange experience. She had never told her own story before. She recalled the first day of the march from Kafaba to Kumase, when she had composed a dirge for herself and her fellow slaves, straight out of her head. That day she had felt as if her spirit had left her body, as if it were floating above her, watching her. Telling her own history now was much the same. It was as if she was telling a story about a stranger, a different person, someone else.

She told him about the rape. It was a long time since she had thought about that day, but as she told the story it all came back to her: the agonising pain in her womb and the humiliation, the degradation of it all. Tomba took her hand and held it in both of his, shaking his head at the terror of it.

"And then?" he pressed her.

She told him about the ride, loaded on Damba's pack horse like a bundle of stolen goods; about the encounter with Itsho; about the failed rescue attempt. She told him about her discovery of Itsho's mutilated body and about how Suba and Damba had helped her to bury him that day.

She told him about Yendi, about Kafaba and Kumase; about the Ya Na and Koranten Péte: and about Akwasi Anoma the drunken bird man who had also raped her. She told him about Minjendo and Esi who were her friends. She told him about the elephants they had met on the way down the Daka river and about her first encounter with the forest on the road to Kumase. She told him about musketeer Mensa and about the magnificence of Kumase and the Asante royals; about the death of Osei Kwadwo and about the coup d'etat which led to the enstoolment of Osei Kwame.

She told him everything but when it came to telling him about her part in the young king's passage to manhood, she was too shy and so she said, "My throat is dry from all this talking and you must be getting bored. It will be dark soon. I think it's time we went back down or Wono will be worried. I'll continue tomorrow if you like."

*****

The wedding of Tomba and Ama was celebrated in a more modest fashion than Williams' and Miranda's.

Tomba ran from the Engenho do Meio to the Engenho de Cima after work on Saturday night just as he did several times a week. Ama had a basin of hot water ready for him to take his bath.

Josef took the part of Ama's father and Olukoya spoke for Tomba. Josef poured libation, speaking to Ama's ancestors, first in their own language, of which, at his own insistence, Ama had taught him a few words, and then in Fanti. Olukoya did the same, speaking in Portuguese so that all could understand. Josef called on the ancestors to bless the union of their daughter with the man she had chosen to be the father of her children. Olukoya had a more difficult task. He and Tomba had become close friends. Tomba had told him about his unusual childhood and about his ignorance as to who his forebears were. He had been brought up without any system of belief and religion played no part in his life. He had no family, except perhaps Ibrahima, and therefore no ancestors. So Olukoya addressed his words to the ancestors of all the African slaves. He spoke of Tomba's struggle against the slave trade in his part of Africa and of his attempt, with Ama, to take control of *The Love of Liberty*. He spoke of his courage and he called on the ancestors to watch over him and his new family, not as a man of this or that nation, but as an African.

They passed the bowl of garapa round and each of the guests drank from it. Then the older women and those who had feigned illness so that they could spend the day cooking, brought in the wedding meal, which they had improvised from bush meat, trapped in the forest, a stolen sheep and the produce of the allotments.

Drums were beaten and there was singing and dancing around the fire.

Benedito came to them after Mass the following day and advised them both, for the sake of their eternal souls, to beg the priest to marry them in church. They promised to consider his advice. Ama asked the Senhora, who had returned to the Engenho de Cima after Miranda's marriage, to speak to the Senhor on her behalf but her mistress thought it better that Ama make her request to the Senhor in person.

The Senhor was playing chess with Father Isaac on the veranda.

"Senhor, Father, I beg permission to make a request," she told them.

"What is it?" grunted the Senhor.

"I want to get married, Senhor."

"Who is the man?" asked the priest.

"His name is João, Senhor."

"I have no slave of that name."

"He belongs to the Engenho do Meio, Senhor."

"Out of the question," replied the Senhor. "Find yourself a man in this *engenho*."

He turned to the priest.

"I won't have my slaves marrying outsiders, Father," he said. "It only causes trouble."

"Senhor, I beg you. Would the Senhor not consider buying João from the *senhor* at the Engenho do Meio; or selling me to the *senhor* there?"

"I will think about it. Now clear these things away."

"I don't mind what the church says," she heard him say as she went through the door, "marriage is not a proper institution for slaves."

Unseen, she paused to hear the rest.

"When they get tired of their spouses, they have a tendency to poison them. Then the poor owner loses a slave through no fault of his own. What do you think, Father?"

"That is certainly a risk, Senhor. I have heard of such cases. The Church, need I say it, is in favour of marriage in principle. In practice the problem is that Africans are so lascivious that once they are married they regularly practice adultery; and that is an affront to the Church."

*****

Though his riding days had long since passed the Senhor could still get excited over the birth of a new foal.

He would raise himself from his rocking chair and waddle ponderously over to the paddock to caress the favourite mare which had so rewarded his loving care and attention. It was much the same with calves and lambs.

When it came to new *peqeniños*, as the Portuguese called black infants, he was less than enthusiastic. For one thing, there was the inevitable decline in the mother's productivity during and after pregnancy. For another, there was the risk of the loss of an asset through the mother's death in labour. And then if a child was born there was the cost of ten years' food and clothing before the new worker could begin to do the simplest useful tasks. In the Senhor's experience, moreover, there was a high probability that the child would not survive to that age. That would mean even more money down the drain. Taking everything into account it made economic sense to extract the maximum labour during the ten years, on average, of a slave's useful working life and then to purchase a replacement, rather than to attempt to breed slaves as he bred livestock.

"A few survive some years beyond their productive period," he had told Williams. "We may not kill them off, of course. We just have to grin and bear the cost of maintaining those survivors: it is just one of the unfortunate circumstances of our sugar economy. Wherever possible we allocate light tasks to the maimed or ill or prematurely aged. That helps to cover at least part of the cost of their upkeep."

Fortunately for the Senhor his economic philosophy regarding *peqeniños* was supported by what appeared to be natural law. The fertility of the slave women was low. The reasons were not far to find, had the Senhor only chosen to look: poor food; long hours of exhausting work; the widespread incidence of venereal and other diseases; and the absence of any form of medical treatment beyond that which the other slave women could provide.

Many of the slave women, moreover, were themselves reluctant to have children. Despair led some to induce abortion as soon as they became pregnant; the others often miscarried anyway; some of those who went to term abandoned their new born babies in the cane fields or in the surrounding bush, leaving them to die in infancy rather than live their lives in bondage. Many of those infants who survived the first hours of life succumbed to what the Brazilians called the seven day illness, which resulted from the unhygienic conditions in which the umbilical cord was cut. Then there were the hazards of measles, whooping cough and diphtheria which forest herbs might or might not cure. Even a child who reached adolescence might be sold by a *senhor de engenho* temporarily strapped for cash. *Why go through all the pain and suffering and heartache?* the women reasoned.

This story was repeated all over sugar Bahia. The *senhores de engenho* argued, *Why go to the trouble and expense of rearing your own stock, when Africa is so much more efficient and economical a slave farm?*

Conditions for the female slaves in the *casa grande* were marginally better than for those in the cane fields and the mill. For one thing the work was not as hard and the diet, supplemented by left overs from the Senhor's table and stolen food, was more nutritious. It is true that the hours were long but on the other hand there was often a chance to take a nap in the afternoon, during the Senhor and the Senhora's own siesta.

But in the *casa grande* the women faced a new and different problem: the father of the unborn child was often white and the pregnancy the fruit of a relationship which invariably had an element of duress. Moreover the mother of a mulatto child might have to face the anger and contempt of the slave men whose potential wife, herself, had been appropriated by the Senhor or his overseers.

All these matters were discussed in depth and at great length when, a year after Tomba's first appearance, Ama discovered that she was pregnant.

"I had a daughter once, a dearly beloved child," Tomba told her. "She was taken from me suddenly and by force, she and her mother, who was the only woman I had loved until I met you. You know the story. I have told it to you before. That loss drove me mad. Who but a madman would have taken it upon himself to launch, single-handed, a campaign to destroy the slave trade? I don't want to be driven mad again and I don't want you to be driven mad either. Let us be content with one another. Take something, I beg you, to abort the pregnancy."

"No, no, no," she replied. "I want to have the child. You do not understand. A woman is not a woman until she has brought forth. Tomba, I beg you too, do not make me do this thing."

This was their first serious quarrel. There was little else for them to quarrel about. They lived apart and though Tomba ran over after his work several times a week, there were no petty domestic issues to divide them. They were united in their hatred of slavery and in their determination to resist it in any way they could. They had the deepest respect for one another; and lying together on the bed Tomba had made for them, they were able to escape, briefly, from the humiliation and harshness of their daily lives.

Tomba's unusual childhood had left him free of the gender prejudices which male dominated societies build into their offspring during their formative years. Of his mother he had no more than the dimmest of memories. Sometimes he wondered whether he really remembered her at all; perhaps he was just recalling what Ibrahima had told him of her. As for Sami, she had been like a beautiful pearl discovered in an oyster, a delicate object to be treasured, a source of constant amazement.

Ama had witnessed Tomba's courage in the most difficult of circumstances and she had also seen how deeply those whom she had known on board as 'Tomba's people' revered him. She loved him with a fierce passion but she also had a deep respect for him.

They resolved the quarrel by agreeing to accept Olukoya's mediation. The *babalorisha* listened to them both. Then he closed his eyes and sat perfectly still, in silence, while they waited.

When he had finished his meditation, he said, "Tomba and Ama, my dear friends. I am sorry that I cannot accept this task. Please forgive me."

"But why not?" they burst out simultaneously and then looked at one another and laughed.

Olukoya laughed too.

"May you always be of one mind," he told them.

He continued, "My problem is that I made up my own mind on this issue long ago, even before Ama arrived here. Because of that I cannot be a fair arbitrator."

"No matter," Tomba told him. "We agreed before we came to see you that we would accept your advice whatever it might be."

"Can you not guess what it would be?"

Tomba said, "No."

Ama said, "I can guess."

Olukoya said, "We need witnesses," and sent his wife to summon Josef and Wono.

When they had all shaken hands, Olukoya explained the circumstances.

Then he said, "Josef, I beg you, pour libation for us. Summon the spirits of all our ancestors and ask them to let me speak with wisdom and compassion."

Olukoya said, "Tomba, my brother, our brother. You have placed yourself in my hands. I thank you for the honour you do me. Ama, you too.

"Tomba, what I have to say might possibly cause you pain. If that is so, it will not be from any malicious intention, please believe me."

Mystified, Tomba nodded.

"The five of us here, Ama, Josef and Wono, Ayodele and I, represent three different nations. Wono and Ayodele and I are all Yoruba. Josef is an Akan. Though Ama is well versed in the customs of the Akan, her own people are called Bekpokpam. I don't have to tell you that.

"There is one thing that the five of us have in common. We all grew up in large families, mothers, sometimes several mothers, fathers, grandparents, brothers and sisters. While we were growing up we witnessed both births and deaths within our families. We all share a belief in the continuity of the living, the dead and those yet to be born. We believe that when we die we go to join our ancestors.

"But in order for us to do so, for our spirits to rest in peace, custom must be performed. The performance of that custom is the work of our children.

"Because of your strange history, which you have shared with us, my brother, and from what you have told me, I know that these beliefs and customs have little meaning for you. That is the reason why I first declined to be your arbitrator. I am not a fair judge. Just look at us. Ayodele and I have two children. So do Josef and Wono."

Tomba made as if to speak but Olukoya held up his hand.

"Wait please," he said quietly, "I have not finished. There is another argument, concerning which there is no difference amongst us, all six of us, and which I believe will carry more weight with you. I know you, and not only by Ama's account, as a man of unsurpassed courage. It would be uncharitable for me to taunt your fear of a repetition of a loss which, as you have told us, affected you so deeply, as a want of courage. We have talked long into the night together, you and I, about what we need to do to regain our freedom. I think we are in broad agreement. But I have to ask you, if we do not produce children, what is the purpose of our plans; and if our generation fails, who will there be to implement our dreams? The Portuguese bring shipload after shipload of our fellows from Africa. Each generation dies out leaving just a small residue of Crioulos and mulattos. Many of them think not like Africans but like their masters or their white fathers. In order to achieve our aims we must create a new generation who know both Africa and Brazil, who are committed to Africa and committed also to the overthrow of slavery and the creation of a new Africa here on this soil."

Tomba bowed his head.

"There are many things I do not know," he said. "You put me to shame."

"Tomba, lift up your head. You know that that was not my intention. Agree to let Ama have this baby. We will give her, and you, all the love and support we can. Ama will teach your child to read and write, as she is teaching us. We will survive together in this country. Africa will survive in Brazil. One day Brazil will become part of Africa, a better Brazil, a better Africa, without slavery and without the wars which feed it. And your child will be part of it."

*****

For the first time since their marriage, Williams brought Miranda home.

Ama was busy preparing their bedroom for them when Miranda walked in. Her face lit up when she saw Ama.

"Ama, *atúù*," she said as they approached, using the Asante which Ama had taught her.

"Senhora Miranda, *awâwâwâ*," Ama replied as they embraced.

They stepped back and held each other at arm's length. Each looked at the other; then, eyes wide, each pointed at the other's belly and giggled. They embraced again. Then they went to sit side by side on the bed.

"Tell me all the news," Miranda demanded. "I want to know exactly what has happened here since I left. My mother tells me nothing; well, nothing of any importance. I didn't even suspect that you were pregnant, let alone married. All of a sudden. Who is he?"

"He is called João. He comes from the Engenho do Meio. But we are not married. Not in church, anyway. The Senhor would not permit it."

She gave Tomba the name by which the Portuguese knew him.

"What nonsense, Ama," Miranda said.

Ama knew the look of concern on her face was genuine.

"Why, in heaven's name?"

Marriage to Williams, or was it living in Salvador, had changed Miranda, Ama noticed. Such a casual profanity would never have passed her lips when she was a child.

"I think it would be better if you asked the Senhor that question yourself, Senhora Miranda," Ama replied, "but it is not really important. Everyone knows we are married. But tell me about yourself. How long are you going to stay?"

"Until my baby is born. Senhor Williams says he needs a break from my extravagant habits. He complains that I am driving him into debt. So my pregnancy has provided him with a convenient excuse to send me home to Mother. For the duration, at least."

"Won't you miss him?"

"Of course, but he has promised to come down at least twice a month. He says he is going to get Josef to teach him how to sail. Oh, Ama. He is such a wonderful husband. Not at all like the stuffy Portuguese men. He has taught me so much. Do you know that I can read and write English now? And speak it a little, too."

"I don't believe you. Show me."

"Heh! Cheeky, cheeky! Speaking to your mistress like that. I'll have to report you to the Senhor."

She saw Ama start at the rebuke, smiled at her little joke and kissed her on the cheek.

"Tchtt! Tchtt! You didn't take me seriously, did you? You see, my little one-eyed beauty, I have penetrated your disguise. I know all your secrets. Senhor Williams has told me everything about you. Everything!"

"Everything?"

"Everything! You wicked girl. Why did you keep so many secrets from me? Don't you see? Now we can talk together in English and when Senhor Williams is not around, no one else will be able to understand a word?"

"I don't think the Senhora would approve of that. Do you?"

"Hmm! Perhaps you are right. I didn't think of that. But at least we can read to each other. Story books. Novels. I love English novels, don't you? They are so much more interesting than those boring Portuguese stories about the saints. Realistic, Senhor Williams says."

"What have you been reading?"

"Tom Jones. Tom Jones is my favourite. And Pamela. She is so brave. Heh! Senhor Williams says that when he knew you before, your name was Pamela. It that true? How many other names do you have, dear Ama, that you have never told me about? You really are a most secretive person. I want you to vow to me that from now on you will have no secrets from me, not a single one. And I will make the same vow to you. Ama, promise!"

"Senhorita Miranda, I mean Senhora, how you have changed! The ideas that just come tumbling out, one after the other!"

"Ama, your vow! Repeat after me, 'I vow that I will never keep another secret from Miranda, so help me God,' and cross your heart."

"Senhora, I cannot do that."

"Why not? Why not? Ama you are not my real friend. I would do anything for you, anything. And when I ask you for just this small favour you refuse. I think I am going to cry."

Ama put her arm around her shoulder and hugged her. Miranda sank her head into Ama's breast. Ama rubbed her back, comforting her as she had done when she was just a girl, before she had married. After a moment Miranda sat up straight.

"I've changed my mind," she said. "I don't think I shall cry. But tell me why you won't take my vow, you little vixen."

"I beg your pardon, Senhora, I am not your little vixen; nor anyone else's for that matter," said Ama.

It struck her that Miranda was acting out the part of a romantic heroine in one of the novels her husband had given her to read. She smiled indulgently, recalling the idle months she herself had spent reading her way through Mijn Heer's library. Then a thought struck her.

"Tell me, tell me," insisted Miranda.

"In a moment," Ama replied. "But first I want to ask you something. Those books which Senhor Williams has been giving you to read, are they brand new, or do they have someone else's name written inside the front cover?"

"How did you know that? My mother always said she suspected you of being a witch. Have you been practising black magic, with your drums and cutting the throats of poor cockerels and things?"

"What was the name?"

"I forget. I've never seen a name like that before. It's not Portuguese and not English."

"Try to remember."

Miranda smiled slyly.

"You tell me," she suggested. "Guess the name and I'll tell you if you're right."

"Pieter de Bruyn," Ama said confidently.

Miranda looked at her, flabbergasted.

"My mother was right," she said. "You are a witch. How could you possibly know that?"

"Now, your vow," said Ama, quickly changing the subject. "Are you going to tell me all the intimate secrets which you and Senhor Williams share? How would he feel about that?"

Miranda put her hand over her mouth and stared at Ama.

"I didn't think about that," she said morosely and then almost at once her face brightened and she continued with a note of triumph in her voice.

"It's simple," she said. "We can leave those out. 'All secrets except those shared with husbands.'"

"You win that one," said Ama. "By the way, has Senhor Williams taught you to play chess?"

"Yes, but I'm not very good at it. It's so boring."

"Let's make it more interesting. I challenge you to a game. Only this time the rules will be different. I will play with the white pieces, but only eight of them: the king and the queen, the knights, the bishops and the rooks; no pawns. You'll play black and you will also have eight pieces, only they will all be pawns. What's more, when it is my turn to move, you must warn me in advance just what move you plan to make next. Oh yes, and since I'm playing white, I'll make the first move."

Miranda looked puzzled.

"Ama, I don't understand you. That wouldn't be fair. I wouldn't have a chance. What are you talking about?"

Ama took her hands.

"Senhora Miranda, I'll give you a clue. It's a parable, like those in the Bible."

Miranda looked her in the eye.

"Senhor Williams told me how you lost your eye," she said. "No, I give up. I never was much good at riddles. Explain it to me."

"It's simple," said Ama. "The black pawns are the slaves, us. Do I have to say more? And you are asking us to tell you all our secrets. You see Senhora Miranda, you are the daughter of the Senhor. I am his slave; I am your slave. I love you dearly and I know that you love me too. But I am still your slave. Can't we just be friends and each decide which of our secrets we want to share with the other?"

Miranda got up and went to the window. She stood there a long time, looking out towards the horses in the paddocks. When she spoke it was in such a low voice that Ama had to strain to hear her.

"Senhor Williams received a new book recently. His uncle sent it from London. It was written by a man called Dr. Adam Smith. It's not a novel. I think it's called *An Inquiry into the Nature and Causes of the Wealth of Nations*, or something long and boring like that. Senhor Williams says it's a wonderful book, but that most of it is much too difficult for me to understand. He is so clever, Senhor Williams. Sometimes I wish I were a man."

She came back and sat on the floor, legs crossed, in front of Ama, looking up at her.

"Dr. Smith says that slavery is stupid and that it is also wicked. He says it spoils the soil. He says it costs us more to keep you all as slaves than it would if we gave you your freedom and paid you a wage, like we do with the overseers and the Tupi. He says the real reason that we keep slaves is not that it makes us rich but that it makes us feel powerful, especially our men. Senhor Williams says that the more he thinks about it, the more he sees the truth in Dr. Smith's arguments."

Ama saw that Miranda was crying. She said nothing but took a handkerchief and wiped the tears from her cheeks.

"Ama," she said. "If one day the Engenho de Cima becomes mine, I will set every slave here free. And you will be the first."

"Hush," Ama replied. "You must not speak of your parents' death like that. I believe you; from the bottom of my heart I believe you. But please don't tell the Senhor the way you feel; nor the Senhora. Let it be a secret between us, just the two of us."

*****

Miranda's child arrived first.

Together, she and Ama had prepared one of the guest rooms for the delivery. When her waters broke they sent down to the *senzalas* for the midwives. The women surrounded her bed, constantly moved her arms and legs around and urged her to "push, push, Senhora." Benedito's wife offered her a crucifix to kiss, put a rosary on her belly and prayed to Santa Miranda to watch over her namesake. The Senhora, Miranda's mother, walked up and down distractedly, giving orders which the women pointedly ignored: for once, it was they who were in charge. Ama sat by Miranda's side throughout; it was she who announced to her that her baby was a girl, she who held the baby while the cord was cut and smeared with oil and pepper, and she who took it upon herself to give the infant her first bath.

Miranda insisted that when Ama's turn came, a week later, she should give birth in the same room. The scene was much the same, except for the absence of the Senhora, who was indisposed, and the reversal of the roles of the two young women. But whereas Miranda's labour had been short, Ama's was long and painful. The child was a boy. Miranda bathed him but by the time she brought him to show to his mother, Ama had fallen into an exhausted sleep.

When she woke, it was evening and the candles had been lit. Miranda sat on an upright chair by her side, holding Ama's sleeping child. Williams, who had arrived some days before, sat in an armchair nearby.

Tomba stood at the end of the bed. He shifted his weight uneasily from one bare foot to the other. Williams had never recognised Ama's João as the Tomba who had been her co-conspirator on board ship but Tomba was always nervous in his presence, fearing that revelation of the past might result in his being sold to a distant *engenho*. He was uncomfortable in the presence of all whites, but Williams more so than others. Miranda, too, had failed to win his confidence, though not from want of trying. Tomba had his reservations about Ama's friendly relationship with her mistress and had tried to persuade her to have her child in her cabin rather than in the *casa grande*; but Ama had persuaded him, with some difficulty, that it would be in the baby's best interest to accept Miranda's kindness.

Now Miranda lifted the baby.

"João, take him and show him to Ama," she commanded.

Tomba did what he was told. Mother and father smiled at one another as Miranda brought a candle closer so that Ama could inspect her child.

"Here, João, won't you sit down?" Miranda said, pulling a chair forward for him.

Tomba shook his head awkwardly.

Williams, sensing their need for privacy, inclined his head in a signal to his wife that they should leave. Miranda rose to go and then hesitated.

"Wait," she said. "There is one thing I must discuss with Ama before we go.

Senhor Williams has to return to Salvador soon. We have decided to have our baby baptised in the chapel on Sunday, a week from tomorrow. We are going to call her Elizabeth, Senhor Williams after an old English queen and me after Santa Elizabeta, mother of John the Baptist. If you will agree I . . . we, would like you to have your baby baptised on the same day. We can discuss it later but I thought you might like to talk about what name you intend to give him while João is here."

She leant down to kiss Ama on the forehead.

"I'll come back and bring you some soup after João has left," she said.

*****

At Miranda's suggestion the boy was baptised under the name of Zacharias.

"Zacharias was the father of John the Baptist, so it's appropriate, since our babies were born so close together. My brother is going to be Elizabeth's godfather and I have persuaded Senhor Williams to be god-father to Zacharias, unless you have someone else in mind, that is."

"Senhora Miranda, are you sure that there will be no objection?"

"About my husband being godfather to your son? From whom? My parents? Just let them object. It is none of their business. And Senhor Williams has already agreed."

"That's not what I was thinking of."

"What then?"

"Zacharias and Elizabeth were husband and wife, you know."

"And that means your Zacharias is going to marry my Elizabeth? What rubbish, Ama. Sometimes I think you are just too sensitive. What made you think of such a thing?"

By the Sunday of the baptism, Ama's son already had a name. On Saturday, the seventh day after his birth, Ama rose very early, an hour before the work bell was due to sound. Josef went from cabin to cabin in the dark, rousing all the slaves. When they had assembled at the usual place, he poured libation, praying briefly in Fanti and then switching to Portuguese so that all could understand.

"Spirits of our forefathers, we greet you. I am Josef from Anomabu. With me are all the Africans of the Engenho de Cima. Spirits of our forefathers, we bring you this drink and beg you to accept it. We have risen early this morning to welcome a new arrival in our midst."

"Who is the mother of this child?" he asked.

"I, Ama."

"And the father?"

"I, Tomba."

"Ancestors of Ama and of Tomba, bear witness, we beg you, to the arrival of their first child. It is a boy. Watch over him, guard him, make him strong and wise, honest and compassionate."

"Tomba, what name do you give to this child?"

"I call him Kwame for the spirit of the day on which he was born; and I call him Zumbi in honour of the great King of Palmares."

There was restrained applause. Josef spilled garapa on the ground.

"Spirit of Zumbi of Palmares, we call upon you. Enter into this our boy-child and make him great, even as you are great."

Josef sat down on a stool and Ama gave him the child.

He dipped his right forefinger into a small bowl of water and used it to wet the tongue of the baby. He did the same again; and then a third time. Then he addressed the child.

"Kwame Zumbi, if you say this is water, let it be water which I place upon your tongue."

Wono offered him another small bowl, this one containing *garapa*. He performed the same custom, saying, "Kwame Zumbi, if you say this is *garapa*, let it be *garapa* which I place upon your tongue."

Finally he said to the child, "Kwame Zumbi, I have shown you the difference between water and strong drink. If you say it is black you see, let it truly be black. If you say it is white you see, let it be white."

He rose and gave the child back to Ama. Tomba drank from the bowl of *garapa* and Ama also took a sip.

"Now we have shown your son to the ancestors," Josef told them, "you are free to bring him out of doors."

The slaves lined up to shake hands. Then the bell rang.

"Just in time," said Josef. "I am sorry we had to rush it so."

*****

Life at the Engenho de Cima was little changed. The annual cycle of the *safra*, of St. John's Day and the feasts of the Virgin Mary and the other saints, of Christmas and Easter, continued in an unbroken succession. Slaves worked the ten years, more or less, which fate had allotted to them, died, and were replaced by fresh purchases from Africa. One year slipped into the next.

In spite of their good intentions, Senhor and Senhora Williams visited the Engenho de Cima only at infrequent intervals.

Williams' expanding business interests kept him occupied and Miranda, encouraged by an indulgent husband, became increasing involved in the high society of Salvador. When they did come, they never brought Elizabeth or her younger brothers and sisters.

"The journey across the bay is too dangerous," Miranda told her parents.

The Senhor became increasingly frail but steadfastly refused to follow his chattels to the grave. The Senhora's hair turned white and she spent more and more of her time in prayer and reading the lives of the saints, leaving the day to day running of the *casa grande* to Ama and the other domestic slaves. Increasingly Jesus Vasconcellos took over the running of the business, although the Senhor, in spite of his decrepitude, never allowed him an entirely free rein.

Kwame's early years were carefree. Ama's access to the kitchen stores ensured that he seldom went hungry. For his first six years he ran naked with his fellows, watched over during the day by ancient Esperança and a band of assistants who were scarcely older than their charges. He was invariably asleep when Tomba arrived at night, so it was only on Sundays and saints' days that he saw his father. The three of them often spent that day working in Ama's allotment. Almost before he could walk, Tomba started to take him to the forest to hunt and trap and fish.

The Christmas after he turned seven Kwame was issued with his first dress, identical to those given to the girls. He wore it with great pride for an hour and then, suffering the discomfort of the coarse cloth in the heat, he threw it off and went to play hide and seek, marbles and horseshoe pitching in his normal state of undress. Ama began with the best of intentions: she would teach him to speak Asante and to read and write Portuguese as well as speaking it; but as time went by her remaining eye began to lose its strength. The stresses of her earlier life were taking their toll on her and she often felt tired. So she told him stories instead. Stories from Africa. Stories of her own childhood. But never stories of the harsh episodes of her journey into servitude.

"Tell him," urged Olukoya.

"Later," she insisted. "He is still too young to understand."

But by the time he was old enough to understand it would be too late to tell him.

Ama never did conceive again: Kwame was her only child.

Tomba seemed to shed his own frustrations during his nightly run from the Engenho do Meio to the Engenho de Cima and remained a kind and supportive husband and an indulgent father. Kwame's fellows were not as lucky. Their fathers, subjected to the constant humiliation of slavery, often found temporary relief in beating their wives and children; or they escaped from the real world with the aid of *garapa*.

They rationalised the beating of their children thus: "In order to stay out of trouble when he grows up, he needs to learn to respect the whites and to obey them without question. Absolute obedience to his father is a first step in that direction."

Olukoya, sustained always by an unwavering conviction of the value of what he had brought with him from Africa and by a vision of a better future, was a continuing source of strength, advising, arbitrating, leading by example; but in spite of Josef's best efforts as a courier, his grand plans came to little.

Old Benedito, on the other hand, was confirmed in his faith by the steady growth in the number of converts. Olukoya was intolerant of human failings, particularly those that caused pain to others; on the other hand Father Isaac, behind the curtain of the confessional, casually dispensed total absolution from the most abominable behaviour at the price of a few Hail Mary's and the admonition to go and sin no more.

The Senhor could no longer walk from his bedroom to his rocking chair on the veranda. Bernardo and Tomás the Hausa blacksmith fashioned a simple wheelchair for him. Then he became too weak to sit up and lay all day and night in his darkened bedroom. Ama fed him, washed him, changed his bedclothes and treated his sores as best she could. The Senhora visited him once a day, prayed, and then left him to the tender mercies of his female slaves. Father Isaac said a perfunctory Mass in his bedroom once a week. Then the Senhor became incontinent. Ama wiped him and washed him and dried him; but try as she might she could not clear the pervasive smell of piss and shit from his room. The Senhora stopped coming to pray by his side. Ama sat down at his desk, found quill and ink and wrote to Miranda. Josef took the letter to Salvador. Miranda sent her reply by word of mouth: she had one or two urgent matters to attend to; she would come as soon as she had dealt with them.

The Senhor was dying. He had not eaten for several days and his breathing was irregular. Ama called the priest. Father Isaac administered the extreme unction, fanning his own face while he did so in an attempt to dissipate the foul smell of illness and death. A pale wraith appeared at the door but did not come in; it was the Senhora. Ama was alone with the old man when he died.

"Senhora," Ama told her, "the Senhor is dead."

She did not appear to hear, so Ama repeated the words, loudly, in her ear.

"I heard you. I may be old but I'm not deaf," she replied and crossed herself three times.

The priest, on hearing the news, made the same sign.

Ama went down to the carpentry shop.

"Bernardo," she told the carpenter in Fanti, "dust off his coffin and send it up. I'm worn out. I'm going to tell Josef to take the news to Salvador and then I'm going to sleep. I'll wash his body when I wake up."

*****

By the time Miranda and her brothers arrived, everything was ready: the grave was dug, Ama had dressed the Senhor's shrunken body in the uniform of a colonel of the militia which she found in his trunk; the coffin had been placed on the veranda under an awning to keep off the sun, the kitchen staff had made their preparations to cope with the mourners expected from the surrounding districts.

Miranda lifted her veil and kissed Ama on both cheeks.

"You don't know how grateful I am for all you have done," she told her.

Williams silently nodded his concurrence.

"Elizabeth, dear," said Miranda, "this is Ama. Remember I told you her son is just a week younger than you are? Ama where is Zacharias? I would love to see him."

The girl was dressed elegantly in black, a miniature copy of her mother. Ama knelt down and took her hands.

"Elizabeth let me look at you. You are so pretty. How old are you now?"

But the child ignored her.

"Mama," she said, "I want to see the horses and the sheep and the pigs."

CHAPTER 35

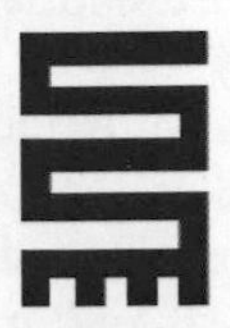

The family met to read the Senhor's will.

Policarpo was given his freedom. But Policarpo was already dead.

The Senhor's property was to pass to the Senhora. The children would inherit only after their mother's death. The Senhora crossed herself and took no further part in the proceedings. It was decided that the eldest son would administer the *engenho*, but since he was running a sugar plantation of his own, and running it successfully, it was necessary to appoint a manager. Jesus Vasconcellos was the obvious choice.

The Senhora would go to live with her daughter in Salvador. The *engenho* would no longer require the services of a resident priest; but fortunately for Father Isaac the *senhor* of the Engenho do Meio was looking for a chaplain.

"Ama, come with me to Salvador," Miranda offered.

"What about Zacharias, Senhora? And João?"

"Of course you would bring Zacharias. But João doesn't belong to us. I would have to talk to Senhor Williams about him."

Williams made an offer to Tomba's master at the Engenho do Meio, but the *senhor* refused to sell. Tomba had become a key man in the running of his mill.

*****

Jesus moved into the *casa grande* as soon as the family had left.

His first action was to have everything removed from the Senhor's room. He set the domestic slaves to scrubbing the floors and whitewashing the walls and ceilings. He consigned all the pictures and mattresses and curtains and upholstery to an outside store. Meanwhile Bernardo scraped every piece of furniture down to the bare wood.

Jesus treated each room in like manner, sending even the cooking utensils to the store. When he had finished, no trace of the Senhor or his family remained in the *casa grande*. He brought his own personal possessions up from the small house he had occupied for so many years. From Salvador he ordered the few things he needed to complete the change, nothing extravagant, just plain cotton curtains and a new mattress.

Next he cut the domestic staff by half, sending maids and seamstresses back to the cane fields or the mill from whence they had once been promoted.

The Senhor's eldest son had set him a target, the net income achieved in the last year of the Senhor's regime. Any surplus he could keep. Jesus leapt at the chance. He knew how inefficiently the business had been run; by tightening up on discipline and implementing a program of austerity, he knew that he could put aside enough in five years to buy the young Senhor out. That was his private dream.

He instructed the overseers to make more liberal use of the whip. He extended the working hours. Saints' days passed unobserved. Sometimes, at the height of the *safra*, he decreed that the next Sunday would be a work day. Children were set to work when they turned nine instead waiting until they were ten. Kwame joined the weeders.

Jesus rearranged the fallow fields so that at the next planting the area of each *tarefa* was increased. He trimmed the slaves' food ration. He cut the prices he paid for the produce which they grew on their allotments. He bought the cheapest supplies in the market, fly-blown meat and grain infested with weevils.

At the same time he carefully favoured the slave drivers, deliberately driving a wedge between them and the other slaves. If anything, the drivers were better off now than they had been in the Senhor's days.

Funerals became more frequent but Vasconcellos would not allow time off for the slaves to bury their dead so they often had to do so late at night. Bernardo was instructed not to supply free coffins, so the dead were buried in cloth.

Jesus kept all the keys himself. He stood by when anything was removed from the stores. Ama no longer had the opportunity to pilfer food from the kitchen. Kwame, now working a full day in the fields, was often hungry.

The talk around the fires on Saturday nights became more and more bitter. Plots were hatched.

One Saturday Jesus announced that the next day would be a working day. That night some person unknown dosed the boiling kettle of *melado* with lemon juice. The syrup failed to crystallise. The day's *tarefa* was wasted. Jesus harangued the mill workers but the direst threats failed to persuade them to point a finger at the culprit. They spent Sunday scrubbing out the kettles. With the mill idle, no cane could be cut; but rather than give the cane cutters the day off, he set them to weeding.

Often hungry and ill, the slaves adopted go-slow tactics. They sabotaged the ox-carts and poisoned the oxen. They adulterated the sugar with sand, knowing that the inspectors in Salvador would reject it.

Jesus berated his overseers. One tried to reason with him and was sacked. Another resigned. Ignacio Gomes, the *cabra* tanner and leather worker, who was a free man, decided at last to abandon the ancient spirits of his land and seek his fortune in the capital.

*****

The field workers returned after dark.

Kwame was so exhausted that he would have fallen asleep without eating if Ama had not forced him to stay awake. She had stopped delivering the produce of her allotment to the *casa grande*: the money was too small and there was invariably an argument about payment. The meat allocation was so worm-ridden that she refused to use it. Tomba brought them whatever he could spare from the slightly better rations at the Engenho do Meio. It was this and the yield of his trapping and fishing that kept them going.

Ama watched over Kwame as he fell asleep. She covered him and rose to return to the *casa grande* to serve Jesus his evening meal.

Leaving the cabin, head bowed, preoccupied with concern about her son's future, she heard the cry, "Fire, fire."

Looking up, she saw a red glow in the sky above the cane fields. Then the work bell rang: the slaves were being summoned to fight the inferno. Undecided as to what to do, Ama went back into the cabin and looked at Kwame's sleeping form. It would be at least an hour before Tomba arrived.

"Kwame, wake up!"

The boy resisted, pulling the blanket back over his head. She grabbed him under the armpits and pulled him to his feet.

"Mama, what is it?" he asked groggily.

"Here take your blanket. You are going to sleep in the cave tonight."

There was a small crevice in the rocks on the hillside where, in earlier days, Ama would go to read. Kwame still loved to hide in it: it was his secret refuge, the only place he could call his own. She pushed him before her, threading her way past the field slaves as they came stumbling out of their cabins in the dark.

*****

Maria Cabinda, the cook, was standing at the kitchen door, looking out at the glow in the dark sky.

She was worried about her husband who would be fighting the fire and about her two young children. If the wind were to turn, the fire might cut the men off from the stream. Then they would be unable to stop the inferno sweeping from the fields, through to the yard and the mill, and on to the *senzalas*.

"Go and bring them up here," Ama suggested but Maria was afraid of Jesus' wrath. She had done that once before when one of them had had a high fever. Finding them asleep in a corner of the kitchen had driven him into a paroxysm of rage.

Ama told her what she had done with Kwame. Maria knew where the cave was.

"If you like, take them there and let them sleep with Kwame. When Tomba comes, I'll ask him to go up and spend the night with them. Don't worry: I cover for you. I'll tell Jesus you have gone to help fight the fire. He could hardly complain about that. And I'll finish the cooking."

*****

The fire turned out to be less serious than had at first seemed likely.

Prompt action confined the damage to three tarefas. Vasconcellos trudged up to the *casa grande*, his face streaked with ash. Ama suppressed a grin and quickly turned her head.

At first Jesus was exhilarated at his success in forestalling a potential catastrophe; but his mood quickly turned to anger. He would have liked to strangle the unknown arsonist. Of course he would impose a stern collective punishment; but that would do little to help him to meet his target this year. Output had declined. If he could not force an improvement his very job might be in jeopardy. It had all seemed so straightforward and simple when he had taken over.

"Rum!" he commanded.

He didn't even notice the absence of the cook. Ama served him his food. By the time he had finished the second course the bottle was half empty. He started to mumble to himself. Returning from the kitchen with the third course, she saw him bang the heavy table with his fist. He turned and glared at her. She averted her eye.

When he had finished eating, she cleared the table. Then she went back to the dining room. He was still sitting there, staring at the empty bottle.

"Will there be anything else, *Senhor*?" she asked quietly.

He turned to stare at her. Then he drained the dregs of the rum from his glass.

"Will there be anything else, *Senhor*?" he mimicked. "Yes, One-eye, there will be something else."

He rose and grabbed her at once by the shoulders, pulling her towards him. She struggled to free herself but he was too strong. He forced her lips apart and drove his tongue into her mouth. She tasted the foulness and the rum. Pulling her arms free she thrust his head from her. Then, almost instinctively, she attacked him at the only place where he was vulnerable: she sank her teeth into his lower lip. He screamed in agony and threw her away so violently that she fell backwards. Her head struck the stone floor. She lay there immobile, stunned. He dropped onto her and ripped her cloth off. Then he was inside her, thrusting away his hatred and frustration.

When he had finished, he rose and stood over her where she lay sobbing on the floor. He said nothing. She turned over on her side, away from him, hiding her face in her hands. He fingered his bleeding lip. Then he drew his right boot back and deliberately, with all his strength, kicked her in the buttocks. Ama screamed and then she lost consciousness.

When she came to, he had gone. Slowly, painfully, she got to her knees. Taking hold of the edge of the table, she pulled herself to her feet. She stood still for a while, dizzy, afraid that she would faint again. Then, step by step, she crossed the open space to the nearest wall. She closed her eyes and rested her weight against the door post. Step by step again, across the kitchen. She went out and, by force of long habit, took the key and locked the door. She met no one on the way. It seemed an age before she reached the *senzalas*. All was quiet: the exhausted fire fighters had dragged their heavy legs back to their hovels and quickly fallen asleep.

Tomba came out of the cabin. He had just arrived. The moon had risen. She could see the sweat glistening on his bare torso.

"Ama," he asked as he saw her approaching, "where's Kwame?"

Then he saw from her crippled gait that something was amiss.

"Ama, what's wrong?" he asked as he went to help her.

"Senhor Jesus," she replied. "He raped me."

"Vasconcellos raped you?" he asked as if in disbelief.

It happened regularly. The women almost accepted it as part of the condition of their life. But it had never before happened to his Ama, not, at least, since they had been married.

"Tomba," she asked him wearily, "bring me water, I beg you."

He ministered to her needs, wiped her face, blew up the embers of a fire and put a basin of water on it. She told him about the fire in the cane fields and what she had done with Kwame. Then she stretched out to try and sleep.

"Have you got a knife?" he asked her.

"Not here," she replied without opening her eye. "In the kitchen."

"Where's the key?" he asked.

She sat up.

"No, Tomba, no!" she commanded, her voice rising.

"Where's the key?" he demanded.

She felt the corner of her cloth.

"I don't have it. I must have left it in the door or dropped it on the way. Tomba don't do it. I beg you Tomba. I beg you."

She was sobbing now.

"Can you walk?" he asked her, gently but firmly forcing her to her feet.

"Tomba, what will you achieve? You will bring tragedy down on all our heads. Think of Kwame. Let it be. You cannot reverse what has been done."

"Come," he told her. "I might need your help."

*****

They didn't find the key and it wasn't in the kitchen door. He whispered instructions to her.

"For the last time, Tomba, I beg you. Remember what we did together on the ship."

"It is because of that, that I must do this," he said. "Now are you ready? Do what I say."

He banged on the jalousie shutters of Jesus' bedroom. At first there was no answer and Ama hoped against hope that in his drunken state the man had fallen asleep somewhere out of earshot. But then they heard his half-awake slurred speech.

"Who the hell is that making that confounded row?"

"Senhor Jesus. It is I, Ama, One-eye."

"Go away. I'll have you whipped to an inch of your life in the morning if you don't stop that row."

"Senhor. The fire has started again. They have set the cane fields on fire."

That woke him up, drunk as he was. They heard him swear as he struggled to pull on his boots. They went round to the veranda. Ama stood a little way off where he would see her in the moonlight as he opened the door. They heard him fumble with the key. The door opened and he stepped out. He was holding a musket at waist height, his hand on the trigger. Tomba, standing beside the door, felled him with a single blow. The gun fell to the floor.

In a moment Tomba had dragged him back into the house.

"Ama, come quickly. Bring the gun and close the door behind you. Now lock it. Do you have a candle? And some rope to tie him with?"

He had already stuffed his cloth into the man's mouth. Now he wound it round and round his head to secure the gag. Then he turned him face down and sat on him.

Ama returned, not with a rope but with a pair of manacles and a pair of leg-irons.

"The keys are in the locks," she told him.

"Excellent," he replied. "Now a knife, the sharpest you can find. Or, better still, a meat chopper or an axe."

"Tomba, I beg you. It is enough. They will torture you before they kill you."

"Never mind. Do as I say."

"What about Kwame? And me?"

"I must do what I must do."

Ama thought, *I cannot reach him. It is as if he has changed into some other person, as if he were mad.* Then she remembered him telling her how the loss of Sami had driven him mad, by his own admission, mad. She shivered and felt she would faint. In the kitchen she sat down, sank her head upon the table and tried to consider her options. She could unlock the front door and run to Olukoya and Josef for help. But by the time they got back Tomba would already have found a weapon and done his worst. Then she would have to live out whatever time remained to her with the knowledge that she had failed him. And what could Olukoya and Josef do but give him up to the militia?

"Well?"

Tomba was standing in the doorway. She pointed to the drawer where the knives were kept. He turned the contents out onto the table.

"Tomba, for the last time."

She put her arm on his naked back and caressed him. He shook her off and continued to examine each of the knives in turn.

She went to the doorway and lay down on the floor, face down, with her head towards him.

"What are you doing?" he asked.

"I am prostrating myself before you, as the Yorubas do before their gods. Kill me, rather."

He stepped over her. She rose and followed him.

He turned the man over and sat down on his stomach. Jesus' manacled hands were behind his back, under him. Tomba put the instruments down beside him. Then he removed the gag.

"You may say your last prayers," he told the manager of the Engenho de Cima.

"Who are you?" Vasconcellos demanded. "I warn you. Release me at once or it will go hard with you."

"It will go hard with me anyway, shit-face. Make your confession and beg for absolution before I cut out your tongue."

Ama was shocked. She had never heard Tomba use foul language before. She hugged herself and rocked from foot to foot. Closing her eye she tried to summon up a vision of Itsho. But all she could see was a dark void.

"Right, Senhor Jesus," said Tomba, "you've had your chance. No prayers."

He forced the man's mouth open and wedged a wooden spoon between his teeth. Then he seized Vasconcellos' tongue with a pair of tongs and pulled it out of his mouth. In a moment he had sliced it off. The blood spurted over him. He stood up. Ama caught a glimpse of the terror in his victim's eyes. Then she vomited.

When she rose to her feet, Tomba had pulled the man's pants down. Now he ripped off his blood-soaked shirt as well. The manager lay naked. Tomba took a cushion from a chair and put it under the man's head.

"I want you to have a good view of this," he told Vasconcellos.

Then, using his knees, he forced the man's legs apart. He grabbed the end of his slack penis with the tongs and pulled. He waved the blood stained knife before the man's eyes.

"Tomba, no, no."

Ama tried to pull him away but he shrugged her off. She ran to the door, turned the key and in a moment was running down to the *senzalas*.

*****

When they reached the *casa grande*, the front door was standing open as Ama had left it.

"Tomba," Olukoya called quietly.

There was no answer. He went inside. Josef followed. Ama had insisted on returning with them. Seeing her state of mind, Josef had told Wono to come too.

"Wono, don't come in. Just look after Ama," Olukoya called back.

"I must see, I must see," Ama cried.

Breaking loose from Wono, she followed them.

Jesus Vasconcellos lay dead in a pool of his own fresh blood. By his side were the severed organs. Tomba sat on the floor with his back against the wall, staring into space. He was still covered with the blood of his victim.

Olukoya spoke to him but he did not reply. Olukoya shook him gently by the shoulders. Tomba did not react. Then Ama knelt before him. She said nothing, just took his limp, bloodstained hands and rubbed them in her own.

"Josef, we may need Wono's help," said Olukoya. "Do you think she can take this?"

"I'll speak to her."

"Lock the door behind you. Then bring her through to the kitchen. We need to talk this out."

*****

Olukoya sat at the kitchen table, his head in his hands.

"Wono. I'm sorry you had to see that. Josef and I need to talk, to make plans. I would like you to join us but I don't think it would be wise to leave Tomba and Ama alone. And we are not ready to take them away. Will you sit and watch them?"

Wono nodded.

Olukoya said, "Josef, my brother, we are in real trouble. We shall be lucky if we come out of this alive. They will miss Tomba at his *engenho* early tomorrow morning. The first thing they will do is to send a messenger to ask after him. We must all be far from here before the messenger arrives."

"What about the body?"

"My first thought was to burn it, and this building, too."

"There's not much here to burn. The building is of stone."

"You are right. And it would delay us too much. We must bury the body in a place where they will never find it."

"What worries me is the overseers," said Josef.

"Yes, that is the first thing. Go down to the *senzalas* and round up ten men we can trust. While you are doing that, I will search the house for arms. Ama may be able to help. Don't waste time telling the men why they are wanted: we can tell them all together when they get here. We'll give them whatever arms we can find. But no more bloodshed, mind; not if we can avoid it. It will only make our situation worse."

*****

"My brothers and sisters," Olukoya told the assembly. "Something has happened tonight which has put us all in great danger. I am going to tell you about it and what I think we must do to save ourselves. I want you to listen to me calmly and quietly. If there are any questions, I will hear them when I have finished."

"Jesus Vasconcellos is dead."

A murmur of shock passed through the crowd. Then there was applause.

"Hallelujah," cried a Christian. "Praise the Lord," and the reply came, "Amen."

Olukoya called for order.

"I will not tell you how he died or by whose hand and I do not want you to ask me. The less each of us knows, the better for all of us."

"As soon as we finish this meeting brother Josef will choose four men to dig a grave. This work is dangerous and those who are asked may refuse. No one will hold it against them. Indeed no one will know who they are.

"While this is going on the rest of us must prepare to leave this place. Go to your allotments and quickly harvest all the ripe crops which you can carry with you. If you have seed, bring that too. Collect together all your important possessions, all you can carry, and bundle them up. There is no need to wake your children, not until the last moment, when we are ready to go. Work in great haste. We must all be away from here well before dawn. I have one more thing to say, but before that: any questions?"

"Where are we going?"

"It would be unwise for me to tell you that. You will understand why in a moment."

"What about the overseers?"

"They are safely tied up, locked up and under guard. None of them has been harmed. We have taken their guns and before we go we will take which ever of their possessions might come in useful to us."

"Shouldn't we take them with us as hostages?"

"Good question. That hadn't occurred to me. But I don't think it would be a good idea. If we took them we might find ourselves having to deal with the army rather than just the militia. No more questions? Good, it seems that I made myself clear.

"Now there may be some of you who, for one reason or another, might be reluctant to join the rest of us. I understand that and I will ask you no questions. All I ask is that for our protection and for your own, you declare your intentions now. Then we will tie you up and lock you up like the overseers so that it will look as if you resisted us. That way there might be less trouble ahead for you; but that is something, of course, that I cannot guarantee."

*****

"Feed your children and yourselves as best you can," Olukoya told them when they reached the clearing. "Then get some sleep. We are all tired out. It will take them some time to get organised so we will take a chance and post no guards until after we wake up. Remember just one thing as you fall asleep. We are no longer slaves. We have thrown off our chains. We are free men and women. May the ancestors watch over our sleep and wake us up well."

"Mama," yawned Kwame as he lay down, "what did Uncle Olu mean? Have we come here to pray to the ancestors?"

Ama searched for an answer but the boy, like his father beside him, was already fast asleep.

She searched Tomba's face, looking for a clue. He was relaxed, his breathing regular, seemingly at peace with the world. For twelve years they had lived together as man and wife. Yet last night she had discovered within him a festering wound whose existence she had never suspected.

She lay down. *I wonder whether Olukoya and Josef have been damaged in the same way*, she mused. She tried to sleep; but sleep would not come. Again and again scenes of the previous night's events passed before her. She summoned the spirit of Itsho; but either he refused to come or he lacked the power to suppress those awful visions.

When she awoke, Olukoya was returning from the shrine. All around, shaded from the midday sun, lay the sleeping forms of their companions.

"Where's Tomba?" Olukoya whispered.

She panicked and leaped to her feet, silently blaming herself: in his despair he must have run away. *He might do himself some damage*, she thought. *I should have stayed awake to watch over him.* But Olukoya had seen him. He beckoned to her and pointed: Tomba was sitting by the stream, fashioning a conical fish trap from reeds.

"Bra Tomba," Olukoya greeted him.

Tomba looked up.

"I thought, 'What are we all going to eat?'" he said and went back to his work.

Olukoya put his hand on Tomba's bare shoulder and squeezed.

"There is one thing I want you to know," he said. "We are all in this together. What you did was long overdue."

Tomba looked up at him but said nothing. He took another reed from the bundle beside him. *I wonder if he remembers anything*, Ama mused. She knelt by his side and hugged him. He turned and looked deep into her eye. Then, again, he went back to his work. *Twelve years we have lived together and now he has become an enigma to me*, she thought.

"It's time to wake up the others," Olukoya said. "There is much to do. Tomba, I have an urgent task which will need your special knowledge; and I don't mean about making fish traps."

Not for the first time Ama was lost in admiration for Olukoya's skill in dealing with people. He was trying to draw Tomba back into the web that held them all together, to make him feel that he was needed. *Is it a natural gift*, she wondered, *or something he learned during his training for the priesthood?*

*****

The altar site was an unsuitable location for a quilombo: it was true that it lay hidden deep in the forest and that it had water; but it was easily approachable on all four sides and there was no height from which a look-out might detect the approach of strangers.

Olukoya sent Tomba out with Josef. He wasn't optimistic. He had made the same search himself many years before and had found nothing suitable. But he thought that there was just a chance that Tomba's past experience might help him to locate a more defensible site.

While they were away he began to organise his people. He had them pool their scant supplies of food. The cooking would have to be done after dark: a plume of smoke would invite detection. They would certainly be pursued: of that he had no doubt; but the militia would have to find them first. He collected the arms which they had appropriated from the *casa grande* and the overseers' houses. Their powder might be spoiled at any time by a shower, so he had a pit excavated on higher ground, lined with leaves and covered with a roof of branches and leaves and soil. It was too early to think of building a more permanent armoury. If they were lucky Tomba would soon return and lead them to a sheltered hillside in some remote wooded valley. There, he told himself, without much conviction, there would be a cave which could serve as a store for their weapons and ammunition.

Olukoya had no illusions about their capacity to resist an attack by a force of any strength. But if they had sufficient warning of the approach of their pursuers, he thought, and if they planned well in advance, they might be able to disperse, to melt away into the forest, leaving the militia without a visible target. The trouble with this strategy was that the fugitives feared the forest, particularly at night. He would have to overcome that fear. He set a ring of day and night guards and sent out scouts.

After defence their most pressing problem was food. What they had brought would last them no more than a few days. Olukoya began to plan a raid on the Engenho de Cima, or on another *engenho* nearby, to steal a few sheep and some bags of grain.

Tomba and Josef returned to report failure. There was no option but to make the best of their present camp. Olukoya set everyone to work: he knew that if he allowed the soldiers in his little army to sit around and talk they would soon become despondent. He invented tasks to keep them fully occupied during all their waking hours. They told him that he was making them work harder than they had ever done as slaves. But they said it with a smile.

That night they all sat around a fire, all except those who stood as sentinels in the dark forest beyond and those who had been sent on an expedition to spy on their former home and steal what food they could find.

Ama had the Bible which Alexandre had stolen for her all those years before. She offered to read a story and the offer was accepted with acclamation. So she lay down on her stomach, with the book close to the fire, and, with her one weak eye, read to them from Exodus.

When she had read the passage in which Moses kills an Egyptian for beating one of his Israelite brothers, and buries the body, she paused and asked for water to wet her throat.

"That Egyptian was called Vasconcellos," came a comment from the dark perimeter.

There was approving laughter.

"And who is our Moses then?" another responded.

"Enough of that," Olukoya interrupted. "No one knows who killed Senhor Jesus. I warned you not to speculate on that matter. It is dangerous talk which could be our undoing. Ama please go on."

She came to the episode where the Pharaoh punished the Israelites for Moses's insolent demands by increasing their *tarefa*, the daily quota of bricks each slave had to make. Again they saw the parallels between the story and their own history.

As Moses visited each of God's plagues upon the Egyptians there were cries of approbation and when he led the Israelites out of bondage Ama had to stop until the cheering subsided.

When she read of Pharaoh's pursuit with his soldiers and horses and chariots the murmurs were more muted. The Israelite fugitives displayed their lack of faith in their leader and their god and there was a cry of "Shame;" but the echo was half-hearted. Ama wondered whether she had selected the wrong story. Yet they cheered again when the Lord parted the waters and Moses led his flock out of Egypt and into the desert and freedom; and Ama's faith was restored.

By this time her eye was watering from the smoke of the fire and her throat was sore.

"I think that's enough for one night," she told them. "If you like, I'll continue some other time."

"Tomorrow," demanded the children.

"Tomorrow," she agreed with a smile.

But that tomorrow never came.

*****

Olukoya assigned Josef, his most able and trusted lieutenant, to lead the raiders.

With great enthusiasm, Pedro, the alcoholic slave-driver, volunteered to join the party. Olukoya had some misgivings about including him. However, having finished off the garapa he had brought with him, Pedro had been sober for several days and had vowed that he was a reformed character. Moreover he would be leaving his wife and daughter behind in the camp and that was surely some sort of guarantee of good behaviour.

Josef and his men returned with the carcasses of two sheep and bad news. Under cover of dark, Pedro had absconded.

Josef woke Olukoya. Tomba and Ama woke too.

"One moment he was there, holding the sheep's head while I cut its throat. A moment later, when I called him to take the carcass on his shoulders, there was no answer. We had no choice but to beat a speedy retreat," Josef reported morosely.

"It is my fault, not yours," replied Olukoya. "I should have listened when the gods spoke to me. Pedro fooled me. The man is ruled by his thirst. He cannot live without the stuff. Are you quite sure that he didn't disappear just to search for a bottle? Perhaps he intended to rejoin you for the return journey?"

"It is possible. But consider my position. I couldn't risk it. He might have returned at any moment with a militiaman. We had to leave at once."

"And as soon as he had laid hands on a bottle he would have been in no fit state to follow you. We have to work on the assumption that he would either give himself up or be captured. It might have happened already or it might happen in the morning. Either way I fear that Pedro would sell us all for a bottle of hooch."

"If they caught him at once, before he had a chance to quench his thirst, they might already be following in our tracks."

"I doubt it. Not at night. They would fear a trap. No, they won't set off until dawn at the earliest. That gives us a little time. We must prepare at once to disperse."

Tomba had listened to all this in silence. Now he spoke.

"Bra Olu, it cannot work. I know. It is not easy to survive in the forest on your own, the more so when you are living in fear of your own shadow. Many of us will get lost. Many will die of hunger."

"You may be right, but what are the alternatives? Stand and fight? Give ourselves up?"

"I will give myself up. I will leave at once, carrying a white flag. That way I will meet them perhaps even before they set off."

"And what will you do when you meet them?"

"Senhor Williams will have arrived by this time. He is the god-father of our Kwame. I will ask to speak to him. I will undertake to reveal the identity of Vasconcellos' executioner, but on certain conditions. First I will tell them what went on at the *engenho* after the Senhor's death. Since I did not suffer Vasconcellos' cruelty myself, Williams might be less inclined to dismiss my testimony. Then I will insist that they promise that only the executioner be punished; and that only after a fair trial. If he agrees to that I will undertake to convince you all to return, but provided only that conditions are improved and that no one but the executioner is punished."

"And if Williams is not there?"

"I will take my chance on that."

"Let's assume that he were to agree. Are you suggesting that we should trust him?'

"What choice do we have? Stand and fight? Die of hunger in the forest? Think of the children, the next generation who are going to fight the battle for real freedom, the way you once told me when we were younger, in a concerted uprising over the whole country. We must be realistic, Bra Olu: Palmares days are over."

"But why should they negotiate? Why not just send in the militia?"

"I can think of two reasons. The first is that this way they will suffer no losses themselves. The militiamen will go home to their wives and children, boasting of their victory without firing a shot. The second is that we are worth money to them. If the *engenho* is to be revived, every one of us who is killed would have to be replaced. Slaves cost them money."

"And you?"

"Me? I have broken their laws. Unlike Moses . . ." he smiled at Ama. "Unlike Moses, I don't have a magic stick. I will tell them what I did and why. Then I will accept my punishment. You only die once."

Ama bowed her head and sobbed. He put his arm around her shoulder and comforted her. The sobbing subsided. She raised her head and wiped the tears from her face with the back of her hand.

"Ama, what do you say?" Olukoya asked her.

"I will go with him," she said.

"No," Tomba objected.

"All that has happened is my fault," Ama insisted. "I was careless. He had never tried anything with me before, so I had dropped my guard. If I had kept a safe distance, I could have got away from him. I shall go with Tomba. If Senhora Miranda is there, I will beg her, for my sake, to forgive Tomba."

"And what of Kwame?"

"He will go with us. He is our son."

CHAPTER 36

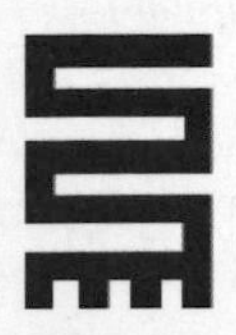

Tabitsha, my mother; Tigen, my father.

It is I, Nandzi, your daughter. I am sitting against the wall of my senzala warming myself in the rays of the early morning sun. I can feel the sun but I cannot see it, for now I have lost the sight of my left eye too. I am completely blind.

My mother and my father, I will be coming to join you soon. Prepare a place for me. The Christians say that we in this country are too far from Africa to join our ancestors when we die, but I do not believe them. When I die my spirit will fly like a bird, back over the sea, back to Africa. Prepare a place for me, I beg you.

Kwame is coming to visit me. Josef brought the message. I am expecting him today. He is a man now. Miranda taught him to read and write. Josef tells me he even knows some English. He is working as a clerk for Senhor William.

He is married and he has a child, a baby girl. He called the child Nandzi Ama. Ama is the name I was given in Kumase. That is what our people call me here. Kwame named his daughter after me. He is bringing his wife and the child to visit his old mother.

Kwame is a free man. It is many years since I have seen him. Miranda took him away to Salvador before they executed Tomba. She said it would not be good for the boy to see his father strung up. Perhaps she was right. They left Tomba's body hanging there for six days. It was only when the flesh began to rot on his bones that they let me take him down and bury him.

Miranda raised Kwame. She calls him Zacharias but to me he is Kwame Zumbi. I have had two husbands in my life. Both were good men and brave. Itsho died trying to rescue me from the Bedagbam. Tomba killed our manager, Senhor Jesus, to punish him for what he did to me. Then he gave himself up to save the slaves at this engenho. Both my husbands were heroes. We gave Kwame the name of a hero too, Tomba and I. We named him Zumbi, after the hero of Palmares. We called him Kwame because he was born on a Saturday and to please Josef. But I had a secret from Tomba, the only secret I ever kept from him. I named my son Kwame also after Kwame Panin the boy who became Osei Kwame, King of Asante and who loved me with such a terrible passion that Koranten Péte had to send me away to Elmina.

Itsho and Tomba, my two husbands. You will be waiting for me too.

My mother I still have the cloth that you gave me. I have kept it all these years. It is torn and threadbare now, but it is all I have left of Africa, all except my spirit, so I treasure it. When they bury me they will put it in my coffin.

I am going to tell Kwame the whole story of my life. Olukoya always urged me to tell him when he was young, but I put it off, thinking there would be plenty of time when he was older. And then he was taken away from me and it was too late. But today I shall tell him. I must tell him; now, before it is too late again.

I shall tell him about you, my mother and about my baby brother Nowu.

I shall tell Kwame how I was left alone when you went to bury my grandfather Sekwadzim; and how I was raped and captured. I shall tell him how Itsho tried to rescue me and got killed in the attempt. I shall tell him how I found Itsho's body and how Damba and Suba helped me to bury him. I shall tell him how Itsho has been coming to me all these years, in my dreams and when I needed him.

I shall tell him about the women who were my friends and who helped through difficult times: about Minjendo, who was with me on the journey to Kumase; about Esi, who taught me everything about Asante and who was sent with me to Elmina because she spoke for me in the court; about Augusta, who was good to me even though she traded in slaves herself; about Nana Esi on the ship The Love of Liberty, whose body was eaten by sharks; about Luiza, who was forced to let men use her body to pay back the money the slave dealer lost when her mother died; about Jacinta, who lost her hands in the mill and the old woman Esperança, who are both now dead; and about Wono and Ayodele who are still my best friends.

I shall tell him about the famous people I have met: the Ya Na and two kings of Asante. Osei Kwadwo said in my presence that if he had been younger he would have taken me as one of his wives. How lucky I was to escape that fate and the worse one of accompanying him when he died! I shall tell Kwame too about Osei Kwadwo's successor, Osei Kwame, after whom I named him; but I shan't tell him everything. There are some things that a mother cannot tell her son.

I shall tell him about the white men I have known; about Mijn Heer, who loved me and might have married me if he hadn't caught the yellow jack at Axim and died; about Jensen who raped Esi, who called him the pig-god; about Van Schalkwyk who gave me English lessons and failed to make a Christian of me; about the Fanti Christian priest, Philip Quaque, who couldn't decide whether he was African or English; about Richard Brew who died on the night of the terrible storm at Anomabu; about Captain Williams whose ship was called The Love of Liberty; about Butcher the surgeon who said he hated the slave trade and George Hatcher, whose bad luck it was to be Tomba's victim; about Knaggs who tried to rape me and who felt the power of my knee in a tender part of his anatomy; about the Senhor, Miranda's father and about Miranda herself and her husband who is also called Williams; and about Jesus Vasconcellos whom Tomba killed.

I shall tell him about the friends who have been my constant support in Bahia; about Josef, Wono's husband and about Olukoya, who speaks to the gods of Africa and looks into the future.

And last but not least I shall tell him the story of his own father, Tomba, who grew up in the African forest and fought many wars against the slave trade; a loving father; a proud man; a man he should be proud to remember.

I shall tell my son Kwame that he should never forget that both his father and mother were Africans; and that he should hold his head up high and be proud of who he is.

After Tomba was executed, Miranda took Kwame away to Salvador. She raised him, she and her husband Senhor William. Then my only contact with my son was through Josef who took messages from me to him and brought me news of how he was doing.

Senhor William often received newspapers from England. As he read them he used to mark the parts he found interesting, mainly the parts about Africa and Brazil and to do with the slave trade. Sometimes Miranda would throw away the old papers. Josef would retrieve them and bring them to me. I would read them, especially the parts which had been marked and I would translate those parts for Olukoya. If there was something important, Josef would take the news back to the brothers in Salvador. The most important news in those times was the war in Haiti. We were all excited. Olukoya thought the time had come for us to follow in the steps of Toussaint L'Ouverture, but nothing came of it. Later Toussaint died a miserable death in a French prison and we mourned him as our brother. By that time I was going blind and I found it more and more difficult to read.. Now we have to rely on others for news of what is going on in the world. Sometimes Miranda tells Kwame something interesting and he passes it on. On his last trip Josef brought the news that the English have stopped the slave trade. And there have been disturbances in the city. But now I am too old to help with such things and since I am blind I can only listen to what they tell me.

The sun has made me sleepy. Sometimes I don't sleep well at night and so I doze during the day. I wonder how long it will be before they arrive. I think I will just take a small nap while I am waiting.

Do you know what is going on in my mind, my mother?

I am hearing the words The Love of Liberty repeated again and again and again.

The Love of Liberty, The Love of Liberty, The Love of Liberty, The Love of Liberty.

The love of liberty . . . love of liberty . . . of liberty . . . liberty . . .liberty. . .

EPILOGUE

In 1807 slaves from Salvador and from the engenhos in the Recôncavo laid a plot. They planned to meet on the outskirts of the city, to attack the whites, capture ships and return to Africa. They were betrayed and their leaders were executed.

There were further abortive insurrections in 1808, 1810, 1813 and 1816.

In 1826 another attempt was made, this time under the leadership of a woman, Zeferina. This too failed; but the slaves were not discouraged: they tried again in 1827 and yet again in 1830.

The most famous rising took place in Salvador in 1835. Again one of the leaders was a woman, Luiza Mahin. This time there was greater unity. Slaves and free blacks, Muslims and non-Muslims, Hausa and Yoruba, Ewe and Nupe all came together under a leadership which was both literate and sophisticated. Only bad fortune denied them victory.

The slave trade was formally abolished in Brazil in 1850, but those who were responsible for implementing the law came from the class of slave owners. It was not until 1888, after widespread disturbances and mass defections by slaves who had lost their patience and were prepared to wait no longer, that the institution of slavery itself was finally outlawed.

In 1891 the Brazilian Minister of Finance decreed the abolition of history: he ordered the destruction of every document which dealt in any way with slavery or the slave trade; a nation-wide burning of the books.

But the clamour of voices from the past drowns out the fiats of forgotten bureaucrats and demands to be heard.

At the end of the twentieth century, the population of Brazil stood at some 165 million. The more than one hundred million Brazilians who are of African descent remain overwhelmingly poor. Political power still rests firmly in the hands of the descendants of the *senhores de engenho.*

Ama is a story of the Slave Trade, a story of Africans who were carried across the Atlantic against their will.

The end of this story has yet to be written.

Acknowledgements

I am indebted to busy friends who made the time to read and criticise the manuscript of *Ama*.

Dr. Robert E. Lee, for many years my dentist and, in spite of that, a good friend, is an authority on the slave trade. I awaited his judgment with the same nervousness which I took to his clinic.

Professor Ama Ata Aidoo, doyenne of Ghana's (and indeed of Africa's) writers, allowed herself to be persuaded to set her own work aside in order to vet mine.

Professor Kofi Anyidoho, poet, critic, teacher, host of the often inspiring African Heritage interviews on Ghana Television, has been supportive in many ways.

Professor Albert Adu Boahen, much-loved Emeritus Professor at the University of Ghana, pioneer historian and courageous politician, ignored pressing deadlines and read the manuscript in a week.

Professor Kwame Arhin (Nana Arhin Brempong), distinguished sociologist and historian, onetime Director of the Institute of African Studies at the University of Ghana, took *Ama* with him on a trip to China at a time when he was the Chairperson of Ghana's National Commission on Culture.

Chantal-Nina Kouoh's unsolicited and unstinting praise and deep commitment to *Ama* persuaded me not to give up the struggle to see the novel published.

Members of my family understood that I would value their criticism as much as their encouragement: my sister Nina, my brother Frank, my cousin Denis (all of them writers themselves) and my son Kwamena.

Without the support of my erstwhile agent and first publisher, Richard Curtis of E-Reads, *Ama* might still be gathering dust in some forgotten drawer.

In April, 2002, *Ama* was awarded the Commonwealth Writers Prize for the Best First Book. The staff of the Book Trust and the Scottish Book Trust organized a stimulating award week. Professor Penina Mlama, chairperson of the judging panel for the African region and the Right Reverend Bishop Richard Holloway, author, former Bishop of Edinburgh and chairperson of the pan-Commonwealth judging panel, chose *Ama* over fine competing debut novels.

Finally, I must thank some two hundred copyright owners for permission to reproduce their writings in the novel's companion website, http://www.ama.africatoday.com. Without their work, *Ama* could not have been written.